History and Examination at a Glance

History and Examination at a Glance

Jonathan Gleadle

MA, DPhil, BM BCh, FRCP (UK)
University Lecturer in Nephrology and Consultant Physician
Oxford Kidney Unit
The Churchill Hospital
Oxford Radcliffe Hospitals
Oxford, UK

Second edition

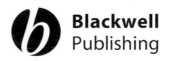

Blackwell
Publishing

© 2007 Jonathan Gleadle
Published by Blackwell Publishing
Blackwell Publishing, Inc., 350 Main Street, Malden, Massachusetts 02148-5020, USA
Blackwell Publishing Ltd, 9600 Garsington Road, Oxford OX4 2DQ, UK
Blackwell Publishing Asia Pty Ltd, 550 Swanston Street, Carlton, Victoria 3053, Australia

First published 2003
Second edition 2007

1   2007

Library of Congress Cataloging-in-Publication Data

Gleadle, Jonathan.
    History and examination at a glance / Jonathan Gleadle. — 2nd ed.
      p. ; cm. — (At a glance)
    Includes bibliographical references and index.
    ISBN-13: 978-1-4051-5518-2 (alk. paper)
    ISBN-10: 1-4051-5518-3 (alk. paper)
    1. Medical history taking—Handbooks, manuals, etc.   2. Physical diagnosis—Handbooks,
manuals, etc.   I. Title.   II. Series: At a glance series (Oxford, England)
    [DNLM: 1. Medical History Taking—Handbooks.   2. Physical
Examination—Handbooks. WB 39 G544h 2007]

RC65.G544 2007
616.07′54—dc22

                                                           2006036290

A catalogue record for this title is available from the British Library

Set in 9.5/12pt Times by Graphicraft Limited, Hong Kong
Printed and bound in Singapore by COS Printers Pte Ltd

Commissioning Editor: Vicki Noyes
Editorial Assistant: Robin Harries
Development Editor: Hayley Salter
Production Controller: Debbie Wyer

For further information on Blackwell Publishing, visit our website:
http://www.blackwellpublishing.com

The publisher's policy is to use permanent paper from mills that operate a sustainable forestry policy,
and which has been manufactured from pulp processed using acid-free and elementary chlorine-free
practices. Furthermore, the publisher ensures that the text paper and cover board used have met
acceptable environmental accreditation standards.

Contents

Preface

The abilities to take an accurate history and perform a physical examination are the most essential skills in becoming a doctor. These skills are difficult to acquire and, above all, require practice. See as many patients as you can and take time to elicit detailed histories, observe carefully for physical signs and generate your own differential diagnoses. Experienced clinicians do not simply ask the same long list of questions of every patient. Instead, they will modify the style of their history taking to elicit the maximum amount of relevant information from each patient. They will also place different emphasis on the importance and reliability of different clinical findings. This book is designed to be used alongside frequent practice of these communication and examination skills with actual patients in order to hone and develop these essential abilities. Once you have taken a history or examined a patient, read the relevant chapters, ask colleagues or other doctors to assess your performance, present your findings to others and check what you did against the communication skills Appendix (p. 202).

The purpose of the history and examination is to develop an understanding of the patient's medical problems and to generate a differential diagnosis. Despite the advances in modern diagnostic tests, the clinical history and examination are still crucial to achieving an accurate diagnosis. However, this process also enables the doctor to get to know the patient (and vice versa!) and to understand the medical problems in the context of the patient's personality and social background.

The book is deliberately concise, emphasizes the importance of history taking and is restricted to core topics. For a complete understanding of any medical condition, you should look at other textbooks such as *Medicine at a Glance* and *Surgery at a Glance*. For detailed descriptions of particular examination techniques watch and learn from an experienced practitioner or from one of the texts below.

This book has four parts. The first section introduces students to key history-taking skills, including relationships with patients, family history and functional enquiry. The second section covers history and examination of the systems of the body and includes chapters on recognizing the ill patient and how to present a clerking. Section three covers history taking and examination of the common clinical presentations whilst section four focuses on common conditions. It thus covers topics in a variety of different ways and this deliberate repetition of important topics is designed to facilitate effective learning.

It is often thought that clinical history and examination is a fixed subject with little change or scientific study. This is incorrect and to emphasize this some subjects have evidence-based sections which have been expanded further in this second edition. These sections do not provide exhaustive coverage of the evidence underpinning aspects of clinical skills but have been included to emphasize the importance of scientific analysis of history and examination. It is hoped that they will act as a stimulus for further reading, study and questioning of the basis of history taking and clinical examination.

Jonathan Gleadle
Oxford

Acknowledgements
I would like to thank the following for their specialist advice on ways to improve on the first edition; Professor Derek Jewell, Dr Maxine Harding, Dr Duncan Young, Dr John Salmon and Dr Bhathiya Wijeyekoon.

Further reading
History and examination
Davey, P. (2006) *Medicine at a Glance*. Blackwell Publishing, Oxford.

Epstein, O., Perkin, G.D., Cookson, J. and Bono, D.P. (2003) *Clinical Examination*. Mosby, St. Louis.

Grace, P.A. and Borley, N.R. (2006) *Surgery at a Glance*. Blackwell Publishing, Oxford.

Sapira, J. and Orient, J. (2005) *Sapira's Art and Science of Bedside Diagnosis*. Lippincott Williams and Wilkins, Philadelphia.

Talley, N.J. and O'Connor, S. (2005) *Clinical Examination: A Systematic Guide to Physical Diagnosis*. Churchill Livingstone, Edinburgh.

Evidence
Clinical Assessment of the Reliability of the Examination (www.carestudy.com/CareStudy).

Clinical Examination Research Interest Group of the Society of General Internal Medicine (www.sgim.org/clinexam.cfm).

McGee, S. (2001) *Evidence-Based Physical Diagnosis*. W.B. Saunders, Philadelphia.

The Rational Clinical Examination Series. Journal of the American Medical Association (1992–2006).

Straus, S.E., Richardson, W.S., Glasziou, P. and Haynes, R.B. (2005) *Evidence-Based Medicine*. Churchill Livingstone, Edinburgh.

List of abbreviations

AA	aortic aneurysm
A&E	Accident and Emergency Department
ACE	angiotensin-converting enzyme
AIDS	acquired immunodeficiency syndrome
ARC	AIDS-related complex
ARDS	adult respiratory distress syndrome
BCG	bacille Calmette-Guérin
BOOP	bronchiolitis obliterans-organizing pneumonia
BP	blood pressure
BS	breath sounds
CABG	coronary artery bypass grafting
CCF	congestive cardiac failure
CI	confidence interval
CNS	central nervous system
COPD	chronic obstructive pulmonary disease
CPAP	continuous positive airway pressure
CRP	C-reactive protein
CSF	cerebrospinal fluid
CT	computed tomography
CTPA	CT pulmonary angiography
CVA	cerebrovascular accident
CVP	central venous pressure
CVS	cardiovascular system
DIP	distal interphalangeal
DIP	desquamative interstitial pneumonitis
DVT	deep vein thrombosis
ECG	electrocardiogram
ENT	ears, nose and throat
FOB	faecal occult blood
GCS	Glasgow Coma Scale
GI	gastrointestinal
GP	general practitioner
GTN	glyceryl trinitrate
HIV	human immunodeficiency virus
ICU	intensive care unit
IgE	immunoglobulin E
IHD	ischaemic heart disease
IP	interphalangeal
IV	intravenous
IVP	intravenous pyelogram
JVP	jugular venous pressure
KUB	kidney – ureter – bladder

LIF	left iliac fossa
LIP	lymphocytic interstitial pneumonitis
LR	likelihood ratio
LUQ	left upper quadrant
LVF	left ventricular failure
LVH	left ventricular hypertrophy
MCP	metacarpophalangeal (joint)
MI	myocardial infarction
MRC	Medical Research Council
NSAID	non-steroidal anti-inflammatory drug
NSIP	non-specific interstitial pneumonitis
OR	odds ratio
PCWP	pulmonary artery capillary wedge pressure
PE	pulmonary embolism
PGL	persistent generalized lymphadenopathy
PIP	proximal interphalangeal (joint)
PMH	past medical history
PN	percussion note
PND	paroxysmal nocturnal dyspnoea
PR	per rectum
PUO	pyrexia of unknown origin
PVD	peripheral vascular disease
RB-ILD	respiratory bronchiolitis associated interstitial lung disease
RIF	right iliac fossa
RIND	reversible ischaemic neurological deficit
RR	respiratory rate
RUQ	right upper quadrant
RVF	right ventricular failure
SIADH	syndrome of inappropriate secretion of anti-diuretic hormone
SLE	systemic lupus erythematosus
STD	sexually transmitted disease
SVC	superior vena cava
TB	tuberculosis
TED	thromboembolic disease
TIA	transient ischaemic attack
TNF	tumour necrosis factor
TURP	transurethral resection of prostate
UIP	usual interstitial pneumonitis
UTI	urinary tract infection
VSD	ventriculoseptal defect

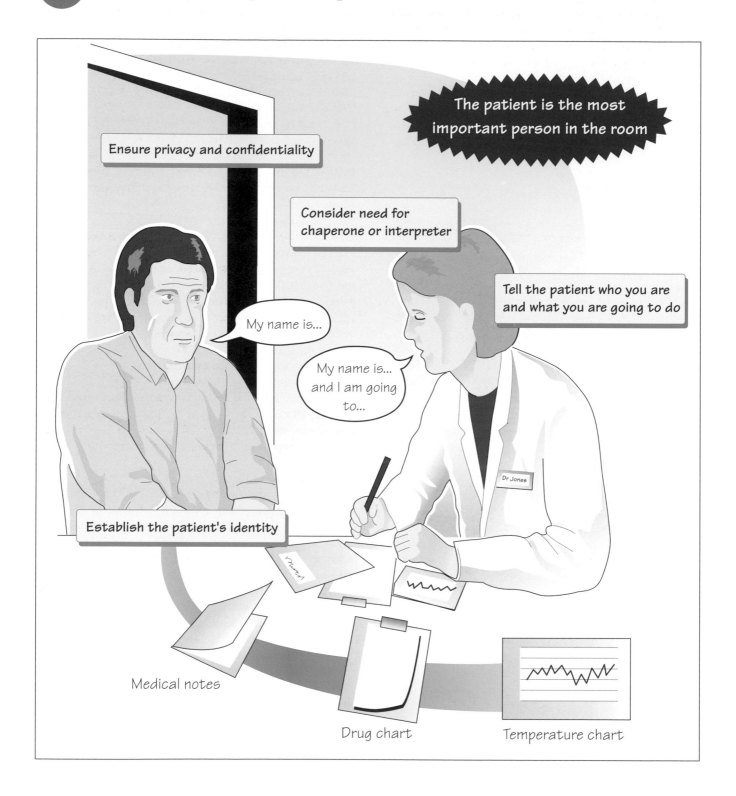

Introduction

When meeting a patient, establish their identity unequivocally (ask for their full name and confirm with their name band, ask for their date of birth, address, etc.) and be certain that any records, notes, test results, etc., refer to that patient.

Often you may wish to shake their hand. You should make eye contact and smile, 'My name is Dr Gleadle. Please come and sit down . . . and you are . . . ?', or 'Your name is . . . ?' and 'Your date of birth is . . . ?', 'Your address is . . . ?' Tell them your name, your title and job and what you are about to do. Always introduce yourself, even if you have met the patient before. For example:

> I am Dr Gleadle, a consultant specializing in kidney medicine and I've been asked to try and work out why your kidneys aren't working properly. I'm going to spend about half an hour talking to you about your medical problems, and then I'll examine you thoroughly. After that I'll explain to you what I think the matter is and what we need to do to help you.

Or you could say, 'I am Jonathan Gleadle, a medical student, and I'd like to ask you some questions about your illness if I may.'

Always be polite, be respectful and be clear. Remember the patient may be feeling anxious, unwell, embarrassed, scared or in pain. Always ensure your hands are washed and that your name badge is clearly visible. Make sure you are fully focused and concentrating on the patient. Ensure you are appropriately prepared by having read the patient's referral letter or notes.

You should be gathering information and observing the patient as soon as you meet them: history taking and examination are not distinct, sequential processes, they are ongoing.

Privacy and comfort

Ensure that there is privacy (this is not always easy in busy hospital wards: make sure curtains are properly closed; see if the examination room is free). Make sure that the patient is comfortable and not hidden by a huge desk or computer screen. These can act as barriers to successful communication. Is the room temperature comfortable?

Language

Establish whether the patient is fluent in the language you intend to use and, if not, arrange for an interpreter to be present.

Relatives, friends, chaperones

Establish who else is with the patient, their relationship with the patient and whether the patient wishes for them to be present during the consultation.

Ask if the patient wishes for a chaperone to be present during the examination and this may be appropriate in any case. Remember that:

THE PATIENT IS THE MOST IMPORTANT PERSON IN THE ROOM!

Remember that all information you gain from your patient or anyone else is **CONFIDENTIAL**. This means that information about the patient should only be discussed with other professionals involved in the care of that patient. You must ensure that patient discussions or records cannot be overheard or accessed by others.

Some guidelines for the use of chaperones

• A chaperone is a third person, (usually) of the same sex as the patient and (usually) a health professional (not a relative).
• When asking a patient if they would like a chaperone to be present, ensure they know what you mean; for example, 'We often ask another member of staff to be present during this examination: would you like me to find someone?'
• If either the patient or the doctor/medical student wish a chaperone to be present then the examination should not be carried out without one.
• Record the presence of a chaperone in the notes.
• A chaperone should be present for intimate examinations by doctors or students examining patients of the opposite sex (vaginal, rectal, genitalia and female breast examination).

Hand washing

The hands of staff are the commonest vehicles by which microorganisms are transmitted between patients and hand washing is the single most important measure in infection control. Whether the hand washing is with alcoholic rubs or medicated soap is less important than that the hands are actually washed. Hands should be washed before each patient contact. Also ensure that your stethoscope is disinfected regularly and other uniforms, such as white coats, are regularly cleaned.

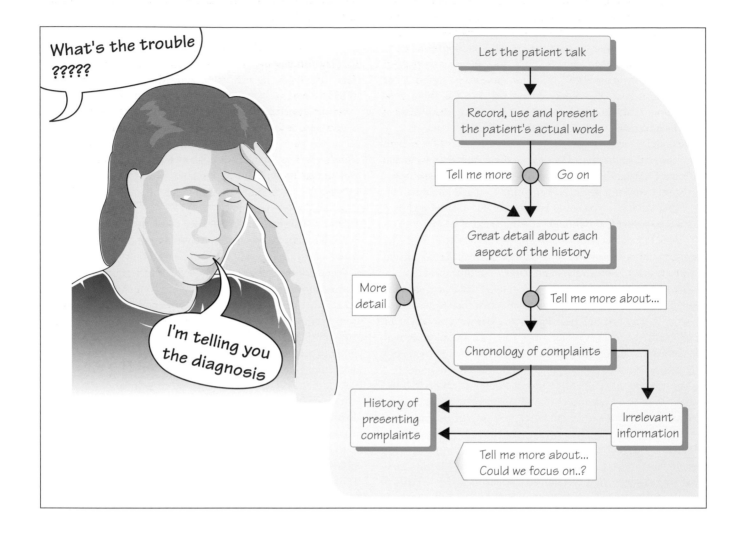

The history of the presenting complaint is by far the most important part of the history and examination. It usually provides the most important information in arriving at a differential diagnosis but also provides vital insight into the features of the complaints that the patient attaches the greatest importance to. It should usually receive the greatest proportion of time in a consultation. The history obtained should be recorded and presented in the patient's own words and should not be masked by medical phrases such as 'dyspnoea' which may mask the true nature of the complaint and important nuances.

If a clear history cannot be obtained from the patient then a history should be sought from relatives, friends or other witnesses. It may be appropriate to seek corroboration of particular features of the history, such as alcohol consumption or details of a collapse.

Let the patient talk

The presenting complaint should be obtained by allowing the patient to talk, usually without interruption. This may be initiated by asking them an open question such as, 'Why have you come

to see me today?', 'What's the problem?' or 'Tell me what seems to be the trouble?' The patient should always be allowed to talk for as long as possible without interruption. Small interjections such as 'go on', or 'tell me more', may help produce more information from a reticent patient. It may be possible to obtain further detail on specific topics by asking about this topic more directly. One strategy is to repeat the last phrase that a patient has voiced in a questioning way; for example, to, 'I'm finding breathing more difficult', you could respond, 'Breathing more difficult?'

Remember that the first complaint may not be the only or the most important concern that the patient has.

More specific questioning

After this, open questions should be addressed to reveal more detail about particular aspects of the history; for example, 'Tell me more about the pain?', 'Tell me in more detail about your tiredness?' or 'You've said that you've been feeling tired?'

More direct questions can then be addressed to gain information about the chronology and other detail of the complaints; for example, 'When exactly did you first notice the breathlessness?',

'Which came first, the chest pain or the breathlessness?', 'What exactly were you doing when the breathlessness came on?'

Directed questions can then be addressed to establish diagnostically important features about the complaints; for example, 'What was the pain like?', 'Was it sharp, heavy or burning?', 'What made the pain worse?', 'Did breathing affect the pain?', 'What about breathing in deeply?', 'How far can you usually walk?', 'What stops you?', 'How do the symptoms interfere with your life (with walking, working, sleeping, etc.)?' If a new symptom or complaint becomes apparent during the interview then it should also be analysed in detail.

It is often helpful to periodically summarize what the patient has told you to verify your own understanding of what the patient has said and invite the patient to correct the interpretation or to provide further information.

Establish the dates and sequence of events

• In some settings, such as during resuscitation of a very ill patient, very focused or abbreviated questioning may be appropriate.
• It may be appropriate to ask the patient what they think is wrong with them, what they think has caused it, and how the problems have affected them (e.g. ability to work, mood, etc.) and their family.

• Other aspects of the history (e.g. PMH or social history) that are conventionally analysed separately, commonly arise during discussion of the presenting complaint and can receive detailed attention at this point.

Focus on the main problems

• Some patients will devote considerable attention to aspects of their illness that are not helpful in achieving a diagnosis or an understanding of the patient and their problems. It may be necessary to interject and divert discussion with phrases such as, 'Could you tell me more about your chest pain?', 'Could we focus on why you came to the doctors this time?' Sometimes there may be a very long list of different complaints in which case the patient should be asked to focus on each in turn.
• Keep in mind the main problems and direct the history accordingly.
• Obtain and record a precise history. Discover exactly how a symptom started, where the patient was, and what they were doing.
• Remember it is the patient's problems that you are trying to understand and record in order to establish diagnoses. Do not force or over interpret what the patient says to fit into a particular diagnosis or symptom, nor simply record what the patient reports other doctors have said.

3 Past medical history, drugs and allergies

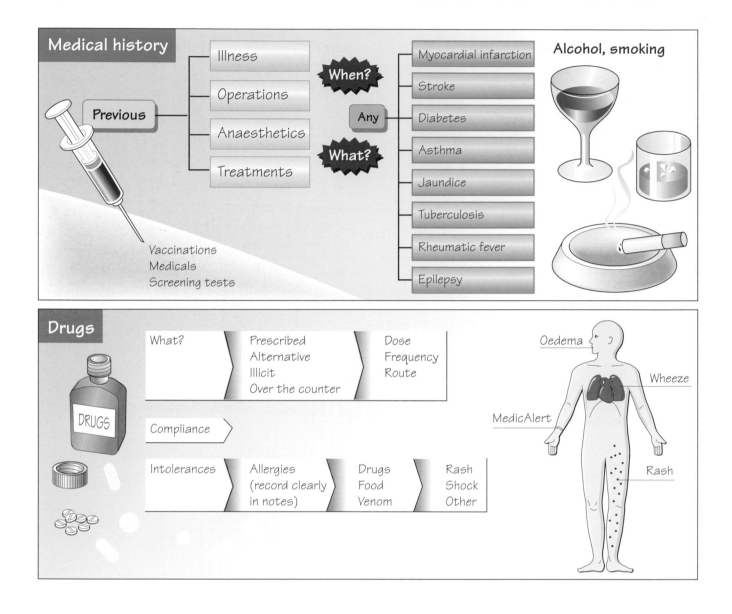

The PMH is a vital part of the history. It is important to record in detail all previous medical problems and their treatment. It is also useful to record this information in chronological order. You could ask, 'What illnesses have you had?', 'What operations?', 'Have you ever been in hospital?', 'When did you last feel completely well?' Ask if there were any problems with operations or anaesthetics, and, if so, what they were. You might turn up a bleeding tendency or an intolerance to particular anaesthetic agents.

If not already discussed in relation to the presenting complaint, specific PMH may need to be enquired about. For example, ask about previous chest pain (angina) in a patient presenting with severe chest pain.

It is conventional to record the occurrence of specific common illnesses, in particular jaundice, anaemia, TB, rheumatic fever, diabetes mellitus, bronchitis, myocardial infarction, stroke, epilepsy, asthma and problems with anaesthesia.

The patient should also be asked about vaccinations, medicals, screening tests (e.g. cervical smear) and pregnancies.

Drug history

- What medication is the patient taking?
- What medication is prescribed and what other remedies are they taking (e.g. herbal remedies, 'over-the-counter' tablets)? Ask to actually see the medication and/or the prescription list.
- Don't forget injections, e.g. insulin, topical treatments, inhalers (patients may not consider them to be drugs).
- What recreational drugs do they/have they taken?

- What is their likely compliance with prescribed medication?
- Is there supervision? A 'dose-it' box?
- What medication have they been intolerant of and why?

Allergies

- It is vital to obtain an accurate and detailed description of the allergic responses to drugs and other potential allergens.
- The patient should be asked if they are allergic to anything. They should be asked specifically whether they are allergic to any antibiotics including penicillin.
- It is also important to elicit the precise nature of the allergy. Was there true allergy with a full-blown anaphylactic shock, an erythematous rash, an urticarial rash, or did the patient only feel nausea or experience another drug side-effect?
- Other important allergies may exist to foodstuffs, such as nuts, or to bee or wasp stings.
- It is also important to elicit other intolerances, such as side-effects, to medication.
- Ensure allergies are clearly recorded in notes, drug charts and, if appropriate, MedicAlert® bracelets.

Smoking

- Does the patient smoke or have they ever smoked?
- If so what type and how many for how long? Smoked cigarettes, pipe or cigar?

Alcohol

- Does the patient drink alcohol? If so what type of alcohol?
- How many units and how often?

- Are there/have there been problems with alcohol dependence (see Chapter 58)?

Evidence

- Many patients recalling a reaction to penicillin are unsure of specific details and are wrongly labelled as penicillin allergic.
- True allergic reactions to penicillin that may produce dangerous reactions on subsequent exposure are characterized by hypotension, anaphylaxis, laryngeal oedema, angiooedema, urticarial rashes and wheezing usually occurring within 1 hour of exposure. Mild maculopapular rashes are very common developing > 72 hours after exposure to penicillin and do not usually indicate a true allergy.
- A detailed history of the patient's drug reaction can help determine whether or not the patient's history is compatible with a true penicillin allergy. Ninety per cent of patients reporting a penicillin allergy are negative for penicillin allergy when assessed by skin testing, meaning that penicillin is withheld from many patients who could safely receive the drug. For patients with a concerning history of penicillin allergy who have a compelling need for penicillin, skin testing should be performed.

Salkind AR, Cuddy PG & Foxworth JW. Is this patient allergic to penicillin? An evidence-based analysis of the likelihood of penicillin allergy. *JAMA* 2001; **285**: 2498–505.

4 Family and social history

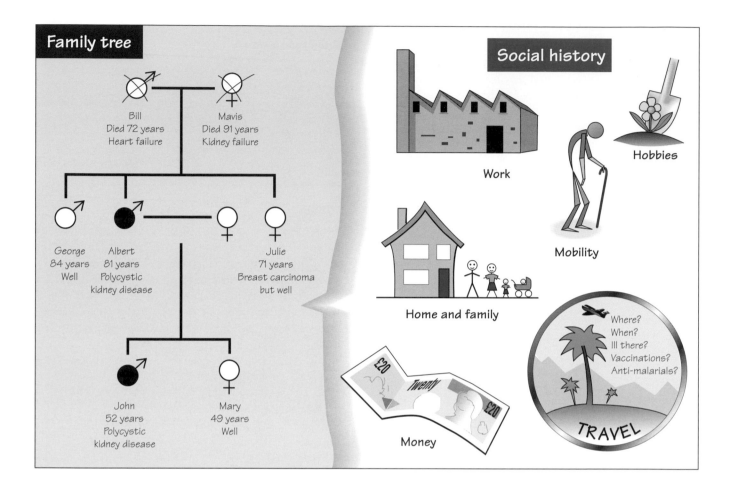

Family tree

Bill
Died 72 years
Heart failure

Mavis
Died 91 years
Kidney failure

George
84 years
Well

Albert
81 years
Polycystic
kidney disease

Julie
71 years
Breast carcinoma
but well

John
52 years
Polycystic
kidney disease

Mary
49 years
Well

Social history

Work

Hobbies

Mobility

Home and family

Money

Where?
When?
Ill there?
Vaccinations?
Anti-malarials?

TRAVEL

Family history

It is important to establish the diseases that have affected relatives given the strong genetic contribution to many diseases:
• What relatives do you have?
• Are your parents still alive? If not, how old were they when they died? What did they die from? Did they suffer from any significant illnesses?
• Have you any siblings, children, grandchildren?
• Are there any diseases that run in the family? (In rare genetic conditions consider the possibility of consanguinity: you can construct a family tree.)
• Are there any illnesses that 'run in the family'?

Social history

It is vital to understand the patient's background, the effect of their illnesses on their life and their family. Particular occupations are at risk of certain illnesses so a full occupational history is important. The following questions should be asked:
• What is your job? What does that actually involve doing?
• What other jobs have you done?
• Who do you live with? Is your partner well? Who else is at home? What sort of place do you live in?

• Do you have any financial difficulties?
• Who does the shopping, washing, cleaning, bathing, etc.?
• What have your illnesses prevented you doing?
• How has it affected your spouse, family?
• Do you get out of the house much? What is your mobility like? How far can you walk? Do you have stairs at home?
• What are your hobbies?
• What help do you get at home? Do you have a home help, 'meals-on-wheels'? What modifications have been made to the house?
• Do you have pets? Are they well?

Travel history

Consider the following questions when taking a travel history from the patient:
• Have you been abroad? Where? When?
• Where did you stop *en route*?
• Where did you visit? Was it rural or urban?
• Did you stay in hotels, camps, etc.?
• Were you well whilst there?
• Did you have specific vaccinations? Have you taken anti-malarial prophylaxis? If so what and for how long?

5 Functional enquiry

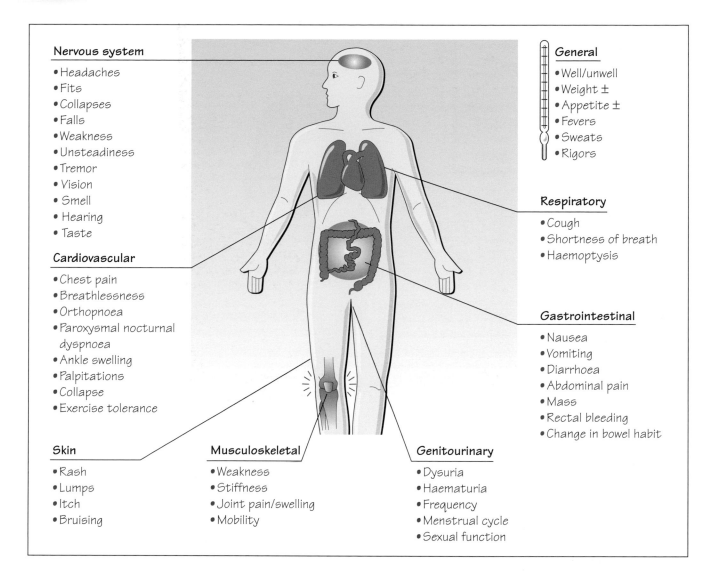

Nervous system

- Headaches
- Fits
- Collapses
- Falls
- Weakness
- Unsteadiness
- Tremor
- Vision
- Smell
- Hearing
- Taste

Cardiovascular

- Chest pain
- Breathlessness
- Orthopnoea
- Paroxysmal nocturnal dyspnoea
- Ankle swelling
- Palpitations
- Collapse
- Exercise tolerance

Skin

- Rash
- Lumps
- Itch
- Bruising

Musculoskeletal

- Weakness
- Stiffness
- Joint pain/swelling
- Mobility

Genitourinary

- Dysuria
- Haematuria
- Frequency
- Menstrual cycle
- Sexual function

General

- Well/unwell
- Weight ±
- Appetite ±
- Fevers
- Sweats
- Rigors

Respiratory

- Cough
- Shortness of breath
- Haemoptysis

Gastrointestinal

- Nausea
- Vomiting
- Diarrhoea
- Abdominal pain
- Mass
- Rectal bleeding
- Change in bowel habit

This part of the history is designed to address any symptoms that have not been elicited from the patient in the history of the presenting complaint. There are obviously a huge number of questions that can be asked. In any given clinical situation these questions will need to be focused depending on the nature of the presenting complaint. The discovery of abnormalities on examination or after investigation may lead to the necessity for further directed questioning. Ask about the symptoms in the figure above.

Other general questions that may be appropriate are asking about heat or cold intolerance or whether there has been any recent injury or falls.

Orthopnoea is breathlessness when lying flat, paroxysmal nocturnal dyspnoea is episodic breathlessness at night. To assess exercise tolerance ask how far the patient can walk on the flat or how many flights of stairs they can climb. Haemoptysis is coughing of blood, haematemesis is vomiting of blood, haematuria is blood in the urine, dysuria is pain on passing urine, dyspareunia is painful intercourse. Ask about erectile dysfunction, the length of the menstrual cycle, period duration, whether periods are heavy, number of pregnancies, age of menarche and menopause.

Is the patient ill?

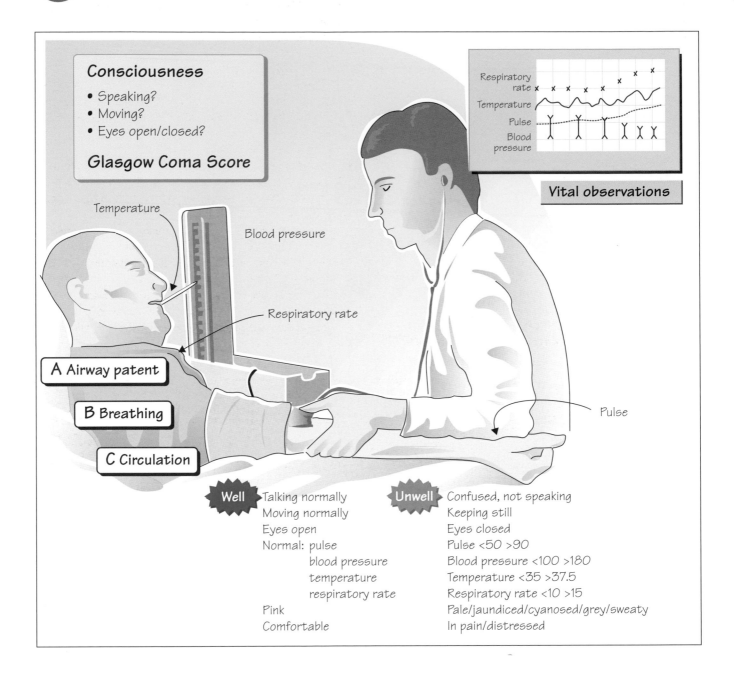

Consciousness

- Speaking?
- Moving?
- Eyes open/closed?

Glasgow Coma Score

Temperature

Blood pressure

Respiratory rate

A Airway patent

B Breathing

C Circulation

Pulse

Respiratory rate

Temperature

Pulse

Blood pressure

Vital observations

Well
Talking normally
Moving normally
Eyes open
Normal: pulse
　　　　blood pressure
　　　　temperature
　　　　respiratory rate
Pink
Comfortable

Unwell
Confused, not speaking
Keeping still
Eyes closed
Pulse <50 >90
Blood pressure <100 >180
Temperature <35 >37.5
Respiratory rate <10 >15
Pale/jaundiced/cyanosed/grey/sweaty
In pain/distressed

One of the most important skills a doctor can gain is the ability to recognize that a patient is ill. There are several features that experienced clinicians notice instantly as warnings that a patient is seriously ill. However, patients may have immediately life-threatening illness without any abnormal findings (e.g. severe hyperkalaemia). In some patients, the history points towards a serious, perhaps life-threatening condition, even in the absence of abnormal physical signs (e.g. the patient who has just had a very sudden onset of the most severe headache they have ever experienced may have had a critical subarachnoid haemorrhage). Experienced nurses and clinicians may also feel that a patient is seriously ill without being able to identify objective abnormalities.

The straightforward *vital observations* of pulse, BP, temperature, respiratory rate and conscious level are essential in assessing ill patients as are trends in those observations (e.g. gradual reduction in blood pressure and increase in pulse rate might indicate the development of hypovolaemia).

If you think the patient is acutely and seriously ill get help from other doctors and nurses.

Airway

- Is the airway patent?
- Is the patient breathing easily and talking comfortably?
- Is there stridor?

Breathing

- Is the patient breathing:
  - slowly
  - rapidly
  - noisily
  - with difficulty?
- Respiratory rate?
- Cheyne–Stokes pattern?
- Is there wheeze?
- Use of accessory muscles?
- Unable to talk because of breathlessness?

Circulation

Check there is adequate circulation:
- Warm/cool peripheries?
- Cyanosis (central/peripheral)?
- Normal/low volume pulse?
- Tachycardia, bradycardia?
- Obvious blood loss?
- Hypotension, postural drop?

Colour

- What is the patient's colour? Is the patient pale (anaemia, shock)?
- What is the temperature? Is the patient pyrexial? Hypothermic?

- Is the patient blue (cyanosed)?
- Is the patient grey? (Combination of cyanosis and pallor?)
- Is the patient clammy? (Sweaty and poor perfusion?)
- Is the patient sweaty?
- Is the patient vomiting?

Consciousness

- Can the patient talk? Does the patient smile? Does the patient make eye contact? Does the patient answer questions appropriately? Does the patient respond to voice, commands? Is the patient drowsy?
- Is the patient comfortable or uncomfortable?
- Is the patient in pain? Grimacing? Appearing abnormally still?
- Is the patient moving normally, restless, paralysed?
- What is the level of consciousness? (Use the Glasgow Coma Score)
- Is the patient alert, reacting to voice, reacting to pain or unresponsive?
- Is the patient moving all their limbs, do his/her eyes open spontaneously?
- Is there abnormal posture, e.g. abnormal extension of limbs (decerebrate), abnormal flexion of arms (decorticate)?
- In any patient, significant changes in these observations may indicate serious deterioration.

Evidence

A modified early warning score (MEWS) derived from five simple observations: systolic BP, heart rate, respiratory rate, temperature and level of consciousness grading is capable of indicating acute medical admissions likely to have an adverse outcome and the patient should receive urgent medical assessment and action.

Scores of five or more on the modified early warning score are associated with increased risk of death (OR 5.4, 95% CI 2.8–10.7) and ICU admission (OR 10.9, 95% CI 2.2–55.6).

Score	3	2	1	0	1	2	3
Systolic BP	< 70	71–80	81–100	101–199		> 200	
Heart rate (b.p.m.)		< 40	41–50	51–100	101–110	111–29	> 130
Respiratory rate (b.p.m.)		< 9		9–14	15–20	21–9	> 30
Temperature (°C)		< 35		35.0–38.4		> 38.5	
AVPU score				Alert	Reacting to voice	Reacting to pain	Unresponsive

Subbe CP, Kruger M, Rutherford P & Gemmel L. Validation of a modified early warning score in medical admissions. *QJM* 2001; **94**: 521–6.

7 Principles of examination

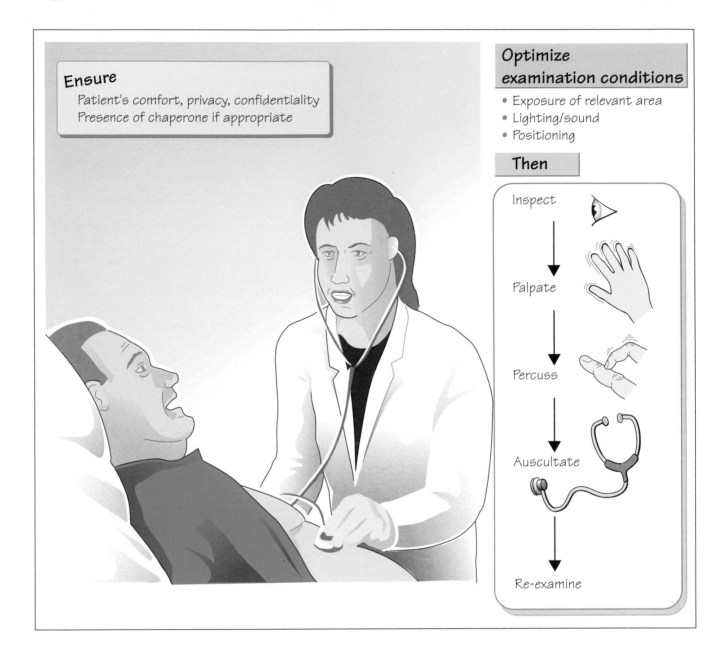

Ensure
Patient's comfort, privacy, confidentiality
Presence of chaperone if appropriate

Optimize examination conditions
- Exposure of relevant area
- Lighting/sound
- Positioning

Then
Inspect
↓
Palpate
↓
Percuss
↓
Auscultate
↓
Re-examine

Explain to the patient what you plan to do. Ensure they are comfortable, warm and that there is privacy. Use all your senses: sight, hearing, smell and touch.

Inspect
- Stand back. Look at the whole patient. Ensure there is adequate lighting.
- Look around the bed for other 'clues' (e.g. oxygen mask, nebulizer, sputum pot, walking stick, vomit bowl).
- Ensure the patient is adequately exposed (with privacy and comfort) and correctly positioned to permit a full examination.

- Look carefully and thoroughly. Are there any obvious abnormalities (e.g. lumps, unconsciousness)?
- Are there any subtle abnormalities (e.g. pallor, fasciculations)?
- Look with specific manoeuvres, such as coughing, breathing or movement.

Palpate
Seek the patient's permission and explain what you are going to do. Ask whether there is any pain or tenderness. Begin the examination lightly and gently and then use firmer pressure. Define any abnormalities carefully, perhaps with measurement. Check if there are thrills.

Percuss

Percuss comparing sides. Listen and 'feel' for any differences. Ensure that this does not cause pain or discomfort.

Auscultate

• Ensure the stethoscope is functioning and take time to listen.

Consider the positioning of the patient to optimize sounds; for example, sitting forward and listening in expiration for aortic regurgitation.

• If abnormalities are found at any stage, try to compare them with the 'normal'; for example, compare the percussion note over equivalent areas of the chest.

8 The cardiovascular system

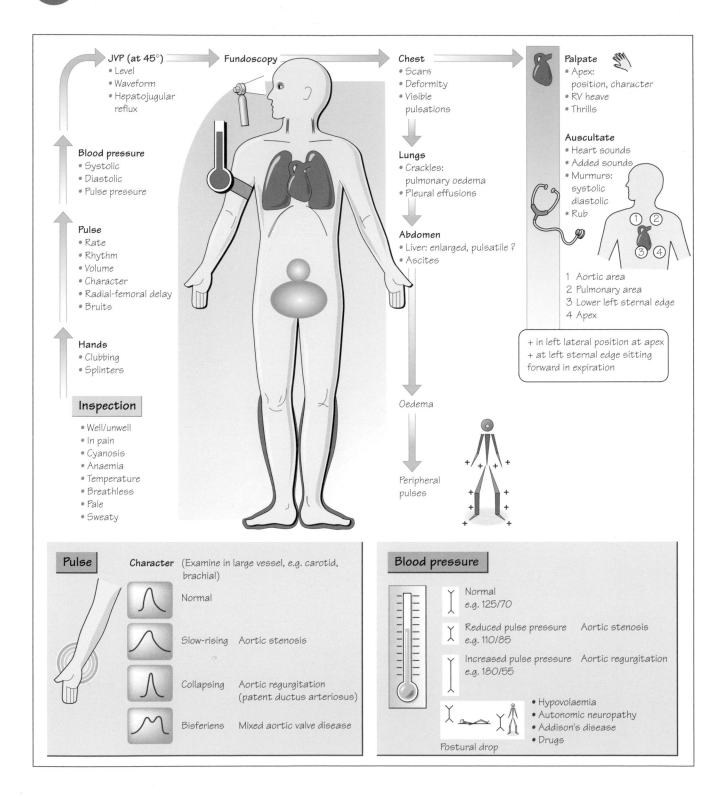

JVP (at 45°)
- Level
- Waveform
- Hepatojugular reflux

Blood pressure
- Systolic
- Diastolic
- Pulse pressure

Pulse
- Rate
- Rhythm
- Volume
- Character
- Radial-femoral delay
- Bruits

Hands
- Clubbing
- Splinters

Inspection
- Well/unwell
- In pain
- Cyanosis
- Anaemia
- Temperature
- Breathless
- Pale
- Sweaty

Fundoscopy

Chest
- Scars
- Deformity
- Visible pulsations

Lungs
- Crackles: pulmonary oedema
- Pleural effusions

Abdomen
- Liver: enlarged, pulsatile ?
- Ascites

Oedema

Peripheral pulses

Palpate
- Apex: position, character
- RV heave
- Thrills

Auscultate
- Heart sounds
- Added sounds
- Murmurs: systolic diastolic
- Rub

1 Aortic area
2 Pulmonary area
3 Lower left sternal edge
4 Apex

+ in left lateral position at apex
+ at left sternal edge sitting forward in expiration

Pulse **Character** (Examine in large vessel, e.g. carotid, brachial)

Normal		
Slow-rising	Aortic stenosis	
Collapsing	Aortic regurgitation (patent ductus arteriosus)	
Bisferiens	Mixed aortic valve disease	

Blood pressure

Normal
e.g. 125/70

Reduced pulse pressure   Aortic stenosis
e.g. 110/85

Increased pulse pressure   Aortic regurgitation
e.g. 180/55

- Hypovolaemia
- Autonomic neuropathy
- Addison's disease
- Drugs

Postural drop

History

Diseases affecting the cardiovascular system can present in a variety of ways:

- chest pain
- breathlessness
- oedema
- palpitations
- syncope
- fatigue
- stroke
- peripheral vascular disease.

Chest pain

- What is the pain like? Where is it?
- Where does it radiate to?
- What was the onset? Sudden, gradual? What was the patient doing when the pain started?
- What brings it on?
- What takes the pain away?
- How severe is it?
- Has the patient had it before?
- What else did the patient notice? Nausea, vomiting, sweating, palpitations, fever, anxiety, cough, haemoptysis?
- What did the patient think it was/is?

Cardiac ischaemia 'Classically' this is central chest pain with radiation to the left arm, both arms and/or jaw (however, it is often 'atypical'). It can be described as pressure, heaviness or as an ache. It is of gradual onset, perhaps precipitated by exertion, cold or anxiety. It can be alleviated by rest, GTN.

Myocardial infarction may additionally have nausea, sweating, vomiting, anxiety (even fear of imminent death).

Pericarditis This is central pain, sharp, with no relation to exertion. It may alleviate on sitting forward. It can be exacerbated by inspiration or coughing.

Pleuritic pain This is a sharp pain exacerbated by respiration, movement and coughing.

Breathlessness

- Breathlessness due to cardiac disease is most usually due to pulmonary oedema.
- The breathlessness is more prominent when lying flat (orthopnoea) or may present suddenly in the night (PND) or be present on minimal exertion.
- It may be accompanied by cough and wheeze and, if very severe, frothy pink sputum.

Oedema (swelling, usually due to fluid accumulation)
Peripheral oedema is usually dependent, commonly affecting the legs and the sacral area. If it is very severe, more widespread oedema can occur.

Palpitations

There may be a sensation of the heart racing or thumping. Establish provocation, onset, duration, speed and rhythm of the heart rate, and the frequency of episodes. Are the episodes accompanied by chest pain, syncope and breathlessness?

Syncope (sudden, brief loss of consciousness)
Syncope may occur as a result of tachyarrhythmias, bradycardias or, rarely, exertion induced in aortic stenosis (it is also seen in neurological conditions such as epilepsy).

- What can the patient remember? What was the patient doing? Were there palpitations, chest pain or other symptoms?
- Was the episode witnessed? What do the witnesses describe? (Was there pallor, cyanosis, flushing on recovery, abnormal movements?)
- Was there tongue biting, urinary incontinence? How quickly did the patient recover?

Past medical history

Ask about risk factors for IHD (smoking, hypertension, diabetes, hyperlipidaemia, previous IHD, cerebrovascular disease or PVD).

- Ask about rheumatic fever
- Ask about recent dental work (infective endocarditis)
- Any known heart murmur?
- Any intravenous drug abuse?

Family history

Any family history of IHD, hyperlipidaemia, sudden death, cardiomyopathy or congenital heart disease?

Social history

- Does or did the patient smoke?
- What is the patient's alcohol intake?
- What is the patient's occupation?
- What is the patient's exercise capacity?
- Any lifestyle limitations due to disease?

Drugs

Ask about drugs for cardiac disease and drugs with cardiac side-effects.

Continued on pp. 24–25.

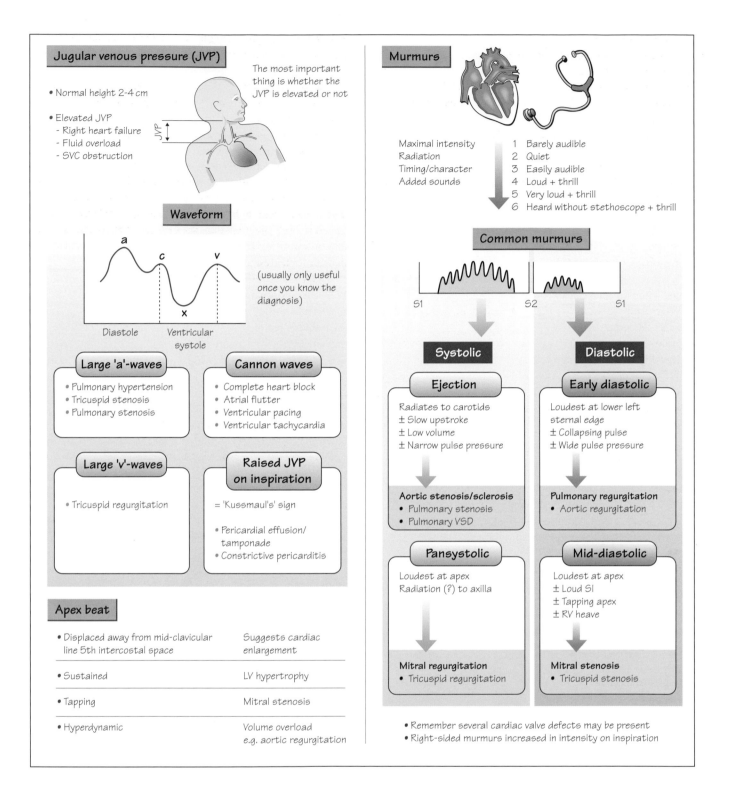

Jugular venous pressure (JVP)

- Normal height 2-4 cm

- Elevated JVP
  - Right heart failure
  - Fluid overload
  - SVC obstruction

The most important thing is whether the JVP is elevated or not

Waveform

(usually only useful once you know the diagnosis)

Diastole Ventricular systole

Large 'a'-waves
- Pulmonary hypertension
- Tricuspid stenosis
- Pulmonary stenosis

Cannon waves
- Complete heart block
- Atrial flutter
- Ventricular pacing
- Ventricular tachycardia

Large 'v'-waves
- Tricuspid regurgitation

Raised JVP on inspiration

= 'Kussmaul's' sign

- Pericardial effusion/ tamponade
- Constrictive pericarditis

Apex beat

• Displaced away from mid-clavicular line 5th intercostal space	Suggests cardiac enlargement
• Sustained	LV hypertrophy
• Tapping	Mitral stenosis
• Hyperdynamic	Volume overload e.g. aortic regurgitation

Murmurs

Maximal intensity	1	Barely audible
Radiation	2	Quiet
Timing/character	3	Easily audible
Added sounds	4	Loud + thrill
	5	Very loud + thrill
	6	Heard without stethoscope + thrill

Common murmurs

S1   S2   S1

Systolic

Ejection

Radiates to carotids
± Slow upstroke
± Low volume
± Narrow pulse pressure

Aortic stenosis/sclerosis
- Pulmonary stenosis
- Pulmonary VSD

Pansystolic

Loudest at apex
Radiation (?) to axilla

Mitral regurgitation
- Tricuspid regurgitation

Diastolic

Early diastolic

Loudest at lower left sternal edge
± Collapsing pulse
± Wide pulse pressure

Pulmonary regurgitation
- Aortic regurgitation

Mid-diastolic

Loudest at apex
± Loud SI
± Tapping apex
± RV heave

Mitral stenosis
- Tricuspid stenosis

- Remember several cardiac valve defects may be present
- Right-sided murmurs increased in intensity on inspiration

Examination

- Is the patient well or unwell? Is the patient comfortable/distressed/in pain/anxious?
- Does the patient need immediate resuscitation?
- Consider the need for oxygen, intravenous access, ECG monitoring.
- Is the patient pale, cyanosed, breathless, coughing, etc?
- What is the patient's temperature?
- Inspect for any scars, sputum, etc.
- Stigmata of hypercholesterolaemia (arcus, xanthelasma) and smoking?

Hands

Is there clubbing, splinter haemorrhages, good peripheral perfusion?

Pulse

- What are the rate, rhythm, volume and character of the radial pulse?
- Assess pulse character at large pulse (brachial, carotid, femoral).
- Are all peripheral pulses present?
- Is there radial–femoral delay?

Blood pressure (see Chapter 36)

- What are the systolic, diastolic and hence pulse pressures?
- Is there a postural fall in BP?
- For diastolic BP use Korotkoff V (when sounds disappear).

Jugular venous pressure

- What is the level of the JVP? (Describe it as centimetres above the sternal angle [or clavicle] when at 45°.)

- Is there hepatojugular reflux (or abdominojugular test)? (The rise in JVP with firm pressure over the right upper-quadrant of the abdomen.)
- Is there an abnormal JVP waveform (e.g. cannon waves)?
- Inspect the mouth, tongue, teeth, praecordium (any scars, abnormal pulsations).
- **Palpate** for position and character of **apex beat**. Any right ventricular *heave*, any *thrills?*
- **Auscultate heart**. Listen for first heart sound, second heart sound (normally split?), added heart sounds (gallop?), systolic murmurs, diastolic murmurs, rubs, clicks, carotid and femoral bruits. Auscultate in left lateral position (particularly for mitral murmurs) and leaning forward in expiration (particularly for early diastolic murmur of aortic regurgitation).
- **Auscultate lungs**. Pleural effusions, crackles?
- **Peripheral oedema** (ankles, legs, sacrum)?
- **Palpate peripheral pulses:**
  - radial
  - brachial
  - carotid
  - femoral
  - popliteal
  - posterior tibial
  - dorsalis pedis.
- **Palpate the liver**. Is it enlarged? Is it pulsatile (suggesting tricuspid regurgitation)? Ascites?
- **Fundoscopy**: changes of hypertension?

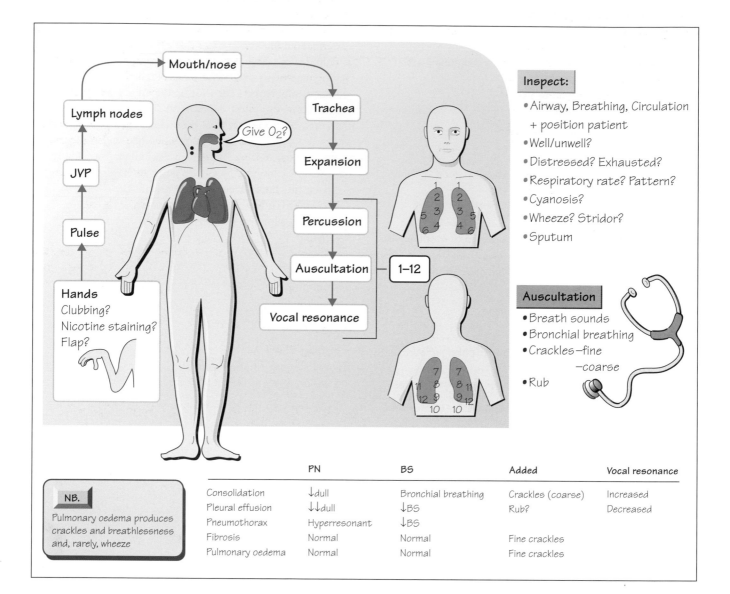

	PN	BS	Added	Vocal resonance
Consolidation	↓dull	Bronchial breathing	Crackles (coarse)	Increased
Pleural effusion	↓↓dull	↓BS	Rub?	Decreased
Pneumothorax	Hyperresonant	↓BS		
Fibrosis	Normal	Normal	Fine crackles	
Pulmonary oedema	Normal	Normal	Fine crackles	

NB.

Pulmonary oedema produces crackles and breathlessness and, rarely, wheeze

History

Diseases affecting the respiratory system may present with breathlessness, cough, haemoptysis, or chest pain.

Breathlessness

• Is the patient breathless at rest, on exertion or when lying flat (orthopnoea)?
• How far can the patient walk, run or climb upstairs?
• Is it a chronic condition or has it occurred suddenly?
• Is it accompanied by a wheeze or stridor?

Cough

• Is it dry or productive?
• If productive, what colour is the sputum? Is it green and purulent? Is blood coughed up (haemoptysis)? Is it 'rusty' (pneumonia) or pink and frothy (pulmonary oedema)?
• Does it occur every winter or is this a new symptom?

Haemoptysis

• How many times? How much blood is expectorated?

Chest pain

• When did it start? What type of pain? Where is it and where does it radiate to? Is it worsened/alleviated by breathing, posture, movement? Is there localized tenderness?
• Disorders affecting the respiratory system commonly produce a 'pleuritic-type' pain that is sharp, localized, exacerbated by breathing and coughing.

Systemic manifestations

• Any weight loss due to, e.g., a bronchial malignancy.
• Any fever, rigors, weight loss, malaise, night sweats, lymphadenopathy, skin rash?
• Are there gaps in breathing (apnoea) accompanied by snoring and/or excessive daytime sleepiness suggesting obstruct-

ive sleep apnoea (especially in the obese with increased collar size)?

Past medical history
• Does the patient have previous respiratory conditions? Asthma, COPD, TB or TB exposure?
• Was the patient ever admitted to hospital for breathlessness?
• Did the patient ever need ventilation?
• Any known chest X-ray abnormalities?

Drugs
• What medication is the patient taking?
• Any recent changes to the patient's medication?
• Any responses to treatment in the past?
• Is the patient using tablets, inhalers, nebulizers or oxygen?

Allergies
Any allergies to drugs/environmental antigens (e.g. pollen, cats, dogs, etc.)?

Smoking
Is the patient currently smoking? Did the patient ever smoke? If so, how many?

Family and social history
• Has the patient been exposed to asbestos, dust or other toxins?
• What is the patient's occupation?
• Any family history of respiratory problems?
• Does the patient own any pets, including birds?

Examination
• Is the patient well or unwell?
• Is there an adequate airway? If not, correct with head position, oral airway, laryngeal mask or endotracheal intubation.
• Is the patient breathing? If not, ensure airway, give supplemental oxygen and ventilate.
• Is the circulation adequate?
• Is the patient cyanosed (peripherally or centrally)? *If there is cyanosis, hypoxaemia on pulse oximetry, respiratory distress or the patient appears unwell give oxygen via face mask.* (Caution with a high concentration of oxygen is only relevant in patients with COPD who may have a hypoxic ventilatory drive.)
• What is the respiratory rate and pattern?
• Is there breathlessness at rest, on moving, getting dressed or getting onto a couch?
• What is the patient's general appearance? Cachexia, thin,

signs of SVC obstruction (fixed elevation of JVP, dilatation of superficial chest veins, facial swelling)?
• Is the patient comfortable, in pain, exhausted, scared or distressed?
• Check for signs of respiratory distress: rapid respiration rate, use of accessory muscles, tracheal tug, intercostal recession, paradoxical abdominal movements, use of pursed lips or respiratory rate falling as patient becomes fatigued.
• Is there audible wheeze (largely expiratory noise) or stridor (principally inspiratory sound)?
• Is there clubbing or wrist tenderness (hypertrophic osteoarthropathy), nicotine staining of fingers or a flap (consistent with carbon dioxide retention)?
• Examine the patient's pulse and the JVP, for lymphadenopathy, the mouth and the nose.
• What is the position of the trachea? Any deviation?

Chest
Examine the chest anteriorly and posteriorly by inspection, palpation, percussion and auscultation. Compare the left and right sides and ensure the examination includes the axillae and lateral parts of the chest.

Inspection
• Shape of chest wall and spine?
• Scars (radiotherapy or surgery)?
• Prominent veins (SVC obstruction)?
• Respiratory rate and rhythm?
• Chest wall movement (symmetrical, hyperexpanded)?
• Intercostal recession?

Palpation
Examine for tenderness, position of apex beat and chest wall expansion.

Percussion
Examine for dullness or hyperresonance.

Auscultation
• Use the diaphragm of the stethoscope.
• Listen for breath sounds, bronchial breathing and added sounds (crackles, rub, wheeze).
• Diminished/absent breath sounds occur in effusion, collapse, consolidation with blocked airway, fibrosis, pneumothorax and raised diaphragm.
• Bronchial breathing can be found with consolidation and collapse.
• Examine for vocal resonance and/or vocal fremitus.

Evidence

There is a paucity of good-quality evidence on the sensitivity and specificity of clinical signs in respiratory disease. Several studies do suggest a low interobserver agreement for chest signs, low sensitivity and specificity in diagnosing pneumonia on examination alone (Spiteri *et al.* 1988; Wipf *et al.* 1999). This emphasizes the need for other investigations, e.g. a chest X-ray, if the patient is unwell.
Spiteri MA, Cook DG & Clarke SW. Reliability of eliciting physical signs in examination of the chest. *Lancet* 1988; **1**: 873–5.
Wipf JE, Lipsky BA, Hirschmann JV *et al*. Diagnosing pneumonia by physical examination: relevant or relic? *Arch Intern Med* 1999; **159**: 1082–7.

10 The gastrointestinal system

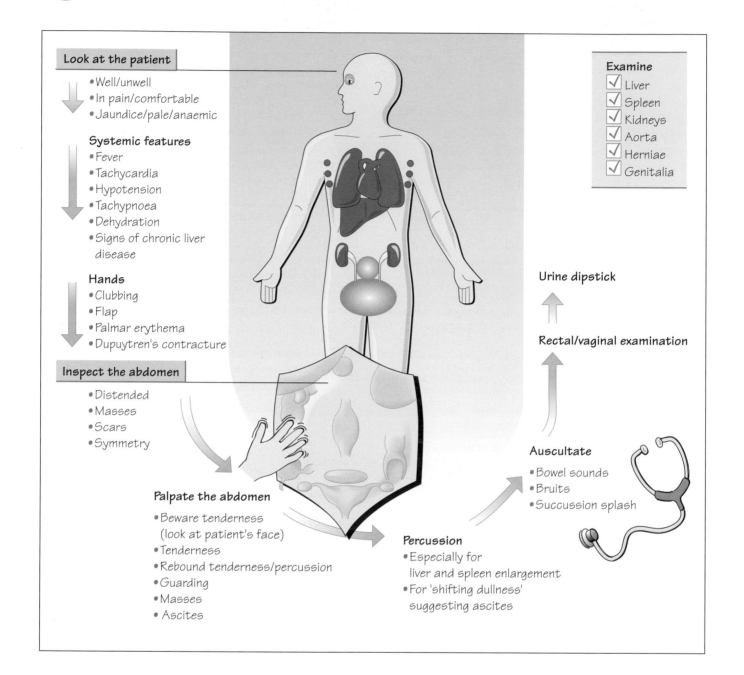

Look at the patient
- Well/unwell
- In pain/comfortable
- Jaundice/pale/anaemic

Systemic features
- Fever
- Tachycardia
- Hypotension
- Tachypnoea
- Dehydration
- Signs of chronic liver disease

Hands
- Clubbing
- Flap
- Palmar erythema
- Dupuytren's contracture

Inspect the abdomen
- Distended
- Masses
- Scars
- Symmetry

Palpate the abdomen
- Beware tenderness (look at patient's face)
- Tenderness
- Rebound tenderness/percussion
- Guarding
- Masses
- Ascites

Percussion
- Especially for liver and spleen enlargement
- For 'shifting dullness' suggesting ascites

Auscultate
- Bowel sounds
- Bruits
- Succussion splash

Urine dipstick

Rectal/vaginal examination

Examine
- ☑ Liver
- ☑ Spleen
- ☑ Kidneys
- ☑ Aorta
- ☑ Herniae
- ☑ Genitalia

History
Disorders affecting the abdomen and GI system may present with a very wide range of different symptoms:
- abdominal pain
- vomiting
- haematemesis (vomiting blood or 'coffee grounds')
- difficulty swallowing (dysphagia)
- indigestion or dyspepsia
- diarrhoea
- change in bowel habit
- abdominal swelling or lump
- reduced appetite
- recurrent mouth ulcers
- weight loss or symptoms due to malabsorption
- melaena (black, tarry stool due to blood from the upper GI tract) or blood per rectum.

It is important to assess both whether there is local disease and whether there are any systemic effects such as weight loss or malabsorption.

Past medical history
- Any previous GI disease?

- Are there any previous abdominal operations?
- Establish the patient's alcohol and smoking history. A detailed alcohol history is essential.
- What drugs has the patient taken?
- Has the patient taken any treatments for GI disease, including any that may be a possible cause of the symptoms (e.g. NSAIDs and dyspepsia)?

Family history
Are there any inherited conditions affecting the GI system?

Examination
Look at the patient
- Is the patient well or unwell, comfortable or in pain, moving easily or lying motionless?
- Is there pallor, jaundice or lymphadenopathy?
- Is the patient thin or obese?
- Look for systemic features of illness (fever, tachycardia, hypotension, postural hypotension, tachypnoea, dehydration and hypovolaemia).
- Look for signs of chronic liver disease (spider naevi, gynaecomastia, bruising, parotid hypertrophy, palmar erythema, leuconychia, Dupuytren's contracture, excoriations and a metabolic flap [asterixis]).

Examine the hands
Is there clubbing, palmar erythema, Dupuytren's contracture or a metabolic flap (asterixis)?

Examine the mouth and tongue
- Look for angular stomatitis, aphthous ulcers, telangiectasia
- Look for supraclavicular and other *lymphadenopathy* (Virchow's node or Troissier's sign—left supraclavicular lymphadenopathy due to spread from abdominal carcinoma).

Examine the abdomen
Ensure patient is warm, comfortable and there is sufficient exposure of the abdomen. The patient should be lying flat with the head supported. Relax the patient.

Inspect the abdomen
- Is it distended, asymmetrical, are there masses, scars, visible peristalsis, stoma?
- Ask the patient to cough, take a deep breath and look carefully.

Palpate the abdomen
- Ask if they have any pain or tenderness: be particularly careful if they have. Look at the patient's face whilst examining for any tenderness or pain. Palpate lightly with fingertips ± ulnar border of index finger and then more deeply. Palpate all areas of the abdomen. Any masses or other abnormalities should be assessed in great detail for size, position, shape, consistency, location, edge, mobility with respiration and pulsatility.
- Is there any tenderness? If so, define the area with care.
- Any rigidity?

- Is there rebound tenderness? (pain on quick removal of examining hand—some clinicians prefer to use percussion to minimize pain).
- Is there guarding?

Auscultate
Auscultate for bowel sounds (absent/present, normal/abnormal, hyperactive, high-pitched, tinkling [suggesting obstruction]).

Is there ascites?
Abdominal distension, flank dullness with shifting dullness?

Examine for specific organs
Examine the liver
- Is it enlarged? Is it palpable below the right costal margin?
- Palpate with ulnar border and pulp of index finger during gentle respiration. Begin in the right iliac fossa.
- Measure. Define the upper extent by percussion. Is the liver smoothly enlarged, tender, pulsatile, hard or irregular (suggesting tumour)? Is there a bruit?

Examine the spleen
- Is the spleen enlarged? Is it palpable below the left costal margin? Begin in right iliac fossa and palpate towards left costal margin. Measure. Define the upper extent by percussion. Is it tender? Bruit? Does it move with respiration?
- Are there any other signs of portal hypertension e.g. ascites, caput medusae, distended veins (determine direction of flow)?

Examine the kidneys
Are the kidneys palpable? Ballottable? Smoothly or irregularly enlarged (consider polycystic kidney disease), bruits?

Examine for an aortic aneurysm
Size, pulsatile, tender?

Examine for inguinal and femoral herniae
Cough impulse, irreducible, tender?

Examine external genitalia
- Any testicular tenderness, lumps, enlargement or penile discharge?
- Are there any vulval lumps, ulcers, discharge or prolapse?

Perform digital rectal examination
Is there tenderness, abnormal masses, prostatic enlargement, stool, blood or mucus present?

Vaginal examination
Consider performing a vaginal examination.

Urine and faeces examination
Consider examining urine (dipstick ± microscopy) and faeces (faecal occult blood).

11 The male genitourinary system

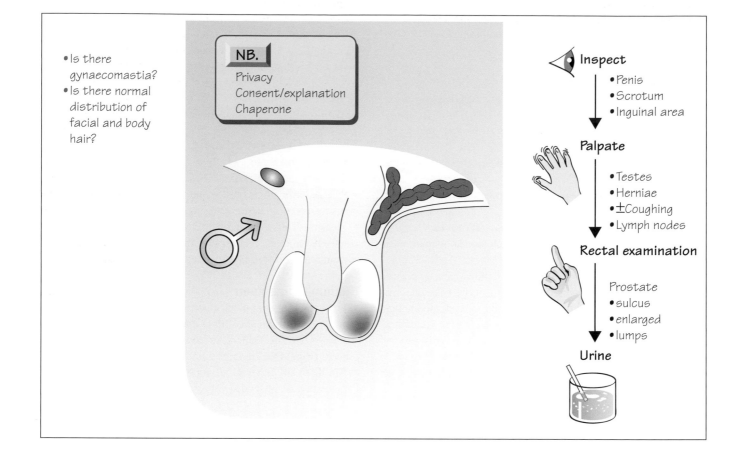

History
Presentations can include:
- dysuria (pain or discomfort on passing urine)
- urethral discharge
- genital ulceration
- erectile dysfunction or other sexual difficulties
- infertility
- testicular pain or lump
- urinary symptoms, such as frequency.

Assess each symptom in detail. A 'permission giving' style of questioning may be helpful when asking about sensitive topics; for example, 'Some men with diabetes find it hard to achieve erections. Have you had any problems like that?' If there is erectile dysfunction, discover when the problem occurs, if normal erections are ever achieved (e.g. in the early morning) and what the patient thinks the difficulty is.

Ask in detail about the urinary stream (hesitancy, frequency, power of stream, terminal dribbling, spraying, nocturia).

Past medical history
- Any previous genitourinary problems? Ask particularly about STDs.
- Any previous UTI, haematuria or calculi?
- Any history of cardiovascular or neurological diseases?

- Any investigations for infertility?
- Any history of testicular disease (e.g. torsion)?
- In a patient with sexual dysfunction consider the possibility of:
  - *diabetes* which can eventually cause impotence in up to half of affected men
  - *depression and psychotic illnesses* which cause loss of sexual desire in a high proportion of men
  - *heart disease*, especially when combined with hyperlipidaemia and arteriopathy, accounts for erectile dysfunction in many men
  - *other hormone deficiencies*, especially thyroid and testosterone, reduce sexual desire
  - *operations and trauma*, especially prostate, can cause problems. Damage to the pelvis or spine is another obvious cause
  - *prolactinoma* may, rarely, present as a loss of sexual desire and headaches in a younger man

Drugs
Consider drugs that might produce erectile dysfunction (e.g. anti-hypertensives).

Alcohol and smoking history
Ask the patient about any history of alcohol or smoking.

Family and social history

- Ask about the patient's sexual activity and orientation.
- Does any partner have any problems or symptoms of STD (e.g. vaginal discharge)?
- What contraceptive measures has/does the patient use?
- Has the patient fathered children?

Functional enquiry

Are there any symptoms of renal disease, depression?

Examination

- Ensure that the patient is comfortable, chaperoned if appropriate, that there is privacy and that they understand fully what the examination will involve. Remember the patient will usually be anxious or embarrassed and the examination may be uncomfortable and should be undertaken gently.
- Expose the genitalia fully.
- Inspect carefully the penis, scrotum and inguinal region.
- Look for any lumps, warts, discoloration, discharge, rashes.
- Inspect the urethral meatus and retract the foreskin to expose the glans.
- Palpate the penis, vas deferens, epididymus and testes.
- If any lumps are apparent you can examine them with trans-illumination for fluid.
- Examine for herniae with coughing.
- Perform a digital rectal examination.

- Examine the anus for any abnormalities. Examine for any rectal lumps and palpate prostate gland. Is there any tenderness? Is the median sulcus preserved? Is the prostate enlarged? Is it hard, irregular, craggy, fixed?
- Examine the urine with dipstick and microscopy for blood, protein, white blood cells and casts.
- If there is erectile dysfunction it may be appropriate to examine carefully for peripheral vascular disease and any neurological deficits. There is dual innervation of the male reproductive system from the sacral roots (S2–4) through the pudendal and pelvic nerves with predominantly somatic and parasympathetic fibres, and from the thoracolumbar roots (T11–L2) through the hypogastric, sympathetic, and pelvic nerves. Tactile (dorsal column) and pinprick (spinothalamic tract) sensation in the perineal and lower limb dermatomes should be assessed. If there is concern about the possibility of neurological deficit the perineal reflexes may be tested, require very careful explanation and can provide evidence of spinal cord dysfunction:
  - *Bulbocavernosus reflex (S2 and S3)*. Firmly squeezing the glans penis provokes a contraction of the bulbocavernosus muscle located between the scrotum and anal sphincter.
  - *Bulbo-anal reflex (S3 and S4)*. Firmly squeezing the glans penis provokes a contraction of the anal sphincter.
  - *Anal reflex (S4 and S5)*. Stroking or scratching the skin adjacent to the anus provokes a contraction of the anal sphincter.

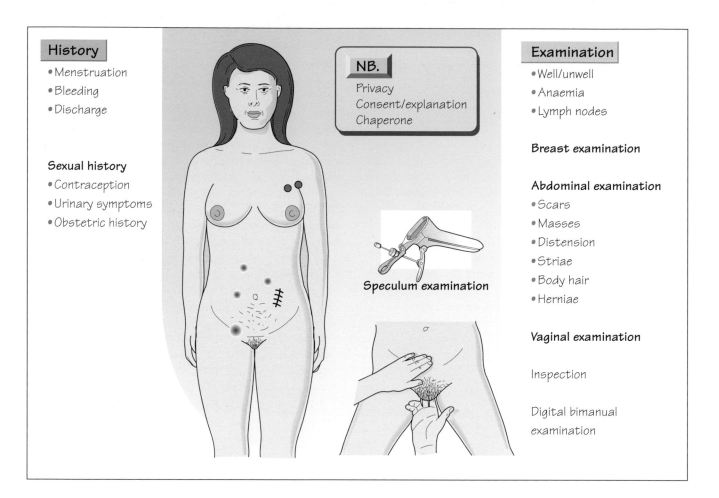

History
- Menstruation
- Bleeding
- Discharge

Sexual history
- Contraception
- Urinary symptoms
- Obstetric history

NB.
Privacy
Consent/explanation
Chaperone

Speculum examination

Examination
- Well/unwell
- Anaemia
- Lymph nodes

Breast examination

Abdominal examination
- Scars
- Masses
- Distension
- Striae
- Body hair
- Herniae

Vaginal examination

Inspection

Digital bimanual examination

Gynaecological problems can present with a variety of symptoms including:
- heavy periods (menorrhagia)
- no menstruation (amenorrhoea)
- vaginal discharge
- suprapubic pain
- vaginal bleeding
- contraceptive problems
- painful sexual intercourse (dyspareunia).

Menstruation
• How often are the patient's periods? How long does the patient's menstruation last? Are the periods regular, irregular? Are they heavy (menorrhagia) (ask about number of pads, tampons and presence of clots)? Are they painful?
- Any intermenstrual bleeding?
- Any postcoital bleeding?
- Any vaginal discharge? If so what is it like?
- When was the last menstrual period?
- Any postmenopausal bleeding?

Sexual activity/contraception/cervix
• Is the patient sexually active? Are there any problems with sexual intercourse?

• Is intercourse painful (dyspareunia)? Does it hurt deep inside or superficially?
• What contraceptive is the patient using?
• What contraceptive measures has the patient used in the past?
• When was the patient's last cervical smear?
• Has the patient ever had an abnormal smear? If so what was done (e.g. colposcopy)?

Urinary symptoms
• Any urinary frequency, dysuria, haematuria, nocturia, urgency or incontinence?
• If there is incontinence, when? With straining, coughing or urgency?
• Does the patient have any sensation of a mass in the vagina or a dragging heavy sensation (e.g. due to prolapse)?

Past medical history
• Has the patient had any previous gynaecological operations, STDs or significant medical conditions?

Past obstetric history
• Has the patient ever been pregnant? If so ask about deliveries, health of any children now, how they were born and what their birth weight was.

- Has the patient had any miscarriages or terminations of pregnancy?
- Did the patient have any major complications during pregnancy or labour?

Drugs
- Does the patient take any regular medications or contraception?
- Does the patient have any allergies?

Family history
Any family history of breast or ovarian carcinoma?

Social history
- Ask about any current relationships. Is the patient married? Does she have any children?
- What is the patient's occupation?

The gynaecological examination
Remember that over a third of women prefer to be examined by a doctor of their own sex and it should be considered if this is possible, and that in some cultures intimate examinations may not be acceptable.

General appearance
- Is the patient well or unwell, thin or overweight?
- Any sign of anaemia or lymphadenopathy?
- Look for secondary sexual characteristics and hirsutism.
- What is the patient's pulse, BP and temperature?

Breast examination (see also Chapters 13 and 46)
- *Inspect* the breasts. Are they symmetrical? Is there an obvious lump, is there tethering of the skin? Is the overlying skin abnormal (e.g. *peau d'orange* appearance, puckering, ulceration)?
- Examine the breast with the patient's arms elevated. Are the nipples normal, inverted, any discharge?
- Lightly *palpate* each quadrant of the breast including the axillary tail of breast tissue. Use the palmar surface of the fingers. Are there any lumps? If so, where and what size? What is their consistency (firm, soft rubbery, craggy, etc.)? Are the lumps tender? Examine the overlying skin for discoloration and tethering. Examine for tethering of the lump to deep structures.
- Examine for axillary and other lymphadenopathy. Are the arms normal or swollen?

Examine the abdomen
- *Inspect* the abdomen for scars, masses, distension, striae, body hair distribution and herniae.
- *Palpate* the abdomen for masses and tenderness. Palpate specifically for masses from umbilicus down to the symphysis pubis. If there are masses, can you get below them or do they seem to arise from the pelvis?
- *Percuss* the abdomen for masses and for shifting dullness.

Vaginal examination
- Ensure a chaperone is present if appropriate and that there is privacy. Remember the patient may feel anxious and embarrassed.
- Explain that you are going to examine the patient internally and that it may be uncomfortable but that it should not be painful.
- Inspect for any lumps, ulcers, discoloration, discharge and obvious prolapse.
- Using lubricating jelly and gloved fingers, gently insert the first two fingers of the right hand into the vagina. Place the left hand above the symphysis pubis and push downwards gently into the pelvis.
- Examine for the cervix, the uterus and the adnexa. Are there any masses, irregularities or abnormal tenderness?

Cuscoe's speculum examination
This is designed to allow inspection of the cervix and vaginal walls.

Ensure the speculum is warmed and lubricated. Insert the speculum with the blades closed and parallel to the labia. Rotate it 90° and then insert it a little further in. Open the blades slowly and ensure the patient is not uncomfortable throughout. It should now be possible to visualize the cervix. Look for irregularities, bleeding and ulceration. A smear may be taken. Slightly withdraw the speculum and partially close it. As the speculum is further withdrawn the vaginal walls may be inspected for abnormalities.

Sim's speculum
This speculum examination is undertaken with the patient in the left lateral position with legs curled up. It can enable better inspection of the vaginal walls and is used in particular if prolapse is suspected.

Rectal examination
A rectal examination may be required, particularly if there is posterior wall prolapse or malignant cervical disease.

13 Breast examination

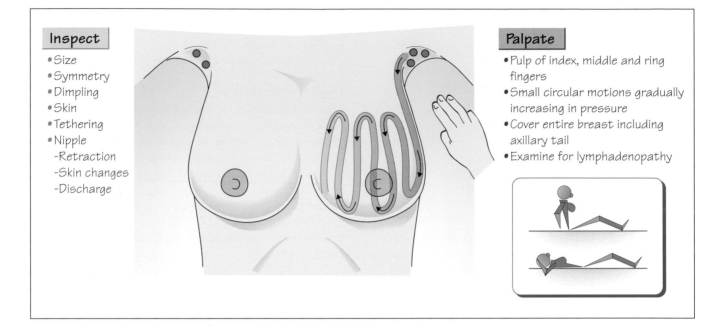

Inspect
- Size
- Symmetry
- Dimpling
- Skin
- Tethering
- Nipple
  - Retraction
  - Skin changes
  - Discharge

Palpate
- Pulp of index, middle and ring fingers
- Small circular motions gradually increasing in pressure
- Cover entire breast including axillary tail
- Examine for lymphadenopathy

History

Diseases of the breast may present with lumps, pain, rash, discharge from the nipple or they may produce systemic symptoms (e.g. fever with breast abscess or weight loss and back pain with metastatic carcinoma of the breast).

Past medical history

Any previous breast disease, lumps, mammography, biopsy, mastectomy, radiotherapy or chemotherapy?

Drugs

- Any use of tamoxifen?
- Any use of oestrogens?

Family history

Any family history of breast cancer?

Functional enquiry

- Patient's menstrual cycle?
- Systemic symptoms that might suggest metastatic disease, such as weight loss, back pain, jaundice or lymphadenopathy?

Examination

- Ensure the patient is comfortable, warm, understands what you are going to do. Also ensure that there is a chaperone present if appropriate and the patient is lying at 45°.
- Inspect the breasts for shape, size, symmetry, skin abnormalities and scars. Look for any obvious lumps, dimpling, skin tethering. Ask the patient to lift their arms above their head and inspect again. Look at the nipples for retraction, any skin changes or discharge.
- Many practitioners then lay the patient flat. Palpate the breasts, gently initially and then more firmly using the pulps of the first three fingers. Use gentle circular motions and examine each quadrant of the breast and the axillary tail. Take time to examine carefully. If any lumps are defined examine them carefully assessing size, consistency, tethering to skin or deep structures. It may be helpful to examine with the arm elevated above the head and with the patient sitting at 45°.
- Palpate for axillary and supraclavicular lymphadenopathy.

Evidence

Barton MB, Harris R & Fletcher SW. Does this patient have breast cancer? The screening clinical breast examination: should it be done? How? *JAMA* 1999; **282**: 1270–80.

14 Obstetric history and examination

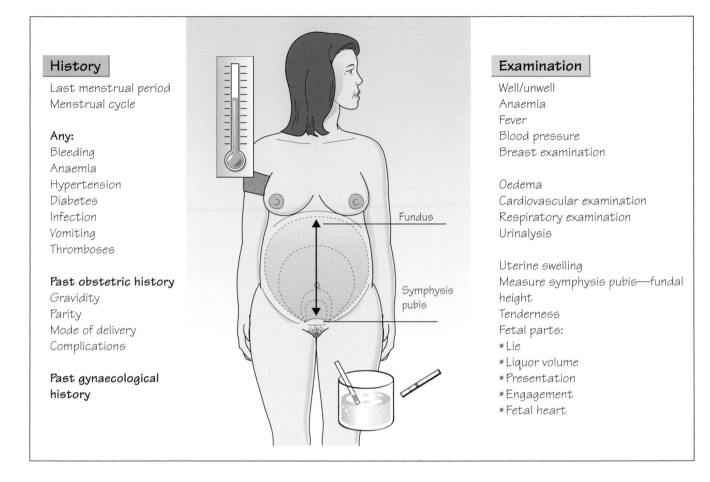

History

Last menstrual period
Menstrual cycle

Any:
Bleeding
Anaemia
Hypertension
Diabetes
Infection
Vomiting
Thromboses

Past obstetric history
Gravidity
Parity
Mode of delivery
Complications

Past gynaecological history

Fundus

Symphysis pubis

Examination

Well/unwell
Anaemia
Fever
Blood pressure
Breast examination

Oedema
Cardiovascular examination
Respiratory examination
Urinalysis

Uterine swelling
Measure symphysis pubis—fundal height
Tenderness
Fetal parts:
• Lie
• Liquor volume
• Presentation
• Engagement
• Fetal heart

The pregnant woman may present routinely for a prenatal check or because of vaginal bleeding, labour, hypertension or pain.

History of present pregnancy
• When was the last day of the patient's most recent menstrual period and what is the normal length of her menstrual cycle?
• How many weeks gestation is she?
• Any bleeding, diabetes, anaemia, hypertension, urinary infection or problems during pregnancy?
• What symptoms have accompanied the patient's pregnancy (e.g. nausea, vomiting, breast tenderness, urinary frequency)?
• Consider the possibility of thromboses (e.g. DVT and pulmonary embolism).

Past obstetric history
• Full details of all previous pregnancies (parity = number of deliveries of potentially viable babies; gravidity = number of pregnancies) to include gestation, mode of delivery, any complications for mother or baby, breast-feeding difficulties, birthweight, sex, name and current health of children, any miscarriages and past gynaecological history.

• Ask in particular about heart disease, murmurs, diabetes, hypertension, anaemia, epilepsy and assess cardiorespiratory fitness.

Obstetric examination
• In the general examination, examine carefully for blood pressure, oedema, urinalysis and hepatic tenderness or enlargement.
• Look for the anticipated uterine swelling, palpate the abdomen lightly and then slightly more firmly.
• Measure the symphysis to fundal height distance (after 24 weeks this should correspond in centimetre to gestation in weeks ±2).
• Examine for fetal parts and determine the lie (longitudinal, transverse or oblique).
• Assess liquor volume: is it normal, reduced (fetal parts abnormally easy to palpate) or increased (tense with difficulty in distinguishing fetal parts)?
• Assess the presentation (the fetal part occupying the lower segment of the pelvis). Is the head engaged?
• Auscultate for fetal heart beat with Pinard's stethoscope (listening usually between fetal head and umbilicus): what is the heart rate? (it should be 110–160 b.p.m.)

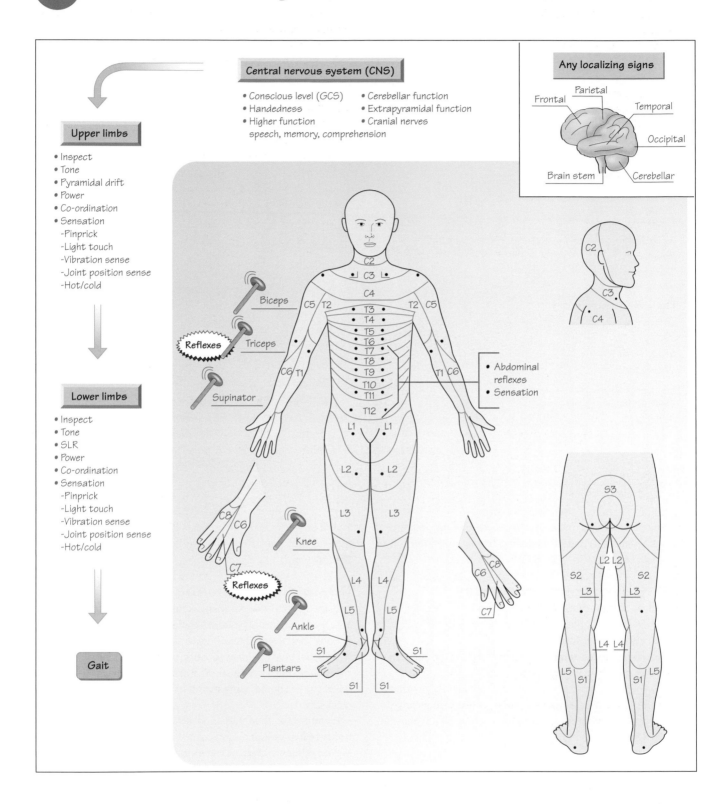

Central nervous system (CNS)

- Conscious level (GCS)
- Handedness
- Higher function
  speech, memory, comprehension
- Cerebellar function
- Extrapyramidal function
- Cranial nerves

Any localizing signs

Frontal
Parietal
Temporal
Occipital
Brain stem
Cerebellar

Upper limbs

- Inspect
- Tone
- Pyramidal drift
- Power
- Co-ordination
- Sensation
  - Pinprick
  - Light touch
  - Vibration sense
  - Joint position sense
  - Hot/cold

Lower limbs

- Inspect
- Tone
- SLR
- Power
- Co-ordination
- Sensation
  - Pinprick
  - Light touch
  - Vibration sense
  - Joint position sense
  - Hot/cold

Gait

Biceps
Reflexes
Triceps
Supinator

Knee
Reflexes
Ankle
Plantars

- Abdominal reflexes
- Sensation

History

Abnormalities of the nervous system can present with a very wide range of symptoms that include:

- headache
- fits, faints or funny turns
- dizziness or vertigo
- problems with vision
- hearing disturbance
- abnormalities of smell/taste
- speech difficulties
- problems swallowing
- difficulty walking
- weakness in a limb(s)
- sensory disturbance
- pain
- involuntary movements or tremor
- problems with sphincter control (bladder/bowels)
- disturbance of higher mental functions, such as confusion or personality change.

Past medical history

- Any previous neurological disorder?
- Any systemic diseases, particularly cardiovascular conditions? (Stroke is a very common cause of neurological deficit.)

Drugs

Consider both treatments of neurological disorders and medications that might be causing symptoms.

Family history

Any family history of neurological disease? (There are many important hereditary neurological conditions, e.g. Huntingdon's chorea.)

Social history

- What are the patient's disabilities?
- What can't the patient do that he/she would like to do?
- Does the patient use any aids for mobility?
- What help does the patient receive?

Functional enquiry

- Consider symptoms of raised intracranial pressure (headache, exacerbated with straining, coughing, waking in morning, visual disturbance).
- Are there any previous neurological symptoms such as visual disturbance, weakness or numbness?

Examination

- In examining the nervous system the key objectives are to reveal and describe the deficits in function and to describe the likely anatomical location of any lesion. Is the problem due to a lesion in the brain, spinal cord, peripheral nerve or muscle?

- What is the *conscious level*? Assess with the Glasgow Coma Score.
- Examine *gait*. Ask the patient to walk, try heel–toe walking, examine for Romberg's sign.
- Is the patient right- or left-handed?
- Look at the patient. Are there any obvious abnormalities of posture, wasting or tremor?

Examine the upper limbs

- *Inspect* for obvious wasting, tremor, fasciculation, deformities and skin changes.
- Examine for pyramidal 'drift'; with arms outstretched, supine and with eyes closed.
- Examine for *tone* at the wrist and the elbow.
- Examine for *power*, comparing sides. Examine shoulder abduction, elbow flexion and extension, wrist extension, grip, finger abduction and adduction, and thumb abduction.
- Use MRC grades(0–5):
  - **0** complete paralysis
  - **1** visible contraction
  - **2** active movement with gravity eliminated
  - **3** movement against gravity
  - **4** movement against resistance
  - **5** normal power.
- Examine *co-ordination* through finger–nose testing, rapid movements of fingers, rapid alternating movements (if difficulty = dysdiadochokinesis in cerebellar disorder), pinch and 'playing piano'.
- Test *reflexes* through biceps, triceps and supinator jerks (with reinforcement if necessary, e.g. clenching teeth).
- Examine *sensation*. Test light touch, pinprick, vibration sense, joint position sense and hot/cold reactions.
- Look for abnormalities that might correspond to dermatomal or peripheral nerve defects. Also test thoracic and abdominal sensation and test for abdominal reflexes.

Examine the lower limbs

- *Inspect* for obvious wasting, fasciculation, deformities and skin changes.
- Examine for *tone* at the knee and, with the 'rolling of the leg' test and straight leg raises, check for possible sciatic nerve compression.
- Examine for *power*, comparing sides. Examine hip flexion, extension, abduction and adduction, knee extension and flexion, plantar flexion, dorsiflexion, inversion, eversion and great toe dorsiflexion.
- Use MRC grades (0–5).
- Examine *co-ordination* through the heel–toe test. Examine *reflexes*. Test knee, ankle and plantar responses, and examine for ankle clonus.
- Examine *sensation*. Test light touch, pinprick, vibration sense, joint position sense and hot/cold reactions.
- Look for abnormalities that might correspond to dermatomal or peripheral nerve defects.

Continued on pp. 38–39.

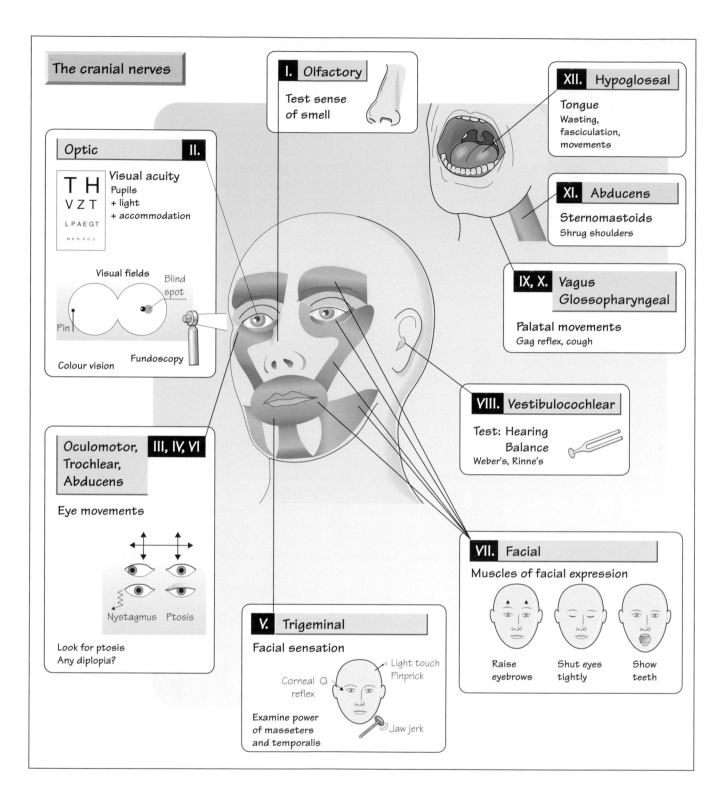

The cranial nerves

I. Olfactory

Test sense of smell

Optic   II.

Visual acuity
Pupils
+ light
+ accommodation

T H
V Z T
L P A E G T
W R N R O Z

Visual fields

Blind spot

Pin

Colour vision   Fundoscopy

III, IV, VI Oculomotor, Trochlear, Abducens

Eye movements

Nystagmus   Ptosis

Look for ptosis
Any diplopia?

V. Trigeminal

Facial sensation

Light touch
Pinprick

Corneal reflex

Examine power
of masseters
and temporalis

Jaw jerk

XII. Hypoglossal

Tongue
Wasting,
fasciculation,
movements

XI. Abducens

Sternomastoids
Shrug shoulders

IX, X. Vagus Glossopharyngeal

Palatal movements
Gag reflex, cough

VIII. Vestibulocochlear

Test: Hearing
Balance
Weber's, Rinne's

VII. Facial

Muscles of facial expression

Raise
eyebrows

Shut eyes
tightly

Show
teeth

Examine the cranial nerves

I Olfactory:
- Test the sense of smell in each nostril

II Optic:
- Test visual acuity
- Test visual fields, examine for blind spot
- Examine pupils and test direct and consensual reactions to light and accommodation
- Examine with ophthalmoscope

III, IV, VI Oculomotor, trochlear and abducens:
- Look for ptosis (drooping of the eyelid[s])
- Examine eye movements and look for nystagmus. Enquire about any double vision

V Trigeminal:
- Examine facial sensation to light touch and pinprick
- Examine power of masseters and temporalis ('clench teeth, open your mouth and stop me closing it')
- Test corneal reflex
- Test jaw jerk

VII Facial:
- Test muscles of facial expression ('raise eyebrows', 'shut eyes firmly', 'show teeth')

VIII Vestibulocochlear:
- Test hearing
- Perform Rinne's test (512 Hz vibrating tuning fork placed on mastoid process and its loudness compared with sound several centimetres from the external auditory meatus. Normally air conduction [AC] is better than bone conduction [BC]. BC > AC suggests conductive deafness. Impaired hearing and AC > BC suggests sensorineural deafness.)
- Perform Weber's test (A 512 Hz vibrating tuning fork is placed in middle of forehead and the patient asked which side the sound localizes to. Normally it is heard centrally: in conductive deafness it is localized to the poor ear and in sensorineural deafness it is localized to the good ear.)
- Test balance (standing with eyes closed, walking along straight line)

IX, X Vagus and glossopharyngeal:
- Examine palatal movements
- Test for gag reflex and cough

XI Abducens:
- Test the power of sternomastoids and shrug shoulders

XII Hypoglossal:
- Examine the tongue for wasting, fasciculation and power
- Examine the tongue at rest, put tongue out and move from side to side

Test higher mental function (Mini Mental Status Examination; see Chapter 110)
- Assess speech
- Examine memory
- Assess comprehension

Localized deficits
Consider the possibility of deficits localizing to any of the following:
- *Cerebellar function.* Examine gait, finger nose co-ordination, nystagmus and dysdiadochokinesis.
- *Extrapyramidal function.* Examine gait, tone, look for tremor, bradykinesia and dystonic movements.
- *Temporal lobe.* Examine memory and language comprehension.
- *Parietal lobe.* Examine object recognition, tasks such as dressing, using toothbrush, writing, reading and arithmetic.
- *Occipital lobe.* Examine visual acuity and fields (NB. in occipital blindness pupillary reflex to light will be intact).
- *Frontal lobe.* Examine higher mental function, sense of smell, affect, primitive reflexes (grasp, pout, palmo-mental reflex). Is there disinhibition and/or personality change?

Are there signs of raised intracranial pressure?
Signs of raised intracranial pressure are:
- depressed conscious level
- false-localizing signs (e.g. III and VIth nerve palsies)
- papilloedema
- hypertension
- bradycardia.

16 The musculoskeletal system

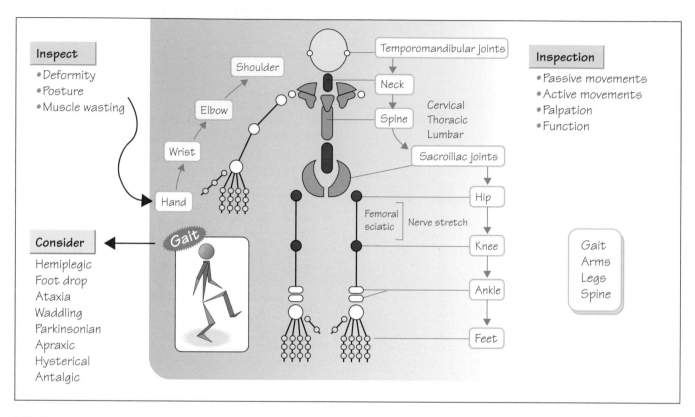

Inspect
- Deformity
- Posture
- Muscle wasting

Consider
Hemiplegic
Foot drop
Ataxia
Waddling
Parkinsonian
Apraxic
Hysterical
Antalgic

Gait

Temporomandibular joints
Neck
Spine
Cervical
Thoracic
Lumbar
Sacroiliac joints

Shoulder
Elbow
Wrist
Hand

Femoral sciatic — Nerve stretch

Hip
Knee
Ankle
Feet

Inspection
- Passive movements
- Active movements
- Palpation
- Function

Gait
Arms
Legs
Spine

History
Disease of the musculoskeletal system can manifest with:
- pain (particularly of joints [arthralgia])
- deformity
- swelling
- reduced mobility
- reduced function (e.g. unable to walk)
- systemic features such as rash or fever.

Past medical history
- Any history of previous joint or bone abnormalities?
- Has the patient had any operations such as joint replacement surgery?

Drugs
Ask the patient about analgesics, NSAIDs, corticosteroids, other immunosuppressants, penicillamine, gold and chloroquine.

Functional enquiry
- Do you have any pain or stiffness?
- Can you dress yourself? Can you climb stairs? When are the symptoms worse? (e.g. symptoms of inflammatory arthritis may be worse in the morning)
- Ask particularly about systemic features of illness such as fever, weight loss, rashes. Ask about dry eyes or mouth (Sjögren's syndrome) and Raynaud's syndrome.
- Consider symptoms of polymyalgia rheumatica (aching and stiffness of muscles of neck, shoulders, hips, thighs) or temporal

arteritis (headache, scalp tenderness, jaw claudication, visual disturbance).
- Any genitourinary or GI disease (e.g. as in Reiter's syndrome)?

Social history
- Discover any functional consequences such as the patient being unable to walk, feed, etc.
- What aids is the patient using (e.g. wheelchair, chair-lift; any home modifications)?

Examination
- Look at the patient for any obvious deformity, abnormal posture.
- Look for obvious muscle wasting: is muscle bulk normal? Look at shoulders, buttocks, hands and quadriceps.
- Look for associated abnormalities; for example, rheumatoid nodules, gouty tophii, psoriasis, or features of systemic rheumatological disease.
- Survey joints for swelling, tenderness, deformity, effusion, erythema and assess the patient's range of active and passive movements. Look for limitation of full extension and flexion.

Examine hand
- Inspect for joint deformities, nail abnormalities, joint tenderness (including a gentle 'squeeze' across the MCP joints) and swelling.
- Look for muscle wasting (e.g. of thenar or hypothenar eminences) and fasciculation.

- Examine movements: flexion, extension, adduction and opposition of the thumb.
- Check flexion, extension, adduction and abduction of the fingers. Make a fist and pinch grip. Test the patient's function (e.g. writing, doing up buttons).

Examine wrist
- Inspect for joint deformities, swelling and tenderness.
- Examine movements of flexion, extension, ulnar and radial deviation.

Examine elbow
Inspect for deformities, rheumatoid nodules, bursae. Examine movements of flexion, extension, pronation and supination.

Examine shoulder and sterno-clavicular joints
- Inspect for joint deformities, swelling and tenderness.
- Examine active and passive movements of abduction, adduction, internal and external rotation, flexion and extension. You can ask the patient to 'put his/her arms behind his/her head'.
- In a patient complaining of pain in the deltoid region, if resisted active movements are painful consider rotator cuff pathology (e.g. supraspinatous trapping, calcification or rotator cuff muscle tear). If there is equal pain with active and passive movements consider capsulitis, synovitis or arthritis of shoulder joint.

Examine temporomandibular joints, neck and spine
Inspect the spine for deformity, abnormal kyphosis, scoliosis and lordosis. Look for the smooth curves of the spinous processes, for any 'steps', and then palpate looking for tenderness and any associated muscle spasm.

Cervical spine Examine active and then passive movements of the neck. Examine flexion, extension, lateral flexion and rotation. Look for the patient's range of movement and pain locally or in the upper limb.

Thoracic spine Examine the patient twisting whilst sitting with arms folded. Examine for chest expansion: the patient should manage > 5 cm.

Lumbar spine Test the patient's range of movement: ask the patient to touch his/her toes keeping his/her knees straight. Assess extension, lateral flexion and rotation.

Sacro-iliac joints Palpate the joints. 'Spring' the joints by firm downward pressure on joint whilst patient prone. With patient supine flex one hip whilst maintaining the other extended.

Nerve stretch tests
- Examine straight leg raising ± dorsiflexion of the foot. Perform the femoral stretch test: with the patient in prone position, flex his/her knee and then extend his/her leg at the hip.
- Examine the leg for muscle wasting and fasciculation.

Examine hip
- Look for differential leg length, abnormal rotation. Stand the patient on one leg and then the other. Examine for flexion, extension, abduction and adduction.
- Perform the Thomas test (flexion of the opposite hip can reveal any fixed flexion deformity of contralateral hip).

Examine knee
- Any deformity or effusion? Perform the patella tap.
- Examine the stability of the joint in the anterior–posterior plane (cruciate ligaments):
  - The Lachmann test (patient lies supine with leg flexed 30°, the femur is fixed with one hand whilst the other hand pulls the tibia forward. The test is abnormal if there is abnormally increased forward movement of the tibia).
  - The anterior drawer test (patient lies supine and leg flexed at 90° and forward movement of the tibia is assessed).
  - The posterior drawer test (examine patient supine with leg flexed at 90° and examine the tibia for posterior subluxation and its correction with anterior movement of the tibia).
- Any joint line tenderness (suggesting meniscal injury)?
- Perform the McMurray test ('popping' and symptoms along the joint line when the knee is extended and internally rotated suggests meniscal injury).
- Examine for flexion and extension.

Examine ankle
Inspect for deformity. Examine for plantarflexion, dorsiflexion, eversion and inversion.

Examine feet
Inspect for deformities; for example, pes cavus, hallux valgus or callosities. Examine the great toe dorsiflexion.

Inspect gait
- Look for steadiness, speed, stride length, arm swing, limping, favouring one leg over the other and ability turning.
- Perform the heel–toe test. Any features of spasticity, footdrop, parkinsonism, apraxia (impairment of complex movements despite normal motor and sensory function), ataxia (unsteady, broad-based gait), etc.?

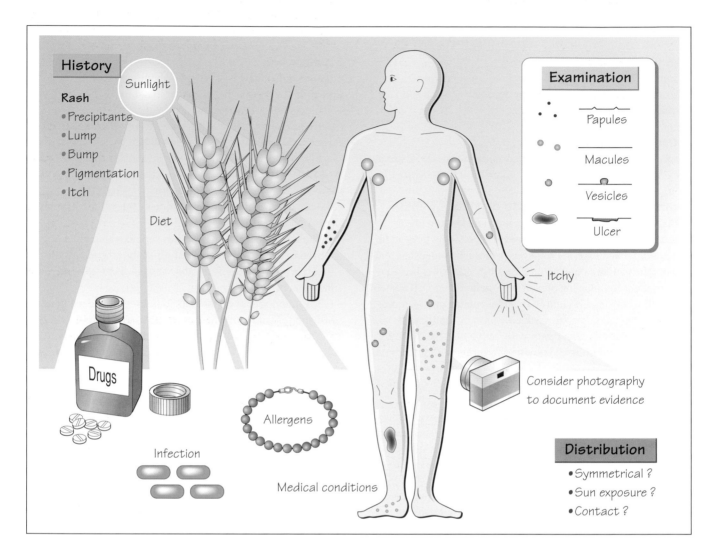

History

An accurate history is vital in establishing the correct diagnosis in conditions affecting the skin. Common presentations include rash, itch, lumps, ulcers, change in skin coloration and incidental observations during presentations with other medical conditions.

• When was the rash first noticed? Where is it? Is it itchy? Were there any precipitants (e.g. medication, dietary, sunlight, potential allergens)?

• Where is the lump? Is it itchy? Has it bled? Has its shape/size/coloration changed?

• Are there other lumps?

• What is the colour change (e.g. increased pigmentation, jaundice, pallor)? Who noticed it? How long ago? Compare with old photographs.

• Are there any associated symptoms suggesting a systemic medical condition (e.g. weight loss, arthralgia, etc.)?

• Consider the possible consequences of serious skin conditions, such as fluid losses, secondary infection, metastatic spread to lymph nodes or other organs.

Past medical history

• Did the patient have any previous skin conditions, rashes, etc.?

• Is there atopic tendency (asthma, rhinitis)?

• Did the patient have any skin problems in childhood?

• Any other significant medical conditions? (Particularly those which may have skin manifestations, e.g. SLE, coeliac disease, myositis or renal transplant.)

Drugs

• A complete drug history is essential of all medications, prescribed and alternative, ingested and topical.

• Any previous treatments for skin disorders?

• Has/is the patient using immunosuppressants?

Allergies

• Does the patient have any allergy to medication? If so, what was the allergic reaction?

• Does the patient know of any other possible allergens?

• Has the patient undergone any patch testing or IgE responses?

Family history

- Any family history of skin diseases or atopy?
- Are there others in the family affected?

Social history

- What is the patient's occupational history: any exposure to sunlight, potential allergens, skin parasites? Any change in washing products, pets, etc.?
- Has the patient travelled abroad recently?
- Any exposure to infectious conditions (e.g. chicken pox)?

Functional enquiry

This should focus particularly on the possibility of any associated systemic disease, such as coeliac disease, parasitic infection, psoriatic arthropathy, SLE, etc.

Examination

- Is the patient well or unwell? Are they pale, shocked, pigmented or febrile? (Serious skin conditions affecting large areas of skin can lead to life-threatening fluid loss and secondary infections.)
- *What* is the skin abnormality? Rash, ulcer, lump, discoloration, etc.:
  - *Macule*—a circumscribed area of change in normal skin colour without elevation or depression of the surrounding skin.
  - *Papule*—a solid elevated lesion < 0.5 cm in diameter.
  - *Plaque*—an elevation above the skin surface that occupies a relatively large surface area in comparison with its height.
  - *Wheal*—a rounded or flat topped, pale red, papule or plaque that characteristically disappears within hours.
  - *Pustule*—a circumscribed elevation of the skin that contains a purulent exudate.
  - *Vesicle/bulla*—a circumscribed elevated lesion containing fluid. Vesicle < 0.5 cm, bulla > 0.5 cm.
  - *Ulcer*—a lesion showing destruction of the epidermis and dermis.
  - *Cyst*—a closed cavity that contains liquid or semi-solid material.
- Is there bruising or petechiae?
  - If so, *where* is the skin abnormality? Completely examine the skin, nails and hair and, in addition, examine the oral cavity and the eyes. Which area of the skin is affected?
- Are there any secondary changes to the skin that are superimposed or consequences of the primary process? For example:
  - *Scale*—desquamating layers of stratum corneum.
  - *Crust*—dried serum, blood or purulent exudate.
  - *Erosion*—an area with circumscribed denudation due to epidermal loss.
  - *Lichenification*—skin thickening that is the result of chronic rubbing or scratching leading to accentuation of normal skin lines.
  - *Atrophy*—epidermal atrophy results from a decrease in the number of epidermal cell layers. Dermal atrophy results from a decrease in the dermal connective tissue.
  - *Scar*—a lesion formed as a result of dermal damage.
  - *Excoriation*—superficial excavations of the epidermis that result from scratching.
  - *Fissure*—a linear, painful crack in the skin.
- What is the *extent* (isolated, localized, regional, generalized, universal) and *pattern* of distribution (symmetrical or asymmetrical, exposed areas, site of pressure, skin creases, follicular)? Does it correlate with clothing, sun exposure or jewellery?
- What is the *colour* of the lesions and what is their *shape* (e.g. round, oval, polygonal, annular, serpiginous, umbilicated)?
- *Palpate* any lesions for temperature, mobility, tenderness and depth. Examine for enlargement of draining *lymph nodes.* Perform a *complete physical examination* to analyse the presence of systemic disease. Could this be a manifestation of a serious systemic condition (e.g. malignancy, SLE)?
- Documenting the skin abnormality accurately is important and can be aided by photography.

18 The visual system

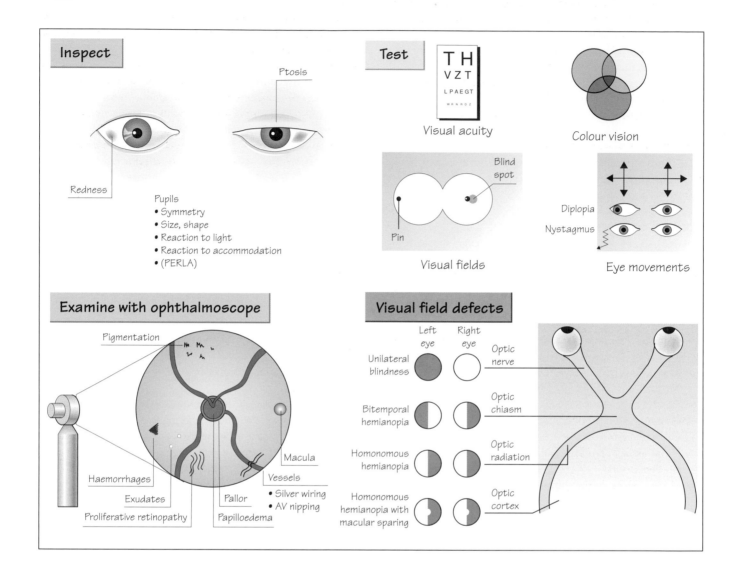

Inspect

Ptosis

Redness

Pupils
• Symmetry
• Size, shape
• Reaction to light
• Reaction to accommodation
• (PERLA)

Test

T H
V Z T
L P A E G T
W R N R D Z

Visual acuity

Colour vision

Blind spot

Pin

Visual fields

Diplopia
Nystagmus

Eye movements

Examine with ophthalmoscope

Pigmentation

Haemorrhages
Exudates
Proliferative retinopathy
Pallor
Papilloedema
• Silver wiring
• AV nipping
Vessels
Macula

Visual field defects

Left eye   Right eye

Unilateral blindness — Optic nerve

Bitemporal hemianopia — Optic chiasm

Homonomous hemianopia — Optic radiation

Homonomous hemianopia with macular sparing — Optic cortex

History
Diseases of the eyes may present with:
• visual impairment or disturbance
• red eye
• painful eye
• double vision.
The eyes are also important windows for detecting systemic disease causing, for example, papilloedema, hypertensive or diabetic retinopathy.

Obtain a very detailed history of the nature of any visual symptom. Most important is whether one or both eyes are affected. Was the onset sudden or gradual? Are there any accompanying symptoms (ocular pain, headache, discharge, etc.)?

Past medical history
• Previous visual problems?
• Diabetes mellitus?

• Hypertension?
• Neurological disease?
• Any specific eye treatments (e.g. laser)?

Drugs
Are there any drugs the patient has taken that might cause visual symptoms or to treat ocular disease (e.g. drops for glaucoma)?

Family and social history
• Any family history of inherited visual problems (e.g. glaucoma)?
• Any family history of eye symptoms (e.g. transmission of infective conjunctivitis)?
• What is the extent of the patient's visual disability?
• Is the patient registered blind?
• Any adaptations to the home?
• Does the patient own a guide dog?

Examination

Inspect the eyes

• Any obvious abnormalities (e.g. proptosis [abnormal protrusion of the globe], redness, asymmetry, obvious nystagmus, ptosis)?

• Look at the conjunctivae, the cornea, the iris, the pupils and the eyelids. Are the pupils symmetrical?

• What size are they? Do they respond normally and equally to light and accommodation?

• Is there ptosis? Check for eyelid closure.

Test the eyes, individually

• Test visual acuity in each eye with, for example, a Snellen chart for far vision and a Jaeger chart for near vision.

• Test colour vision; for example, using Ishihara charts.

• Test visual fields with confrontation and examine for blind spot.

• Test eye movements: ask about diplopia and look for nystagmus.

Examine the eyes with an ophthalmoscope

The ophthalmoscopic examination of the eye is a vital part of the complete physical examination. It can reveal the effects of systemic conditions such as hypertension and diabetes mellitus, causes of visual dysfunction such as optic atrophy, and reveal conditions such as raised intracranial pressure by demonstrating papilloedema. The ocular complications of conditions such as diabetes mellitus may be asymptomatic until sight-threatening complications have developed; hence the importance of screening examinations.

Optimize the conditions for fundoscopy. Both patients and examiner need to be comfortable. Examine the patient in a darkened room with a good ophthalmoscope producing a bright light and, if necessary use pupillary dilatation (contraindicated only in recent head injury when serial pupillary examinations are essential or where there is a risk of acute angle closure glaucoma). If you need to dilate, warn the patient of possible photophobia and visual blurring which will prevent driving.

Ask the patient to fix their gaze on a distant object. Examine their right eye with your right eye and their left eye with your left eye.

Examine from a distance looking initially for the presence of the red reflex and, if absent, consider lens opacities such as cataracts. Then examine the optic disc (shape, colour, edge, physiological cup), the peripheries of the retina following the main vessels outwards from the disc (vessels, venous pulsation, haemorrhages, exudates, pigmentation) and, finally, the macula.

The presence of papilloedema, haemorrhages or exudates, or presentation with loss of vision, requires explanation.

A full examination with particular emphasis on the cardiovascular and neurological systems may be required.

Common, important abnormalities

1 Diabetic retinopathy:
   • microaneurysms
   • 'dot and blot' haemorrhages
   • soft exudates
   • proliferative changes
   • laser treatment scars.
2 Hypertensive retinopathy:
   • silver wiring
   • arteriovenous nipping
   • haemorrhages and exudates
   • papilloedema.
3 Papilloedema:
   • blurred elevated disc margin
   • there may be accompanying haemorrhages
   • loss of venous pulsation, sometimes tortuous vessels
   • the disc may be pink (hyperaemic)
   • there may be enlargement of blind spot.
4 Optic atrophy:
   • pale optic discs.
5 Retinitis pigmentosa:
   • retinal pigmentation.

19 Examination of the ears, nose, mouth, throat, thyroid and neck

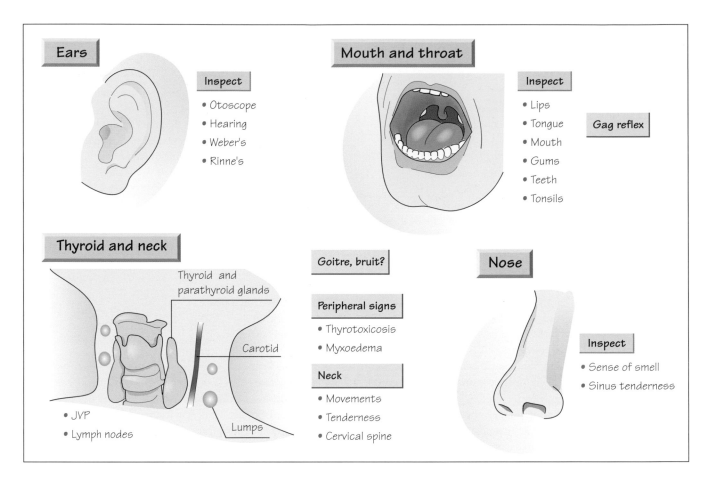

Ears
- Inspect the ears for abnormalities (e.g. tophii, skin cancers).
- Examine with an otoscope: look for pus, wax, other obstruction and tympanic membrane.
- Test hearing, balance and look for nystagmus.

Nose
- Inspect the nose for any previous fracture, 'saddle' nose or rhinorrhoea. Examine nares, inferior turbinates and assess nasal airflow.
- Test for sense of smell and sinus tenderness by percussion.

Mouth and throat
- Inspect with aid of torch and tongue depressor, lips, tongue, gums and teeth.
- Look for angular cheilitis, telangiectasia, pigmentation, wasting or fasciculation of tongue. Ask the patient to stick his/her tongue out and touch the roof of his/her mouth.
- Consider the possibility of dental abscess.
- Examine tonsils, uvula and posterior wall, salivary glands. Ask the patient to say 'aah'. Any inflammation, exudate, enlargement or growths? Palpate any visible abnormalities with a gloved finger.

Neck
- Inspect anteriorly, posteriorly and laterally for masses, pulsations, lumps, deformity. Define the relationship of any lumps to the skin, muscles, trachea and thyroid. Assess movement of any lumps with swallowing.
- Not all lumps in the neck are lymph nodes. Consider the possibility of: branchial cyst; branchial fistula; carotid body tumour; cystic hygroma; pharyngeal pouch; cervical rib; thyroglossal cyst; thyroid lump or goitre.
- Examine active and passive movements of flexion, extension, rotation and lateral flexion. Examine for tenderness of the cervical spine.
- Examine carotid arteries and jugular venous pressure.

Thyroid
- Look for peripheral signs of thyrotoxicosis and myxoedema.
- Inspect the neck: any goitre? Is there tenderness? Diffuse enlargement, single nodule? Is it hard, nodular?
- Ask the patient to swallow water and inspect again. Palpate for thyroid enlargement. Auscultate for bruit. Examine for any associated lymphadenopathy. Percuss upper sternum for retrosternal extension of goitre.

20 Examination of urine

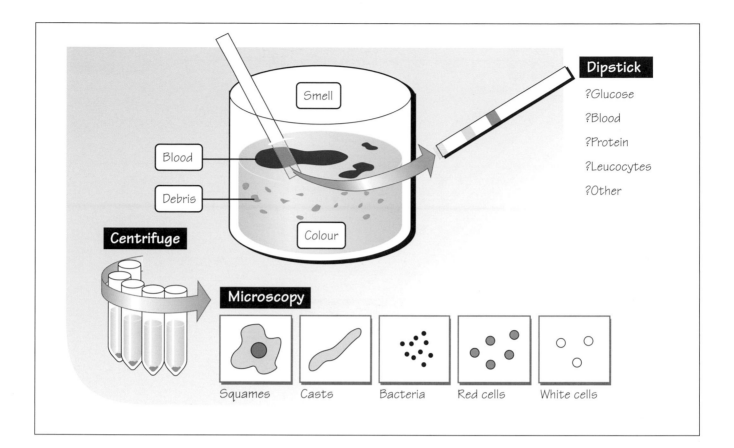

- Is the urine abnormally coloured, containing blood (a small amount of blood can give the urine a 'smoky' appearance or a rosy coloration), cloudy or containing solid matter?
- Ideally collect a mid-stream urine specimen (a 'clean catch').
- Check if the urine specimen has an abnormal smell.
- Dipstick the urine for the presence of protein, blood, glucose (and, with sophisticated dipsticks, leucocytes, nitrites, etc.). If positive for leucocytes and/or nitrite send for microbiological culture.
- Centrifuge the urine at 2000 r.p.m., resuspend the pellet in small volume and analyse under a microscope. Look for red blood cells, white blood cells, bacteria, casts and crystals.

Table 20.1 Common causes of urine abnormalities.

Glucose	Diabetes mellitus
	Renal glycosuria
Red cells	Lesion (tumour, stone) anywhere in renal tract (kidney, ureter, bladder, urethra)
	Glomerulonephritis
	Urinary tract infection
	Menstruation
	Trauma
Proteinuria	Glomerulonephritis
	Other causes of renal damage (e.g. diabetes, renovascular disease)
Leucocytes	Urinary tract infection
	Tuberculosis
	Urethritis
	Interstitial nephritis
Nitrite	Urinary tract infection
Red cell casts	Glomerulonephritis

The psychiatric assessment

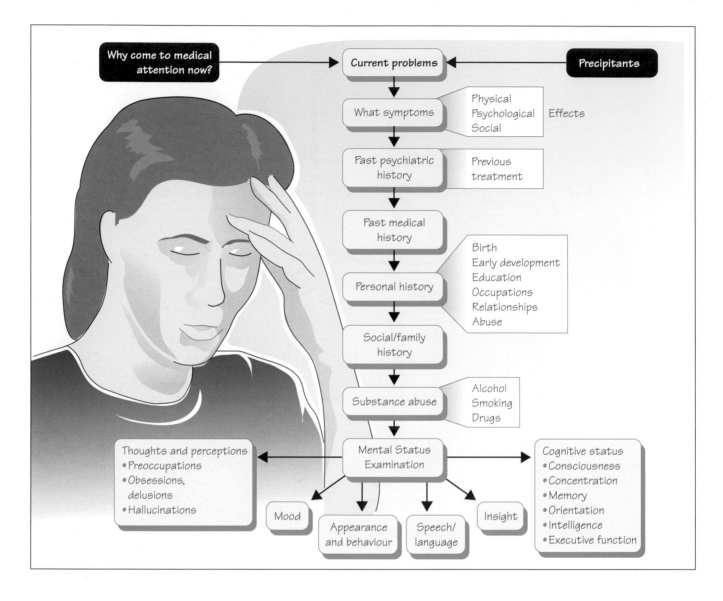

In making a psychiatric assessment, always ensure that there is privacy and explain to the patient who you are and why you are seeing them.

History
- What is the patient's problem?
- If the symptoms are long standing, why are they seeking medical attention now?
- How have they come to medical attention (e.g. self-referral, suicide attempt, found wandering and confused)?
- What is their status with respect to the Mental Health Act?

History of the present illness
- What are the current symptoms (e.g. feeling low, hearing voices, frightened, confused, wanting to die)? Explore the main symptom(s) in detail and discover any associated physical, psychological and social effects.

- What treatments have been tried so far, with what effect?
- What does the patient believe to have precipitated, aggravated, or modified the illness?
- When did the symptoms begin?
- What have others noticed (friends, relatives, other professionals)?

Past psychiatric history
Gather a chronological summary of all previous episodes of mental illness and treatment including hospitalization, previous contact with GP, psychiatrist, psychologist, counsellors, etc.

Also ask about the dose, duration of treatment, efficacy, side-effects, and patient's adherence to previously prescribed medications.

Ask about previous suicide attempts or other self-destructive behaviour.

Past medical history and medication and allergies

Find out what medication is being prescribed and what is actually being taken. Ask if there are any side-effects.

Personal history

The personal history reviews the stages of the patient's life. Ask about the following:
- Birth and any complications.
- Early development.
- Childhood (including separations during childhood, the home environment).
- Education and qualifications (including relationships with peers and teachers).
- Occupations (the sequence of jobs held by the patient, reasons for job changes, job satisfaction, relationships with colleagues and the patient's current or most recent employment).
- Relationships (including marriages, parents and children), sexual history and an assessment of the patient's past and present levels of functioning in family and social roles (e.g. marriage, parenting, work, school).
- Cultural and religious influences.
- Any history of physical, emotional, sexual, or other abuse or trauma.
- Any arrests or convictions?

Premorbid personality

Explore the following:
- Character (usual mood and its stability, sociability, motivation, perfectionism).
- Interests (e.g. hobbies).
- Beliefs (religious, moral and political views).

Social history

Ask about the patient's living arrangements and any current important relationships.

History of substance use

- Ask about the use of alcohol, smoking and other drugs (e.g. marijuana, cocaine, opiates, sedative-hypnotic agents, stimulants, solvents, and hallucinogens).
- Ask when it was first used, the amounts consumed and the routes of administration.
- Any evidence of dependence (craving, tolerance, inability to stop or control use, physiological withdrawal state, drug-related harm, reduction of interests and activities unrelated to drug use)?
- Ask about periods of abstinence and related offences.

Family history

Draw out a family tree. Include available information about general medical and psychiatric illness in close relatives. This information should include any history of mood disorder, psychosis, suicide and substance-use disorders.

Review of systems

The review of systems includes current symptoms not already identified in the history of the present illness. Particularly relevant are sleep, appetite, systemic symptoms such as fever and fatigue, and neurological symptoms.

Physical examination

A physical examination is needed to evaluate the patient's general medical (including neurological) condition.

Mental Status Examination

The Mental Status Examination is a systematic collection of data based on observation of the patient's behaviour during the interview.

The purpose of the Mental Status Examination is to obtain evidence of current symptoms and signs of mental disorders from which the patient might be suffering. Further, evidence is obtained regarding the patient's insight, judgement and capacity for abstract reasoning, to inform decisions about treatment strategy and the choice of an appropriate treatment setting. The Mental Status Examination contains the following elements:

1 **The patient's appearance and general behaviour.**
  Assess:
  - manner
  - rapport
  - eye contact
  - facial expression
  - clothing
  - cleanliness
  - self-care (e.g. grooming, make up)
  - posture
  - motor activity (agitated or retarded?)
  - abnormal movements (tremor, stereotypy, tics, chorea)
  - gait abnormality
  - obvious physical abnormalities (e.g. evidence of self-harm, drug use).

2 **Characteristics of the patient's speech and language:**
  - e.g. rate, rhythm, structure, flow of ideas and pathologic features such as perseveration, vagueness, incoherence, pressure of thought, thought block or neologisms.

3 **Mood:**
  - What is their predominant mood?
  - Do they appear depressed, elated, euphoric, anxious, fearful, suspicious, angry?
  - Is there increased variability of mood (lability) or decreased (reduced reactivity)?
  - Is the apparent mood congruent with speech content?
  - What is their subjective interpretation of their mood? Ask 'How are you feeling at the moment?', 'How are your spirits?'

4 **The patient's current thoughts and perceptions, including the following:**
  - Any preoccupations, worries, concerns, thoughts, impulses and perceptual experiences.
  - Cognitive and perceptual symptoms of specific mental disorders, usually elicited by specific questioning including hallucinations, delusions, ideas of reference, obsessions and compulsions.

Continued on p. 50.

- Suicidal, homicidal, violent or self-injurious thoughts, feelings and impulses. If these thoughts are present, elicit their intensity and specificity, when they occur and what prevents the patient from acting them out.
- Abnormal beliefs, delusions, feelings of external control, depersonalization and derealization.

5 The patient's insight of his or her current situation and willingness to accept treatment.

6 The patient's cognitive status, including:
- level of consciousness
- orientation (day, date, time)
- attention and concentration
- language functions (naming, fluency, comprehension, repetition, reading, writing)
- memory (long- and short-term, immediate recall)
- fund of knowledge (appropriate to age, social and educational background)
- calculation
- drawing (e.g. copying a figure or drawing a clock face)
- abstract reasoning (e.g. explaining similarities or interpreting proverbs)
- executive (frontal system) functions (e.g. list making, inhibiting impulsive answers, resisting distraction, recognizing contradictions)
- quality of judgement.

Functional assessment

Functional assessment should include assessment of the physical activities of daily living; for example, eating, using the toilet, transferring, bathing and dressing. It should also include assessment of the more sophisticated activities of daily living; for example, driving or using public transportation, taking medication as prescribed, shopping, managing one's own money, communicating by letter or telephone and caring for a child or other dependent.

'Biological' features of depression

'Biological' features of depression are:
- low energy
- poor sleep (early morning wakening)
- reduced appetite
- weight loss
- anhedonia
- low libido.

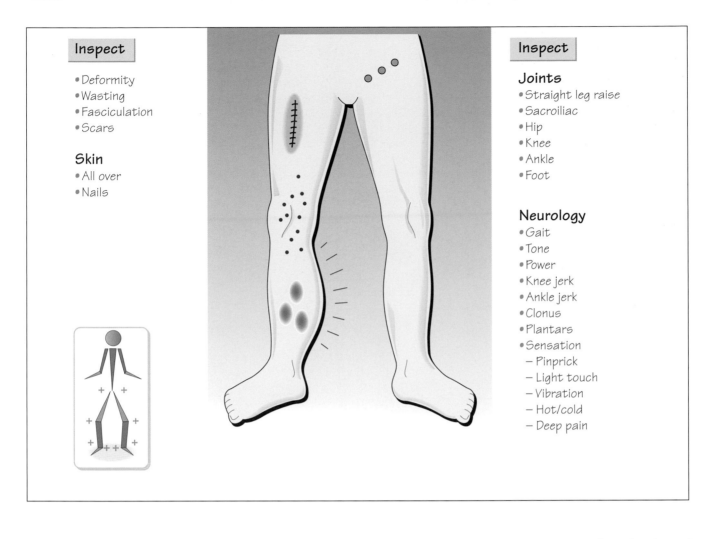

Inspect

- Deformity
- Wasting
- Fasciculation
- Scars

Skin
- All over
- Nails

Inspect

Joints
- Straight leg raise
- Sacroiliac
- Hip
- Knee
- Ankle
- Foot

Neurology
- Gait
- Tone
- Power
- Knee jerk
- Ankle jerk
- Clonus
- Plantars
- Sensation
  - Pinprick
  - Light touch
  - Vibration
  - Hot/cold
  - Deep pain

Examination of the legs is an important and sometimes neglected part of the examination and can feature as an instruction in clinical examinations.

Inspection

Ensure complete exposure of the lower limbs. Are there any obvious abnormalities? Look specifically for deformity, abnormal posture, wasting, scars, joint swelling, rashes, skin discoloration and oedema.

Examine the skin

- Inspect all surfaces of the legs including the toes and between the toes and nails.
- Are there any rashes, discoloration, varicose eczema, ulceration, lumps or scars?

Examine the vascular supply

- Is there good perfusion? Are the toes warm, cyanosed? Is there good capillary return?
- Palpate for peripheral pulses: femoral, popliteal, dorsalis pedis and posterior tibial.

- Palpate for popliteal aneurysms, auscultate for femoral bruits.
- Examine for oedema, calf swelling, tenderness, varicose veins and lymphadenopathy.

Assess the neurology

- Examine gait.
- Inspect for abnormal posture, wasting, fasciculation.
- Assess tone.
- Assess power.
- Assess co-ordination, e.g. heel–shin.
- Examine knee and ankle jerks, plantar reflexes and look for clonus.
- Test sensation to light touch, pinprick, vibration sense, joint position sense and hot/cold.

Examine the musculoskeletal system

Having already assessed gait, muscle power:
- Test straight leg raise
- Examine the joints:
  - Inspect the passive and active range of movements.

23 General examination

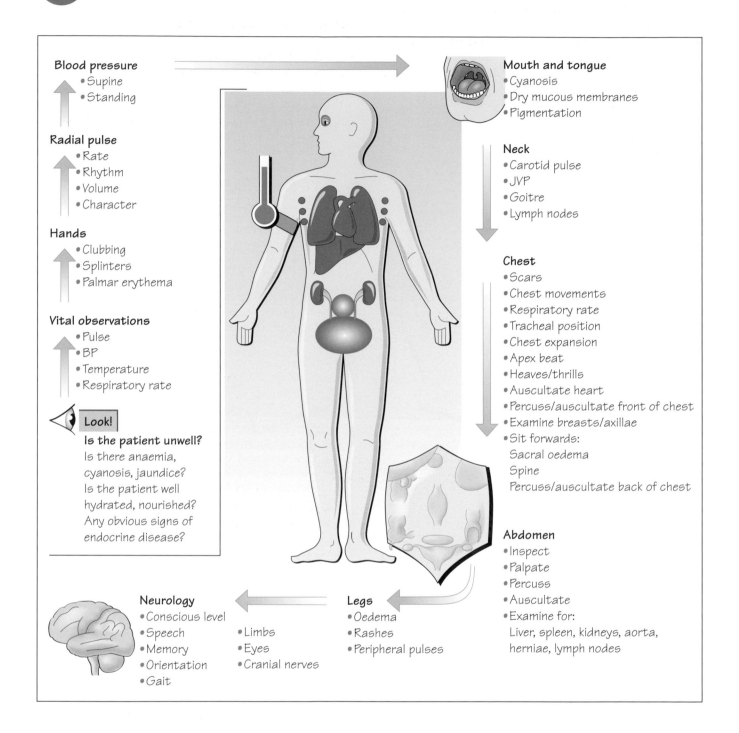

Blood pressure
- Supine
- Standing

Radial pulse
- Rate
- Rhythm
- Volume
- Character

Hands
- Clubbing
- Splinters
- Palmar erythema

Vital observations
- Pulse
- BP
- Temperature
- Respiratory rate

Look!

Is the patient unwell?
Is there anaemia, cyanosis, jaundice? Is the patient well hydrated, nourished? Any obvious signs of endocrine disease?

Mouth and tongue
- Cyanosis
- Dry mucous membranes
- Pigmentation

Neck
- Carotid pulse
- JVP
- Goitre
- Lymph nodes

Chest
- Scars
- Chest movements
- Respiratory rate
- Tracheal position
- Chest expansion
- Apex beat
- Heaves/thrills
- Auscultate heart
- Percuss/auscultate front of chest
- Examine breasts/axillae
- Sit forwards:
  Sacral oedema
  Spine
  Percuss/auscultate back of chest

Abdomen
- Inspect
- Palpate
- Percuss
- Auscultate
- Examine for:
  Liver, spleen, kidneys, aorta, herniae, lymph nodes

Neurology
- Conscious level
- Speech
- Memory
- Orientation
- Gait
- Limbs
- Eyes
- Cranial nerves

Legs
- Oedema
- Rashes
- Peripheral pulses

- Ensure the patient is comfortable, has privacy and understands what you are going to do.
- **STEP BACK AND LOOK** at the patient. Are there any obvious abnormalities?
- Is the patient well or unwell? In pain or comfortable? Do they need immediate resuscitation?
- Are there other diagnostic 'clues' (e.g. vomit bowl full of blood, sputum pot)?
- What are their vital observations? Check the pulse, BP, respiratory rate and temperature.
- Is there anaemia, cyanosis, jaundice, rash?
- Is the patient well hydrated?
- Does the patient look well nourished, wasted or obese?

Examination

Examine the hands
- Look for clubbing, palmar erythema, Dupuytren's contracture, clubbing and splinter haemorrhages.
- Examine the radial pulse-rate, rhythm, volume and character.
- Whilst doing this look again for features of endocrine disease; for example, thyroid, acromegaly, Cushing's syndrome, abnormal pigmentation and syndromes such as Marfan's syndrome.
- Measure the BP (supine and standing).

Examine the mouth and tongue
Look for central cyanosis, dry mucous membranes, dentition and pigmentation.

Examine the neck
- Examine for cervical and supraclavicular lymphadenopathy.
- Look for an enlarged thyroid gland (goitre).
- Is the JVP elevated (at 45°)?
- Examine the carotid pulse: character and volume.

Examine the chest
- Inspect the chest. Look for scars, symmetry of chest movement, use of accessory muscles, respiratory rate and pattern, intercostal recession, sputum pot and abnormal pulsations.
- Palpate for tracheal position and examine for chest expansion.
- Examine for the apex beat: both position and character.
- Feel for heaves and thrills.
- Auscultate the heart, listen sitting forward in expiration for the murmur of aortic regurgitation. Roll the patient onto their left side to listen for mitral murmurs, listen for carotid bruits.
- Percuss then auscultate the front of the chest.
- Sit the patient forward, look at the skin and spine for any abnormalities and examine for sacral oedema. Percuss and then auscultate the chest. Listen for vocal resonance.

Examine the breasts and axillae

Examine the abdomen
- Lie the patient flat, head supported by one pillow. Inspect and ask patient to cough and to take a deep breath. Lightly palpate and then palpate more deeply (watching patient's expression).
- Examine specifically for aorta, liver, spleen, kidneys, herniae, inguinal lymphadenopathy, ascites.
- Auscultate for bowel sounds and bruits.

Examine the genitalia
Consider performing rectal and vaginal examinations.

Examine the legs
- Look for oedema, rashes, ulcers and discoloration.
- Examine for peripheral pulses and perfusion.

Examine the joints and skin
Inspect and examine in more detail if there are any abnormalities on inspection.

Examine the nervous system
- Assess the patient's conscious level and mental state.
- Examine the patient's speech and memory (e.g. the Mini Mental Test Examination).
- Examine the patient's gait.

Examine the limbs
- Examine upper limbs for drift, inspection, tone, power, co-ordination, reflexes and sensation.
- Examine lower limbs for inspection, tone, power, co-ordination, reflexes, plantar responses and sensation.

Examine the eyes
Test visual acuity, visual fields, pupils and their response to light. Examine the fundi and eye movements.

Examine the face
Examine the face for sensation and power, test jaw jerk and corneal reflex.

Examine the patient's hearing

Examine the patient's palatal movements, gag reflex, tongue and tongue movements

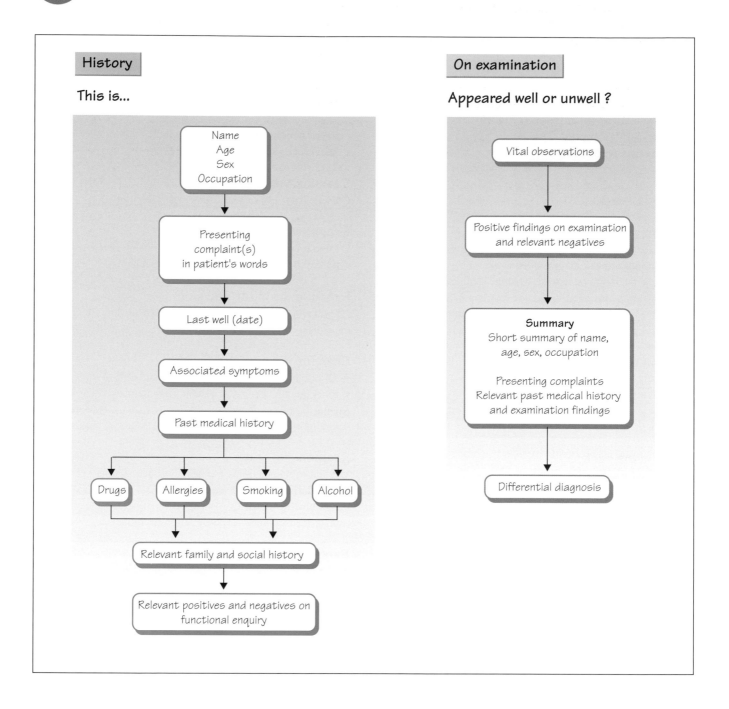

The detail required will vary markedly depending upon the case, the context and the audience. It is imagined here that a patient has just been clerked on take by a junior doctor and is now to be presented to a consultant on the post-take ward round. In general, be concise and omit negative pieces of information but important, relevant negatives should be included.

The priorities are to communicate the patient's name, gender and age, to describe in detail the presenting complaint(s), to describe the significant past medical history, family history, medication and allergies, any relevant positive findings in functional enquiry and place the current presentation in the context of the patient's social circumstances. The presentation of the history should be complaint or problem led. Then, if possible, use the patient's words to describe the presenting complaint. Avoid the use of medical terms, such as dysuria, or medical jargon. In a complex case with several complaints these should be listed and then each presented in detail. A common mistake is insufficient emphasis on the presenting complaint.

The patient should be described as well or unwell in appearance, the vital observations given and positive and relevant negative examination findings described. Be certain about definite findings; for example, 'The BP was 142/78.' If you are uncertain about a finding, say so and why; for example, 'I could not feel a liver edge but there was a fullness in the right upper quadrant with dullness to percussion.' If the CNS examination was normal, say it was normal—do not describe every normal neurological sign that was demonstrated. However, if the main complaint is weakness of the left arm then normal reflexes in that arm is an important finding that should be mentioned. Admit if you didn't perform a part of the examination, rather than give the implication of normality.

Summarize the case in a few sentences, list the differential diagnosis and the relevant available investigations.

Many times other professionals will be 'presented' with your findings in the form of your case notes. Ensure that the *notes* are:
• dated
• timed
• signed
• legible
• clear
• detailed.
In addition:
• minimize jargon and abbreviations
• explain your thoughts (e.g. differential diagnosis, plan of investigations and treatments) and what you have told the patient and their relatives in writing.

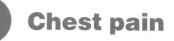
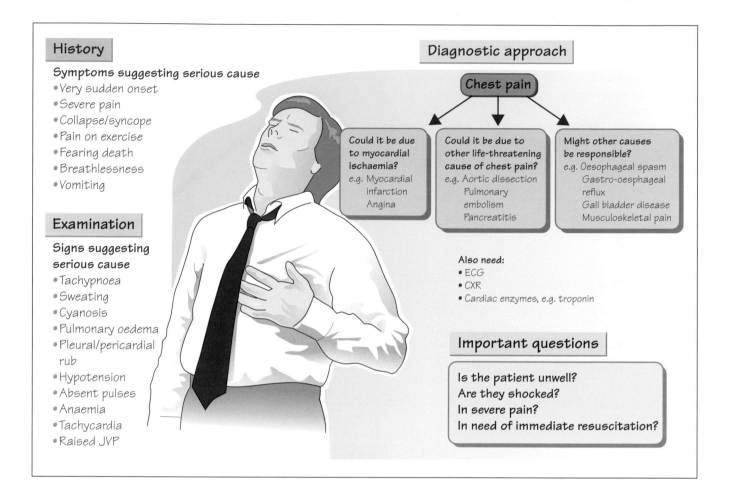

History

Symptoms suggesting serious cause
- Very sudden onset
- Severe pain
- Collapse/syncope
- Pain on exercise
- Fearing death
- Breathlessness
- Vomiting

Examination

Signs suggesting serious cause
- Tachypnoea
- Sweating
- Cyanosis
- Pulmonary oedema
- Pleural/pericardial rub
- Hypotension
- Absent pulses
- Anaemia
- Tachycardia
- Raised JVP

Diagnostic approach

Chest pain

Could it be due to myocardial ischaemia?
e.g. Myocardial infarction
Angina

Could it be due to other life-threatening cause of chest pain?
e.g. Aortic dissection
Pulmonary embolism
Pancreatitis

Might other causes be responsible?
e.g. Oesophageal spasm
Gastro-oesophageal reflux
Gall bladder disease
Musculoskeletal pain

Also need:
- ECG
- CXR
- Cardiac enzymes, e.g. troponin

Important questions

Is the patient unwell?
Are they shocked?
In severe pain?
In need of immediate resuscitation?

Chest pain is an important and common presentation of serious illnesses such as myocardial infarction, angina, pulmonary embolus and pneumothorax.

History

Let the patient describe what has happened in great detail. Use the patient's words, 'What was *it* like?', 'Tell me more about the *pain*.' They may often describe pressure or tightness rather than pain. Once you have allowed the patient to describe the symptoms in full then consider the following directed questions:

- Ask about *onset*. Ask 'What were you doing when the pain started?' 'How quickly did it come on?' (Instantaneous, over minutes, seconds?)
- What is the *character* of the chest pain? Tightness, gripping, crushing, pressing, like a weight (often used to describe myocardial infarction), sharp, stabbing, like a knife (often used to describe pain arising from pleural irritation)?
- Ask about the *severity*. Ask if it was the worst pain ever? Ask the patient the score out of 10 compared to the worst pain they have ever experienced.
- What was the *duration*? Seconds, minutes, hours? When was the first time you ever had this pain?

- What was it *relieved* by? Rest, posture, nitrates, oxygen, analgesia?
- What was it *exacerbated* by? Exertion, breathing, movement, coughing?
- Ask about *location*. Across upper chest, epigastric, sternal? Can you point to the area with one finger?
- Ask about *radiation*. Arms, back, throat, jaw, teeth, abdomen?
- Were there *accompanying symptoms*? Dizzy, faint, syncope, palpitations, sweaty, nausea, vomiting, anxiety, hyperventilation, acid reflux, fever, haemoptysis, abdominal pain?
- Was there any relation to exertion, posture or breathing?
- Ask if the patient ever had it before. Is it similar/better/worse than previous pains/myocardial infarction/angina?
- What does the patient think it is?
- Ask about treatment already received (e.g. aspirin, GTN).
- Establish the character of the pain, its location, onset, radiation, precipitating, exacerbating and alleviating features and accompanying symptoms.

Past medical history

- Any history of ischaemic heart disease, angina, myocardial infarction or cardiac operations?

- Any history of pulmonary disease?
- Any history of systemic disease (e.g. malignancy)?
- Ask about the risk factors for atherosclerosis: smoking, family history, hypertension, hyperlipidaemia and diabetes mellitus.

Examination

Does the patient need immediate resuscitation?

- Check the patient's airway and the patient's breathing. If possible give oxygen and obtain intravenous access, ECG monitor and a 12-lead ECG.
- Does the patient look unwell? Is he/she in pain, distressed, comfortable, vomiting, anxious, sweaty, pale, febrile, cyanosed or tachypnoeic? Are there any surgical scars (e.g. from CABG)?
- Is the patient well perfused or with cool peripheries?
- *Pulse*: rate, rhythm, volume, character peripheral pulses present? Are they equal?
- *BP*: are both arms equal?
- Is the *JVP* elevated?
- *Chest movements*: symmetrical expansion, exacerbation of pain?
- *Apex* beat position?
- Pain reproduced/exaggerated by chest wall pressure?
- *Percussion*: any dullness?
- *Auscultation*: check lung fields for added sounds—crackles, rub or wheeze?
- *Heart sounds*: are there any murmurs, a pericardial rub or gallop?
- Check for peripheral *oedema*, ankles and sacrum.
- Any *urine* output?
- *Abdomen*: any tenderness, guarding, rebound, bowel sounds, organomegaly or aneurysm?
- *CNS*: any weakness or focal deficits?
- An **ECG**, **chest X-ray** and **cardiac enzymes** such as troponin are invaluable in the diagnosis of chest pain.

Table 25.1 The differential diagnosis of chest pain.

Cause of chest pain	Frequency	Common symptoms	Common signs	Important diagnostic investigations
Myocardial infarction	Common	Tight, heavy, crushing central chest pain Nausea, vomiting, anxiety, sweating Radiation to arms, jaw	In pain, sweaty, tachycardia (may have signs of MI complications, e.g. shock, heart failure) **(But may have none)**	ECG Chest X-ray Cardiac enzymes/troponin
Angina	Very common	Tight, heavy central chest pain Radiation to arms, jaw Precipitated by exertion Alleviated by rest, GTN	May have none	ECG Exercise test Coronary angiogram Troponin
Pulmonary embolus	Common	Central or pleuritic chest pain Sudden onset shortness of breath Haemoptysis	Tachycardia Tachypnoea Raised JVP Hypotension Shock Pleural rub **(But may have none)**	ECG Chest X-ray Blood gases V/Q scan CTPA Troponin
Aortic dissection	Rare	Very sudden onset 'tearing' chest or back pain Collapse Nausea, sweating, vomiting	Hypertension BP difference between arms Absent pulses Neurological deficits **(But may have none)**	Chest X-ray ECG CT chest Echocardiogram
Pericarditis	Rare	Burning, aching or heavy chest pain Relieved by sitting forwards	May have pericardial rub	ECG Echocardiogram
Musculoskeletal	Very common	Localized pain Exacerbated or reproduced by movement, breathing, coughing	Localized tenderness	Normal ECG Chest X-ray
Dyspepsia/oesophageal reflux	Very common	Central, epigastric, substernal sharp or burning pain Can radiate to back Relief with antacids	Epigastric tenderness (**or none**)	Normal ECG Chest X-ray
'Pleurisy' may be due to pneumonia, viral infections, malignancy, PE	Common	Sharp, localized, stabbing pain Exacerbated by breathing, coughing, movement	Pleural rub May have signs of consolidation Fever	Chest X-ray

Abdominal pain

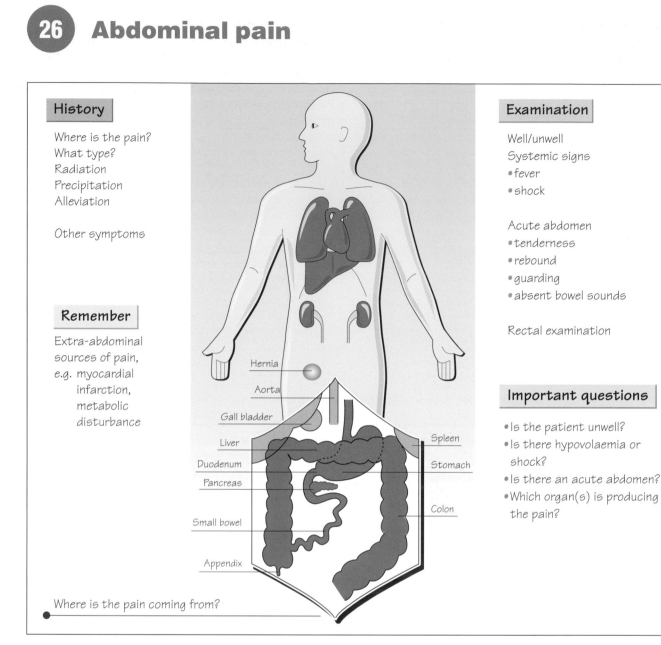

History

Where is the pain?
What type?
Radiation
Precipitation
Alleviation

Other symptoms

Remember

Extra-abdominal
sources of pain,
e.g. myocardial
infarction,
metabolic
disturbance

Where is the pain coming from?

Hernia
Aorta
Gall bladder
Liver
Duodenum
Pancreas
Small bowel
Appendix
Spleen
Stomach
Colon

Examination

Well/unwell
Systemic signs
• fever
• shock

Acute abdomen
• tenderness
• rebound
• guarding
• absent bowel sounds

Rectal examination

Important questions

• Is the patient unwell?
• Is there hypovolaemia or
 shock?
• Is there an acute abdomen?
• Which organ(s) is producing
 the pain?

Abdominal pain is a common and important complaint. It may represent a life-threatening disease, such as a perforated peptic ulcer, or a mild, self-limiting illness, such as gastroenteritis. More rarely it may be a presentation of extra-abdominal disease, such as myocardial infarction, or metabolic disturbance, such as diabetic ketoacidosis.

History
• When did the pain start? Did it start gradually or suddenly?
• What sort of pain is it? Aching, sharp, burning, etc.
• Is it constant or variable? Is it 'colicky' (waxes and wanes in cycles)?
• Where is the pain? Does it radiate? Does it radiate to the back?
• What exacerbates/precipitates the pain (movement, posture, eating)?

• What alleviates the pain?
• Are there any associated symptoms (vomiting, diarrhoea, acid reflux, back pain, breathlessness, GI bleeding, dysuria, haematuria)?
• Have there been previous episodes? When do they occur and how frequently?
• Any recent change in bowel habit? Are there any symptoms of indigestion, steatorrhoea or weight loss?

Past medical history
• Find out the PMH of any significant medical conditions.
• Ask if there is any history of previous abdominal surgery.

Drugs
• Ask about any medication that might cause pain (e.g.

NSAIDs and peptic ulceration) or mask abdominal signs (e.g. corticosteroids).
• Consider alcohol as a cause of the pain (e.g. pancreatitis).

Examination
• Is the patient well or unwell? Comfortable or uncomfortable? Still or restless?
• Eyes open (fearfully watching the doctor's abdominal examination?) or closed and relaxed?
• Is there fever, anaemia, jaundice, lymphadenopathy, evidence of weight loss, malnutrition, foetor, ketosis?

• Are they dehydrated, shocked, hypovolaemic?
• Do they have an acute abdomen? (See Chapter 89)
• Could there be obstruction (distension, vomiting, absolute constipation, high-pitched tinkling bowel sounds)?
• Is there tenderness, guarding, rigidity, rebound, visible peristalsis?
• Might there be enlargement of aorta, liver, kidney, spleen, gallbladder, herniae, other masses?

Table 26.1 The differential diagnosis of abdominal pain.

Cause of abdominal pain	Frequency	Common symptoms	Common signs	Important investigations
Appendicitis	Common	Central abdominal pain, then localizing to right iliac fossa Fever, anorexia	Right iliac fossa tenderness, rebound, guarding	
Infective gastroenteritis	Very common	Vomiting, diarrhoea, diffuse abdominal pain	Dehydration Diffuse abdominal tenderness	Stool culture
Peptic ulcer	Very common	Epigastric pain Can radiate to back Increased certain foods Alleviated antacids	Epigastric tenderness Acute abdomen if perforation	Upper GI endoscopy
Oesophageal reflux	Very common	Burning retrosternal, epigastric pain Alleviated antacids Exacerbated at night, lying flat	None	Upper GI endoscopy
Biliary colic	Rare	Sudden onset, severe upper abdominal pain May have vomiting Can radiate to back/right shoulder	Right upper quadrant tenderness	Abdominal ultrasound
Cholecystitis/cholangitis	Common	Right upper quadrant or epigastric pain Can radiate to back/right shoulder Exacerbation with fatty foods	Right upper quadrant tenderness Fever	Abdominal ultrasound
Pancreatitis	Common	Severe, epigastric pain Can radiate to back Vomiting	Epigastric tenderness Signs of acute abdomen May have shock, breathlessness	Amylase Abdominal CT
Bowel obstruction	Common	Vomiting Absolute constipation Abdominal pain	Abdominal distension Generalized tenderness Tinkling bowel sounds	Abdominal X-ray
Diverticulitis	Common	Pain especially left lower quadrant Fever Change in bowel habit	Fever Tenderness Acute abdomen if perforation	Abdominal CT
Aortic aneurysm	Common	Central abdominal pain Back pain Sudden and severe with ruptured aneurysm	Expansile, pulsatile mass Shock with ruptured aneurysm	Abdominal CT Abdominal ultrasound
Renal colic	Common	Sudden onset, severe pain in loin radiating to groin or testis Pain may wax and wane Haematuria	Loin tenderness Dipstick urine positive for blood	Plain KUB X-ray IVP Ultrasound

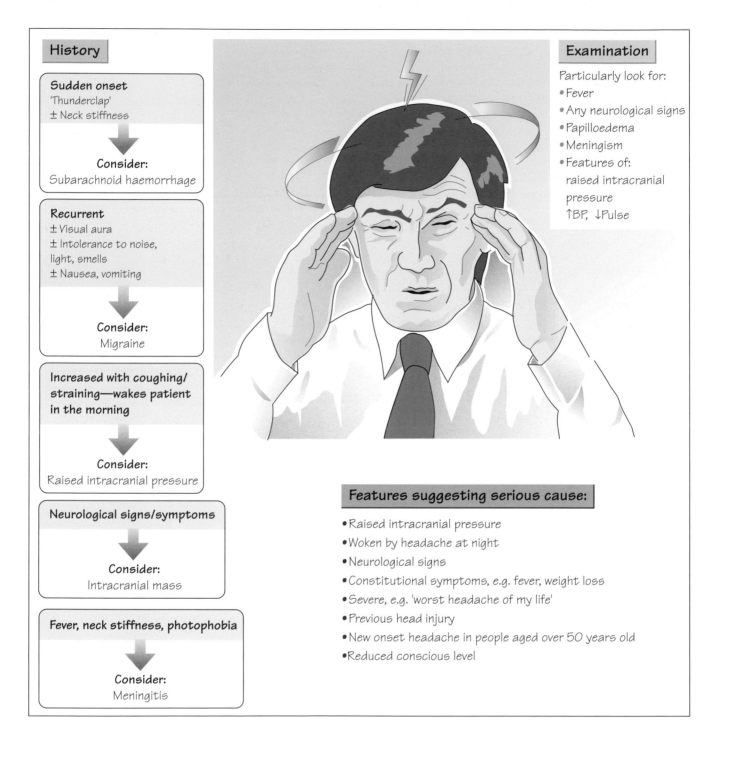

History

Sudden onset
'Thunderclap'
± Neck stiffness

↓

Consider:
Subarachnoid haemorrhage

Recurrent
± Visual aura
± Intolerance to noise,
light, smells
± Nausea, vomiting

↓

Consider:
Migraine

**Increased with coughing/
straining—wakes patient
in the morning**

↓

Consider:
Raised intracranial pressure

Neurological signs/symptoms

↓

Consider:
Intracranial mass

Fever, neck stiffness, photophobia

↓

Consider:
Meningitis

Examination

Particularly look for:
• Fever
• Any neurological signs
• Papilloedema
• Meningism
• Features of:
  raised intracranial
  pressure
  ↑BP, ↓Pulse

Features suggesting serious cause:

• Raised intracranial pressure
• Woken by headache at night
• Neurological signs
• Constitutional symptoms, e.g. fever, weight loss
• Severe, e.g. 'worst headache of my life'
• Previous head injury
• New onset headache in people aged over 50 years old
• Reduced conscious level

Headache is a very common symptom that is rarely due to serious disease. It is thus vital to assess the symptom of headache with care, try to reach an accurate diagnosis of the cause of the headache and establish whether there are any features suggesting a sinister cause of headache.

History

• What does the patient mean by headache? Is there pain? What is it like (e.g. throbbing, stabbing or aching)?
• How did it start? Did it start gradually or suddenly? What precipitated it?
• Have there been any accompanying symptoms (e.g. visual disturbance, vomiting, nausea, fever, photophobia, neck stiffness, rhinorrhoea or neurological deficit)?
• Is it similar to previous headaches? How often does the patient experience these headaches?
• What usually precipitates the headaches? Tension, anxiety, etc?
• How does this headache differ from previous headaches?
• Any history of trauma?
• Are there features of raised intracranial pressure? Is the headache exacerbated by coughing or straining? Is the headache waking the patient early in the morning?
• Any suggestion of meningitis? Accompanying neck stiffness, photophobia, fever, drowsiness?
• Any history of very sudden onset of headache suggestive of subarachnoid haemorrhage?
• Any accompanying neurological symptoms?
• Any change in personality, deterioration in mental abilities? History from relatives may be very informative.

Past medical history

• Previous headaches, especially migraines (with detailed description)?
• Previous neurological conditions?
• Does the patient suffer from hypertension?

Drugs

Any treatments taken for headaches?

Family history

• Any family history of headaches, especially migraines?
• Any family history of cerebral haemorrhage, subarachnoid haemorrhage or meningitis?

Examination

• Is the patient well or unwell? Is the patient in obvious discomfort, vomiting, photophobic?
• Look for pyrexia, neck stiffness and Kernig's sign.
• Are there any neurological abnormalities on full CNS examination?
• Look particularly for gait abnormalities, lateralizing signs and signs of raised intracranial pressure (e.g. papilloedema, bradycardia, hypertension, cranial nerve palsies).

N.B. Significant intracranial mass lesions may be present without papilloedema or other neurological signs. Therefore persisting headaches without a clear alternative diagnosis require further investigation.

Meningism = headache + neck stiffness + photophobia

Table 27.1 The differential diagnosis of headache.

Type	Headache	Other symptoms	Examination
Tension headache	Generalized	Neck aches/stiffness	Normal
Migraine	Throbbing Unilateral Recurrent	Vomiting Visual aura Photophobia	Normal (but rare 'hemiplegic' migraine)
Cluster	Localized to eye Recurrent	Eye watering	Conjunctival injection
Subarachnoid	*Very* sudden onset	Neck stiffness Photophobia	Meningism Subhyaloid haemorrhages
Meningitis	Severe	Neck stiffness Fever Drowsy Photophobia	Meningism Fever
Raised intracranial pressure or space occupying lesion (SOL)	Worse with straining/coughing Early morning headache	Neurological symptoms	Papilloedema Focal neurological signs
Temporal arteritis	Generalized, scalp tenderness	Jaw claudication Polymyalgia rheumatica	Temporal artery tenderness

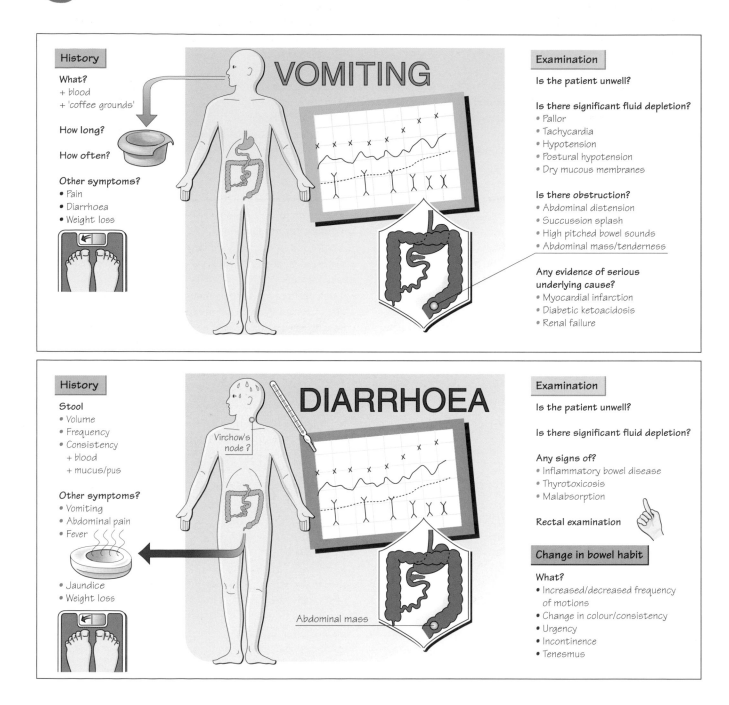

Vomiting

Vomiting is a very common symptom of both serious and benign self-limiting conditions. Causes range from structural problems with the GI tract, such as small bowel obstruction, metabolic disturbances, such as uraemia, myocardial infarction, intoxication with alcohol or drugs, motion sickness, migraine, bulimia nervosa, severe pain, or viral gastroenteritis.

Address the following questions:
- What is the cause of the vomiting?
- Is there substantial fluid depletion or blood loss?
- Are there any features suggesting a serious underlying cause, e.g. metabolic disturbance, cardiopulmonary emergency (e.g. myocardial infarction) or bowel obstruction?

History
- What does the patient actually mean by vomiting (retching or nausea or actual vomit)?
- How often have they been vomiting? What have they been vomiting (altered food, blood, 'coffee grounds') and for how long? Are they managing to drink and keep any fluids down?

- Does anything precipitate the vomiting? Movement or eating?
- What are the accompanying symptoms? Abdominal pain, other pains or diarrhoea?
- Does the patient have vertigo?
- Has there been reduced appetite? Weight loss?
- Any possibility of intoxication or of pregnancy?
- Are there any symptoms of neurological disease?
- Any history of GI disorders (e.g. pancreatitis, known bowel malignancy), previous abdominal surgery, previous episodes of bowel obstruction due to, for example, adhesions, medication (especially chemotherapy or opiates), diabetes mellitus, renal failure or excess alcohol intake?

Examination

- Does the patient appear unwell? Are they in pain or febrile? Patients who are vomiting often appear pale and there may be strong vagal activation producing, for example, bradycardia.
- Is there evidence of significant fluid depletion? Is there pallor, tachycardia, hypotension or postural hypotension?
- Is there evidence of intestinal obstruction (abdominal distension, succussion splash, high-pitched bowel sounds and abdominal tenderness)?
- Is there a smell of ketones (due to 'starvation' or diabetic ketoacidosis)?
- Are there any neurological signs (e.g. of raised intracranial pressure or nystagmus)?

Diarrhoea

Diarrhoea can be due to self-limiting illness, due to infections or be a manifestation of serious disease, such as ulcerative colitis, bowel malignancy or malabsorption.
Try to establish:
- If there is substantial fluid or electrolyte depletion or blood loss.
- If there are any features suggesting a serious underlying cause, for example, inflammatory bowel disease, subacute bowel obstruction or evidence of malabsorption.

History

- What does the patient mean by diarrhoea? Frequent stools? Loose stools? Liquid stools? Is there actually increased stool volume? Is it extremely watery? Is there undigested food in the stool?
- How frequently does diarrhoea occur? For how long does the diarrhoea occur? Is there urgency or tenesmus?
- What is the colour and consistency of the stool? Any blood, mucus or pus? Are the stools pale, do they float (due to steatorrhoea)?
- If there is blood, is it mixed with stool, coating the surface or usually only present on toilet paper (this would suggest haemorrhoids)?
- Consider the possibility of 'overflow' diarrhoea due to constipation.
- Are there other associated symptoms such as recurrent mouth ulcers, vomiting or abdominal pain?
- Are there any symptoms of fluid depletion (e.g. faintness, postural dizziness)?
- Any systemic symptoms such as fever, rash or athralgia?

- Has there been recent change in bowel habit? Any constipation?
- Any features suggesting malabsorption (e.g. weight loss, symptoms of anaemia)?
- Any contact with others with diarrhoea and vomiting?
- Any history of previous diarrhoea, known GI disease or abdominal operations?
- Any foreign travel?
- Are there any drugs that the patient is taking that might be causing the diarrhoea? Has the patient taken any drugs for the treatment of diarrhoea?
- Any family history of inflammatory bowel disease or gut malignancy?

Examination

- Is the patient well or unwell? Does the patient have a fever?
- Is there evidence of fluid depletion (tachycardia, postural hypotension, hypotension, dry mucous membranes)? Are there signs of weight loss, anaemia, angular stomatitis or koilonychia?
- What is the patient's body mass index (weight [kg])/height [metres squared])?
- Are there any signs of inflammatory bowel disease?
- Are there any signs of thyrotoxicosis?
- Is there abdominal tenderness, masses or rectal tenderness?
- Are bowel sounds normal, hyperactive or high-pitched tinkling (suggesting obstruction)?
- Any blood, mucus or masses on rectal examination?
- If there is blood rectally or if there is failure of symptoms to resolve the patient will probably require a sigmoidoscopy.

Change in bowel habit

A change in bowel habit represents an important symptom as it may be due to a GI lesion, such as a rectal carcinoma, an adenomatous polyp or be due to malabsorption. However, a change in bowel habit can occur in benign conditions, such as irritable bowel syndrome.

History

- What has the patient noticed? Increased frequency of motions? Change in colour, consistency of motion? For how long has this occurred?
- Are there any other symptoms such as diarrhoea, vomiting or flushing?
- Are there any features suggesting malignancy or malabsorption (e.g. blood, weight loss, abdominal mass, pain on defecation, jaundice or anaemia)?
- Any clear precipitation by particular foods?
- Any history of GI disorders (e.g. previous bowel carcinoma, inflammatory bowel disease or thyroid dysfunction)?
- Any family history of bowel malignancy?

Examination

- Is the patient well or unwell?
- Are there any signs of weight loss, jaundice, anaemia, lymphadenopathy (including Virchow's node)?
- Any abdominal mass or herniae?

Continued on p. 64.

Rectal examination

The patient is likely to need sigmoidoscopic examination.

Intestinal obstruction

Intestinal obstruction should be considered in any patient with prolonged vomiting or unexplained abdominal pain.

The symptoms of bowel obstruction may include colicky abdominal pain, vomiting, absolute constipation (no faeces or flatus).

Consider features in the history pointing towards a cause of the obstruction (e.g. known bowel malignancy, previous abdominal surgery, metabolic disturbance leading to ileus).

On examination look for:
- signs of hypovolaemia (see Chapter 61)
- abdominal distension
- high pitched tinkling bowel sounds (but absent in ileus)
- succussion splash
- signs of bowel malignancy (e.g. mass, weight loss, anaemia, hepatomegaly)
- scars from previous operations suggesting adhesions as a possible cause
- digital rectal examination ± sigmoidoscopy for obstructing mass.

Table 28.1 The differential diagnosis of vomiting.

Cause of vomiting	Frequency	Symptoms	Signs
Gastroenteritis	Very common	Nausea Diarrhoea	Dehydration Abdominal tenderness
Intoxication (e.g. with alcohol)	Very common	Nausea Unsteadiness	Drowsy Smells of alcohol
Bowel obstruction	Common	Nausea Absolute constipation (no faeces or flatus)	Dehydration Abdominal distension Tinkling bowel sounds
Ileus	Common (postoperatively)	Vomiting	Absent bowel sounds
Metabolic disturbance (e.g. renal failure, ketoacidosis)	Rare	Nausea Vomiting	Active bowel sounds
Raised intracranial pressure	Very rare	Headache Neurological deficits	Papilloedema Hypertension Neurological signs
Pancreatitis	Rare	Abdominal pain	Abdominal tenderness Acute abdomen

Table 28.2 The differential diagnosis of diarrhoea.

Cause of diarrhoea	Frequency	Symptoms	Signs	Important investigations
Gastroenteritis	Very common	Abdominal pain Vomiting Blood unusual Self-limiting	Abdominal tenderness Dehydration	Stool culture
Inflammatory bowel disease	Common	Abdominal pain Weight loss Blood, pus, mucus	Abdominal tenderness Active bowel sounds	Sigmoidoscopy
Malabsorption	Uncommon	Steatorrhoea Weight loss	Rarely neuropathy Anaemia	Blood tests: albumin, full blood count Endoscopy
Bowel malignancy	Common	Weight loss BP	Abdominal mass Rectal mass Anaemia	Endoscopy Barium examinations

29 Gastrointestinal haemorrhage

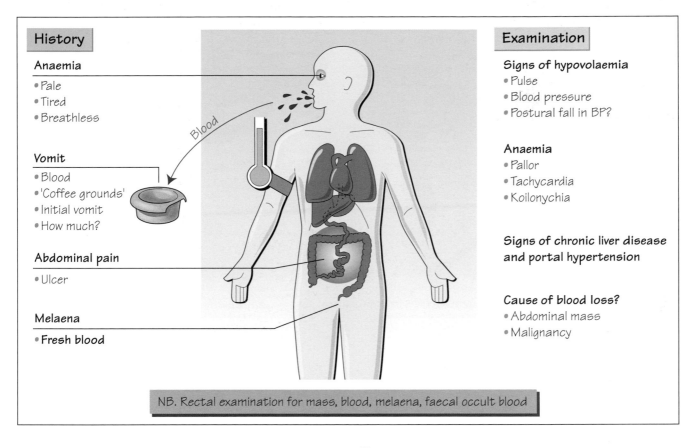

History

Anaemia
- Pale
- Tired
- Breathless

Vomit
- Blood
- 'Coffee grounds'
- Initial vomit
- How much?

Abdominal pain
- Ulcer

Melaena
- Fresh blood

Blood

Examination

Signs of hypovolaemia
- Pulse
- Blood pressure
- Postural fall in BP?

Anaemia
- Pallor
- Tachycardia
- Koilonychia

Signs of chronic liver disease and portal hypertension

Cause of blood loss?
- Abdominal mass
- Malignancy

NB. Rectal examination for mass, blood, melaena, faecal occult blood

This may present acutely with vomiting of blood (haematemesis) or passing of blood per rectum, which may be altered by passage through the GI tract and appear as melaena (black, tarry stool). Chronic GI haemorrhage may lead to anaemia and iron deficiency without obvious blood loss.

History
- Has the patient been vomiting blood or 'coffee grounds'?
- How much, how many times and for how long has the patient vomited?
- Did the first vomit contain blood or only subsequent ones? (Consider the possibility of Mallory–Weiss tear—bleeding due to oesophageal tear following vomiting.)
- Any indigestion, heartburn, acid reflux or abdominal pain?
- Any blood loss per rectum or melaena (which suggests upper GI haemorrhage)? Blood mixed with stool or separate from it? Present on paper? Any change in bowel habit? Any pain on defecation? Any mucus, diarrhoea?
- Does the patient feel faint or dizzy, especially with sitting/standing upright?
- Are there symptoms suggestive of chronic anaemia (reduced exercise tolerance, fatigue, angina, breathlessness, etc.)?

Past medical history
Any history of previous GI blood loss, anaemia, bleeding tendency, liver disease (consider varices)?

Drugs
- Is the patient taking aspirin, NSAIDS, anticoagulation drugs or iron (produces black stools)?
- Ask about the patient's smoking and alcohol history. If the patient's alcohol intake is excessive, consider alcohol-induced gastritis, ulcers or even variceal haemorrhage.

Family history
Is there history of bowel malignancy, colitis or rare hereditary conditions, such as Osler–Weber–Rendu syndrome?

Examination
- Is the patient well or unwell? About to die because of hypovolaemic shock?
- Is the patient hypovolaemic? (See Chapter 61.) If so resuscitate the patient, obtain intravascular access and give fluids.
- Check the pulse, BP, postural BP, JVP and for pallor. Are they cold and clammy?
- Examine the patient's stool and any vomit bowl. Assess the volume of blood lost.
- Are there any signs of chronic liver disease?
- Does the patient have anaemia, koilonychia or telangiectasia? Are there any signs of heart failure?
- Check the abdomen for tenderness, distension or masses.

Indigestion and dysphagia

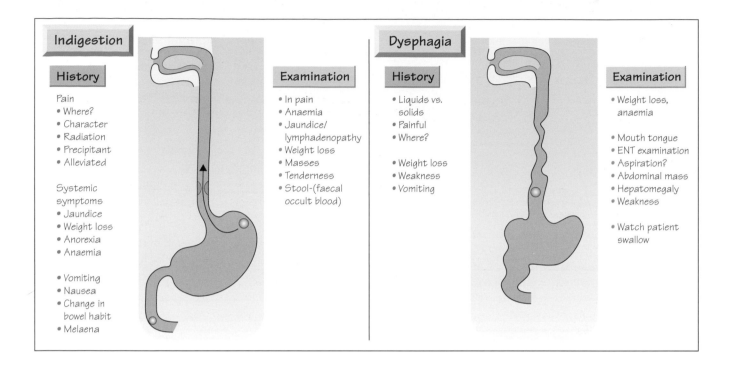

Indigestion

Indigestion is a very common symptom but it means different things to different people. It can mean abdominal pain, difficulty swallowing, acid reflux, retrosternal pain, etc. It can be a symptom of many important diseases, including peptic ulceration, gastric carcinoma and oesophageal reflux.

History

• What does the patient actually mean by indigestion?
• How do they use their hands to describe the symptom?
• What is the character of any pain or discomfort (e.g. burning, aching, stabbing)?
• What does it feel like? Where do they feel it?
• Does the pain or discomfort radiate (e.g. to the back)?
• When are the symptoms apparent (after meals, after certain foods, after alcohol, at night)?
• Does anything relieve the symptoms (e.g. sitting upright, antacids, drinking milk)?
• Any relationship with exertion? (Consider a cardiac source of the symptom)
• Any weight loss, anorexia, jaundice, symptoms of anaemia?
• Any vomiting, nausea, change in bowel habit, dark/black stools, haematemesis?

Past medical history

• Are there any previous episodes of indigestion?
• Any history of peptic ulcers?
• Any previous endoscopies?

• Any treatment with H_2 antagonists or proton pump inhibitors?
• Any stomach operations (e.g. vagotomy and pyloroplasty, gallstones)?

Drugs

• Are there any treatments (e.g. H_2 antagonists, proton pump inhibitors), *Helicobacter pylori* eradication or other possible causes of indigestion (e.g. NSAIDs)?
• Ask about the patient's alcohol and smoking history.

Examination

• Is the patient well or unwell? In pain or comfortable?
• Any anaemia, jaundice, lymphadenopathy, clubbing?
• Well nourished or signs of weight loss?
• Are there any signs of blood loss?

Examine abdomen

• Any masses, abdominal tenderness, abnormal bowel sounds?
• Give rectal examination and haemoccult test.

Frequency of GI symptoms in dyspepsia-related diseases

Table 30.1 illustrates the difficulty in establishing a diagnosis in dyspepsia from history alone. Diseases with a significant difference in symptom frequency are shown in **bold** type. Weight loss and GI haemorrhage are features that increase the likelihood of an underlying gastric cancer. The table emphasizes the importance of careful history, examination and investigations, such as

Table 30.1 Percentage frequency of GI symptoms in dyspepsia-related disease.

Symptom	Functional dyspepsia	Oesophagitis	Duodenal ulcer	Gastric ulcer	Irritable bowel syndrome	Gallstone disease	Alcohol-related dyspepsia	Gastric cancer
Anorexia	40	35	47	56	35	29	55	**64**
Nausea	39	17	34	39	33	28	37	**48**
Vomiting	24	22	34	34	**11**	23	**59**	49
GI haemorrhage	12	14	**26**	23	5	7	32	**34**
Heartburn	20	**64**	32	23	12	19	25	22
Weight loss	23	20	26	34	**16**	32	33	**72**

Adapted from Spiller RC. ABC of the upper GI tract. Anorexia, nausea and vomiting. *BMJ* 2001; **323**: 1354–7.

endoscopy, in reaching a precise diagnosis of the cause of indigestion.

Dysphagia

Dysphagia means difficulty swallowing. It is usually due to structural disease of the oesophagus, such as a benign stricture, oesophagitis or oesophageal carcinoma, although extrinsic compression by a tumour or aneurysm, tumours of the oropharynx and neuromuscular disorders, such as myasthenia gravis, bulbar palsy (e.g. motoneurone disease), stroke, achalasia or pharyngeal pouch, may be responsible.

History

• Is there difficulty swallowing liquid and solids? How has this developed? (Difficulty swallowing both fluids and solids from the beginning suggests a motility disorder.)
• Is it difficult to make a swallowing movement (consider bulbar palsy)?
• Is swallowing painful (odynophagia)? (Consider malignancy or oesophagitis)
• Is there bulging of the neck or gurgling? (Consider pharyngeal pouch)
• Where does the patient feel things are sticking?
• Any coughing or choking with swallowing? (This would suggest a neuromuscular cause)
• Any weight loss?
• Any evidence of weakness elsewhere?
• Any haematemesis, vomiting or regurgitation?

Past medical history

• Any history of ulcers, systemic illnesses (e.g. scleroderma) or neurological disorders (e.g. myasthenia gravis)?
• Any history of operations for reflux (e.g. fundoplication)?

Drugs

• Any treatment such as proton pump inhibitors?
• Any drugs that might cause or exacerbate oesophagitis (e.g. NSAIDs)?
• Ask about the patient's smoking and alcohol history.

Examination

• Is the patient well or unwell?
• Any signs of anaemia, lymphadenopathy or jaundice?
• Evidence of weight loss?
• Any abnormalities of the neck? Is there a goitre?
• Examine the mouth and tongue.
• Consider specialist ENT examination of pharynx and larynx.
• Any cardiovascular or respiratory signs?
• Look for signs of aspiration.
• Any abdominal masses? Any hepatomegaly or epigastric tenderness?
• Perform a neurological examination. A full examination is necessary with particular focus on any muscular weakness, fasciculation, the tongue and gag reflex.
• Watch the patient swallow fluid. Any choking, coughing or neck swelling?

31 Weight loss

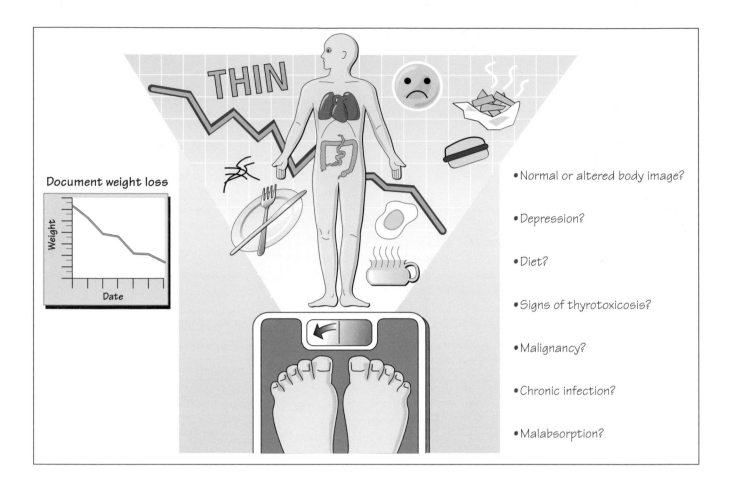

Document weight loss

- Normal or altered body image?
- Depression?
- Diet?
- Signs of thyrotoxicosis?
- Malignancy?
- Chronic infection?
- Malabsorption?

Weight loss may be a sole presenting complaint or accompanied by other symptoms. It may represent serious physical or psychological illness.

History
- How much weight has the patient lost and over how long?
- Are there objective measures of weight loss (e.g. clinic recordings, patient's measurements)?
- Has there been loosening of clothing, tightening of belts?
- Is the appetite normal or reduced?
- Are there any symptoms suggesting malabsorption (diarrhoea, abdominal pain, vomiting, steatorrhoea)?
- Are there any symptoms suggesting thyrotoxicosis (tachycardias, tremor, etc.)?
- Are there any features of depression (lowered mood, early morning wakening, suicidal ideation, etc.)?
- Are there any symptoms suggesting malignancy or chronic infection?
- Are there any symptoms of uncontrolled diabetes mellitus (e.g. polyuria, thirst, polydipsia)?
- Are there any symptoms suggesting major organ dysfunction (e.g. of heart failure)?

- What is the patient's perception of the weight loss? Do they regard it as abnormal? Do they think they look thin or normal?

Past medical history
- Any history of previous serious illnesses?
- Any history of previous malignancy, thyroid disease, anorexia nervosa, malabsorption or depression?

Drugs
Is the patient taking any diuretics, laxatives or 'slimming' drugs (e.g. amphetamines)?

Examination
- Does the patient look well or unwell?
- Any evidence of weight loss? (Have you weighed the patient?) Does the patient have a gaunt appearance with lax skin?
- Is there anaemia, jaundice, lymphadenopathy, pigmentation, hypotension or fever?
- Are there any signs of thyrotoxicosis?
- Are there any signs of malignancy or chronic infection?
- Are there any features of GI illnesses (e.g. Crohn's disease or ulcerative colitis)?

Table 31.1 The differential diagnosis of weight loss.

Cause of weight loss	Symptoms	Signs
Malignancy	Malaise Symptoms of specific malignancy (e.g. change in bowel habit, cough)	Anaemia, clubbing, lymphadenopathy, jaundice, hepatomegaly
Thyrotoxicosis	Anxiety, tremor, palpitations, heat intolerance, normal appetite	Tremor, goitre, thyroid eye disease, tachycardia
Malabsorption	Diarrhoea, abdominal pain, vomiting, steatorrhoea	Anaemia, neuropathy, bruising, proximal myopathy
Cardiac cachexia	Fatigue, breathlessness, leg swelling	Raised JVP, peripheral oedema, hypotension, cardiac enlargement, enlarged tender liver
Depression	Low mood, sleep disturbance, poor appetite	Of depression
Anorexia nervosa	Altered body image	Often profoundly thin
Chronic infection including HIV disease	Fever, malaise, rigors, night sweats	Fever, lymphadenopathy
Dietary inadequacy	Poverty, alcohol excess	

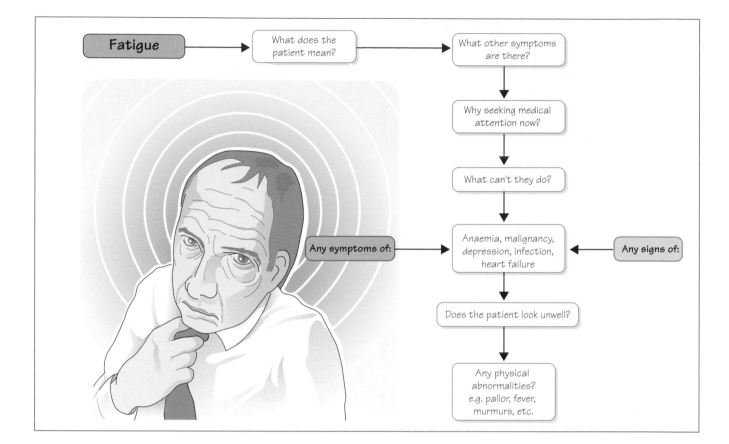

Fatigue or tiredness is a very common presentation and can be a manifestation of many different physical illnesses. However, it can also be a manifestation of social stresses or depressive illness. In many cases no identifiable organic disorder or psychiatric illness is found. It is particularly important to look hard for any clues concerning organic physical or psychiatric illness. Features suggesting an organic physical illness include weight loss, fevers, night sweats, specific pains, persistent symptoms of new onset and increasing age.

History

• What does the patient mean by fatigue or tiredness?
• Is the patient feeling tired the whole time? Does he/she mean they are unable to exercise, have exertional breathlessness or are fed up?
• When were the symptoms first noticed? What seemed to precipitate it? Are there any other physical symptoms? Any significant social changes at this time?
• Why have they sought medical attention now?
• What does the patient think the problem is?
• Any breathlessness? Is there weight loss, fever or loss of appetite? Are there any other physical symptoms?
• Are there any features of anaemia, hypothyroidism, Addison's disease, underlying malignancy, renal failure, cardiac failure, chronic infection or obstructive sleep apnoea?

• What are they unable to do that they would like to? What do they do (are they working a 10-hour day and looking after three children or staying in bed all day long)?
• Are there any features of psychiatric illness (depression, anorexia, lowered mood, anhedonia, early morning wakening, suicidal ideation, etc.)?

Past medical history

• Any history of previous illnesses, psychological problems, psychiatric illness or previous episodes of fatigue?
• A full **family and social history** is essential.

Examination

• Does the patient look well or unwell? Are there any physical abnormalities?
• Look particularly for anaemia, heart failure, hypothyroidism, Addison's disease.
• If symptoms are severe and there is no clear explanation, investigations such as a full blood count, thyroid function, CRP, etc., are likely to be required.
• Focus in detail on any symptoms other than the fatigue, any objective features, such as weight loss, and any abnormal physical signs.

Chronic fatigue syndrome
Definition

Clinically evaluated, unexplained persistent or relapsing chronic fatigue that is of new or definite onset (i.e. not life-long), is not the result of ongoing exertion, is not substantially alleviated by rest, and results in substantial reduction in previous levels of occupational, educational, social or personal activities. Together with the concurrent occurrence of four or more of the following symptoms: substantial impairment in short-term memory or concentration, sore throat, tender lymph nodes, muscle pain, multi-joint pain without swelling or redness, headaches of a new type, pattern or severity, unrefreshing sleep or postexertional malaise lasting more than 24 hours, the symptoms must have persisted or recurred during 6 or more consecutive months of illness and must not have predated the fatigue.

Conditions that exclude a diagnosis of chronic fatigue syndrome

- Any active medical condition that may explain the presence of chronic fatigue, e.g. untreated hypothyroidism, sleep apnoea and narcolepsy, and iatrogenic conditions, such as side-effects of medication, malignancies and chronic infection.
- Previous or current diagnosis of a major psychiatric disorder.
- Alcohol or other substance abuse.
- Severe obesity.

Table 32.1 The differential diagnosis of fatigue.

Cause of fatigue	Frequency	Symptoms	Signs	Important investigations
Anaemia	Common	Exertional breathlessness Angina	Pallor Signs of cardiac failure	Full blood count
Depression	Common	Sleep disturbance (especially early morning wakening) Low mood Anhedonia Poor appetite Suicidal ideation	Of depression	
Chronic fatigue syndrome	Common	Memory difficulties Headaches Myalgias Sore throat with fatigue of over 6 months	None	Full blood count Liver function Renal function
Hypothyroidism	Rare	Weight gain Cold intolerance Constipation Menorrhagia	Goitre Hair loss Puffy complexion Anaemia Slow relaxing reflexes	Thyroid function tests (TSH)
Heart failure	Rare	Exertional breathlessness Peripheral oedema	Raised JVP Gallop rhythm Enlarged liver Oedema Ascites	Chest X-ray ECG Echocardiogram
Addison's disease	Rare	Dizziness Poor appetite Vomiting	Pigmentation Hypotension (postural)	Electrolytes Synacthen test
Chronic infection	Rare	Fever Rigors Night sweats Poor appetite Weight loss	Fever Stigmata of endocarditis Other local findings in infection (e.g. empyema)	CRP
Renal failure	Rare	Polyuria Nocturia Itch Nausea Vomiting	Pigmentation Hypertension Haematuria Proteinuria Anaemia	Creatinine
Malignancy	Rare	Weight loss Reduced appetite Local symptoms (e.g. cough) Haemoptysis Breast lump	Lymphadenopathy Anaemia Jaundice Cachexia	Chest X-ray Full blood count
Obstructive sleep apnoea	Common	Snoring Frequent wakening at night Breathing pauses during sleep	Obesity Large collar size	Sleep study with oximetry

History

From:
- Relatives
- Friends
- Witnesses
- Ambulancemen
- Police
- Medical notes
- GP

Episodes
- Current
- Past
- Previous

Drugs
Alcohol
Social history

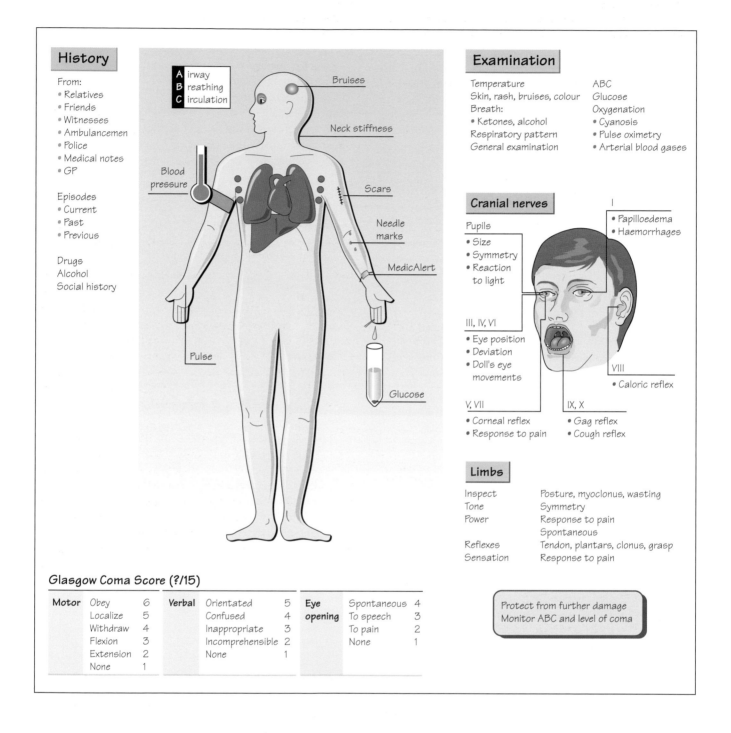

Airway
Breathing
Circulation

Bruises

Neck stiffness

Blood pressure

Scars

Needle marks

MedicAlert

Pulse

Glucose

Examination

Temperature
Skin, rash, bruises, colour
Breath:
- Ketones, alcohol
Respiratory pattern
General examination

ABC
Glucose
Oxygenation
- Cyanosis
- Pulse oximetry
- Arterial blood gases

Cranial nerves

Pupils
- Size
- Symmetry
- Reaction to light

III, IV, VI
- Eye position
- Deviation
- Doll's eye movements

V, VII
- Corneal reflex
- Response to pain

I
- Papilloedema
- Haemorrhages

VIII
- Caloric reflex

IX, X
- Gag reflex
- Cough reflex

Limbs

Inspect   Posture, myoclonus, wasting
Tone   Symmetry
Power   Response to pain
                 Spontaneous
Reflexes   Tendon, plantars, clonus, grasp
Sensation   Response to pain

Protect from further damage
Monitor ABC and level of coma

Glasgow Coma Score (?/15)

Motor			Verbal			Eye opening		
Obey	6		Orientated	5		Spontaneous	4
Localize	5		Confused	4		To speech	3
Withdraw	4		Inappropriate	3		To pain	2
Flexion	3		Incomprehensible	2		None	1
Extension	2		None	1			
None	1						

History

- **A history can and should always be obtained concerning an unconscious patient.**
- Interview relatives or friends (if not present attempts should be made to contact them and history obtained by telephone if necessary).
- Interview any witnesses of the circumstances in which the patient became unconscious. Detailed descriptions of the process of loss of consciousness can be very helpful in reaching a diagnosis.
- Interview other sources for the history may include ambulance reports, ambulance officers, the police, the GP and any medical notes that can be obtained.
- Just as one takes a history from a patient, similar questions should be addressed to relatives and witnesses. The following features in the history are particularly important:
  - detail of events surrounding the loss of consciousness
  - any recent medical or psychological problems
  - drug history (both illicit and prescribed)
  - history of alcohol intake
  - allergies
  - any previous episodes of loss of consciousness
  - any past medical history of significant cardiorespiratory symptoms, neurological or metabolic disorders
  - any recent medical symptoms such as of headache, fever or depression.
- A review of systems can often be obtained in surprising detail from relatives or friends.

Examination

The priorities in examination of the unconscious patient are to ensure that there is an adequate *Airway*, the patient is *Breathing* and that there is an adequate *Circulation*.

Urgent resuscitative measures should be enacted to ensure this and will usually include:
- nursing the patient in the recovery position
- maintenance of the airway often with endotracheal intubation
- administration of oxygen
- if trauma is possible and could have produced spinal injury, immobilize the cervical spine manually, with collars and splinting
- intravenous access and fluids.

Measures should be undertaken to ensure that the patient sustains no further damage as a consequence of their coma.

The possibility of hypoglycaemia should always be entertained in the unconscious patient, a rapid bedside blood glucose test performed and intravenous glucose administered if hypoglycaemia is present or if there is uncertainty.

Once the need for resuscitation has been addressed the examination should establish the depth of the coma, its likely aetiology and possible consequences.

Continual observation is essential to ensure that the 'ABC' is maintained.

The depth of coma is often assessed using the *Glasgow Coma Score*.

The examination should look specifically for:
- hypothermia (measure rectal temperature)
- fever
- MedicAlert® bracelets or necklaces
- scars
- smell of ketones or alcohol
- bruises or evidences of fractures with particular attention to the head and neck
- neck stiffness and Kernig's sign (but not if trauma possible)
- the presence of rashes compatible with infection (e.g. meningococcal septicaemia) or drug consumption, or injection marks
- pupil size, symmetry and response to light.

The ears and mouth should be examined.

Injuries to the tongue or evidence of urinary incontinence may suggest recent epileptic fit.

Full cardiovascular, respiratory, abdominal and musculo-skeletal examinations should be undertaken: there may be evidence of systemic illness (e.g. chronic liver disease) or the consequences of being unconscious (e.g. aspiration pneumonia).

As for history taking, it is sometimes wrongly assumed that the neurological examination can only be very limited in the unconscious patient, but a detailed examination is possible and may yield vital diagnostic information and must be performed.

- The patient should be inspected for abnormalities of posture, abnormal movements, such as myoclonus and muscle wasting.
- The tone of limbs should be examined, a grasp reflex sought and limb power assessed if necessary in response to painful stimuli.
- The tendon reflexes should be assessed, clonus sought and the plantar responses examined looking especially for asymmetry.
- The response to sensory stimuli, often pain, should be assessed in the limbs and trigeminal nerve distribution.
- As detailed in the figure opposite, each cranial nerve should be examined. Particular attention should be paid to eye movements or deviation, pupil size, symmetry and response to light. A careful fundoscopic examination is necessary and the presence of papilloedema should be looked for. The presence of gag and corneal reflexes should be sought and if absent ensure that the airway and eyes are protected.

> ### Evidence
>
> In comatose survivors of cardiac arrest the following signs at 24 hours were associated with death or poor neurological outcome: absent corneal reflexes (LR, 12.9), absent pupillary response (LR, 10.2), absent withdrawal response to pain (LR, 4.7) and no motor response (LR, 4.9).
> Booth CM, Boone RH, Tomlinson G & Detsky AS. Is this patient dead, vegetative, or severely neurologically impaired? Assessing outcome for comatose survivors of cardiac arrest. *JAMA* 2004; **291**: 870–87.

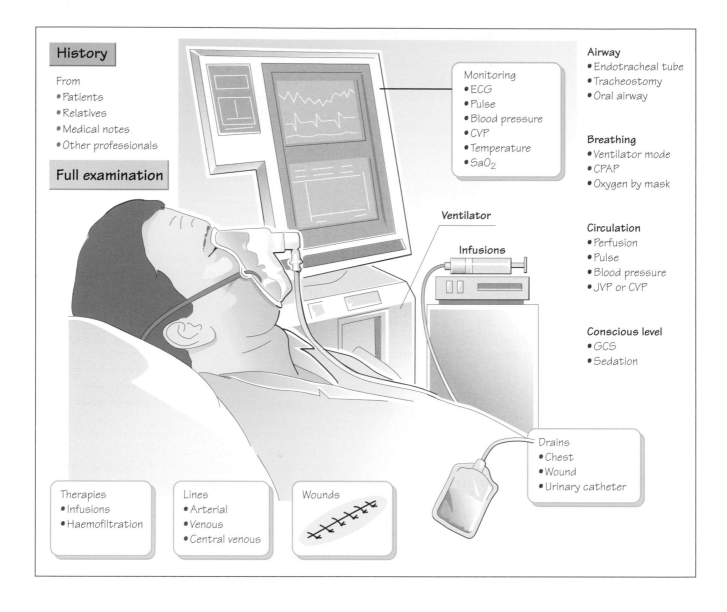

History

From
- Patients
- Relatives
- Medical notes
- Other professionals

Full examination

Monitoring
- ECG
- Pulse
- Blood pressure
- CVP
- Temperature
- SaO_2

Airway
- Endotracheal tube
- Tracheostomy
- Oral airway

Breathing
- Ventilator mode
- CPAP
- Oxygen by mask

Ventilator

Infusions

Circulation
- Perfusion
- Pulse
- Blood pressure
- JVP or CVP

Conscious level
- GCS
- Sedation

Drains
- Chest
- Wound
- Urinary catheter

Therapies
- Infusions
- Haemofiltration

Lines
- Arterial
- Venous
- Central venous

Wounds

It is important to take a history and carefully examine all patients, and those in the ICU are no exception. Whilst sophisticated monitoring, frequent blood tests and X-rays will reveal many important abnormalities, they will fail to demonstrate many vital clinical findings. Clinical signs such as the purpuric rash of meningococcal septicaemia, a new heart murmur, a drain bottle filling up with blood, a pleural rub, ileus, or hemiplegic weakness are just some examples that may only be detected by clinical examination and could critically alter diagnosis and management.

Similarly, despite the unconsciousness of many ICU patients it is still vital to obtain a full history from relatives, other witnesses and medical and nursing staff. Not only is this required to achieve precise diagnoses but details of previous illnesses, current medication, allergies and social history are all likely to be central to successful patient management.

Examination
- **Airway**: How is the patient's airway maintained (nasal/oral endotracheal tube, tracheostomy, oral airway)?
- **Breathing**: How is the patient ventilated (self-ventilating, CPAP, machine ventilation [what modality])?
- **Circulation**: Is the patient well perfused? What are the patient's pulse, BP and CVP/JVP?
- What is the level of responsiveness? What sedation/analgesia has been administered? Document with the Glasgow Coma Score. What are the pupil size, symmetry and responses?
- **Despite apparent deep coma, it is good practice always to treat the patient as if they can hear and understand everything that you say and experience all that you do.**
- What monitoring is in place? What is the blood glucose? What is the urine output?

• What treatments are being administered through which routes?

• How long have central lines, chest drains, etc., been in place? Are they still functioning?

• What is the patient's temperature, skin colour (jaundice, anaemia, cyanosis)?

• Examine the skin from head to toe for rashes, pressure areas and wounds.

• Full examination of cardiovascular, respiratory, abdominal and CNS systems should be undertaken. This may require additional sedation to ensure the patient's comfort and temporary pausing of the ventilator to aid auscultation.

• Integrate the clinical observations with the monitoring. Are they concordant?

Evidence

Scoring systems based upon physiological abnormalities have been developed in attempts to predict hospital mortality of ICU patients and as research tools. The most widely used are the Acute Physiology and Chronic Health Evaluation (APACHE) Score which uses vital observations, arterial blood gases, biochemistry, haematology, urine output, Glasgow Coma Score, age, chronic health conditions, length of pre-ICU in hospital stay and admission diagnosis.
Zimmerman JE, Kramer AA, McNair DS & Malila FM.
   Acute Physiology and Chronic Health Evaluation
   (APACHE) IV: hospital mortality assessment for today's
   critically ill patients. *Crit Care Med* 2006; **34**: 1297–310.

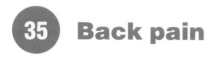

35 Back pain

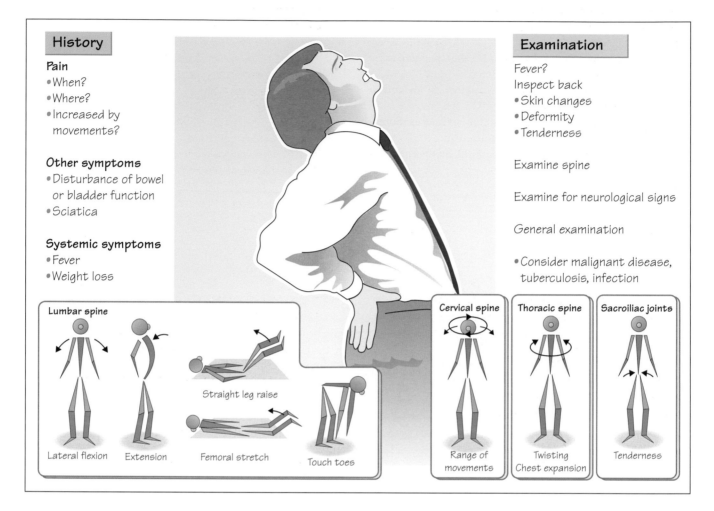

History

Pain
- When?
- Where?
- Increased by movements?

Other symptoms
- Disturbance of bowel or bladder function
- Sciatica

Systemic symptoms
- Fever
- Weight loss

Examination

Fever?
Inspect back
- Skin changes
- Deformity
- Tenderness

Examine spine

Examine for neurological signs

General examination

- Consider malignant disease, tuberculosis, infection

Lumbar spine

Lateral flexion Extension Femoral stretch Straight leg raise Touch toes

Cervical spine — Range of movements

Thoracic spine — Twisting Chest expansion

Sacroiliac joints — Tenderness

Back pain is a very common symptom producing considerable morbidity. It may be due to benign muscle strains, significant structural problems, such as disc prolapse or vertebral collapse, or, more unusually, a presentation of malignant disease, such as myeloma or bony metastases, or of intra-abdominal pathologies, such as aortic aneurysm or pancreatitis.

History

- When did the pain start? Did it start suddenly or gradually? What was the patient doing?
- Where is the pain? Is the pain exacerbated by movement?
- Is there pain at night? (When low back pain is due to infection or cancer the pain is usually not relieved when the patient lies down.)
- Are there any associated symptoms (e.g. symptoms of cord compression, disturbance of bowel or bladder function, weakness, sensory disturbance)?

- Are there any symptoms of sciatica? Do these symptoms increase with straining or coughing? (This suggests disc herniation.)
- Are there systemic symptoms (e.g. fever, weight loss, rigors)?
- Are there any other symptoms (e.g. morning stiffness)?

Past medical history

- Any history of back problems or operations?
- Any history of any known malignant disease, arthritis, TB or endocarditis?

Drugs

Is the patient receiving analgesics, NSAIDs or corticosteroids?

Family and social history

- What is the patient's occupation?
- Does the patient do manual work?
- Has the patient taken time off work?

Examination

- Is the patient in pain or comfortable?
- Any fever?
- Is there evidence of systemic disease (e.g. anaemia, weight loss, jaundice, lymphadenopathy)?
- Examine the back and spine fully. Inspect the spine carefully looking for any skin changes, deformity, abnormal kyphosis, scoliosis, lordosis. Look for smooth curves of the spinous processes, for any 'steps' and then palpate looking for tenderness and any associated muscle spasm.
- *Cervical spine*: examine active and then passive movements of the neck. Examine flexion, extension, lateral flexion and rotation. Look for range of movement, pain locally or in the upper limb. Examine again with gentle pressure on vertex of skull.
- *Thoracic spine*: examine twisting whilst sitting with arms folded. Examine for chest expansion: the patient should manage > 5 cm.
- *Lumbar spine*: test the range of movement. Ask the patient to touch his/her toes, keeping his/her knees straight. Assess extension, lateral flexion and rotation.
- *Sacro-iliac joints*: palpate the joints. 'Spring' the joints by firm downward pressure on joint whilst patient prone. With the patient supine, flex one hip whilst maintaining the other extended.
- *Nerve stretch tests*: Examine straight leg raising ± dorsiflexion of the foot. Carry out a femoral stretch test: with patient in prone position, flex the knee and then extend leg at the hip.
- Perform a full examination of cardiovascular, respiratory, abdominal and neurological systems.
- Examine particularly for abdominal masses, aortic aneurysm and sites of primary tumours such as breast, testis, prostate or lung.
- Examine for any signs of neurological deficit.
- Look particularly for any other joint abnormalities.

Worrying ('red flag') features of back pain

1 *Cancer as a cause of back pain:*
  - history of cancer
  - unexplained weight loss
  - age > 50 years or < 20 years
  - failure to improve with therapy
  - pain persists for more than 4 weeks
  - night pain or pain at rest
  - thoracic spine pain.

2 *Infection as a cause of back pain:*
  - fever
  - history of intravenous drug abuse
  - recent bacterial infection
  - history of TB
  - immunocompromised.

3 *Cauda equina syndrome as a cause of back pain* (due to large central disc protrusion or other cause of lumbar canal stenosis):
  - urinary incontinence or retention
  - saddle anaesthesia
  - anal sphincter tone decreased or faecal incontinence
  - bilateral leg weakness or numbness
  - progressive neurological deficit.

4 *Significant disc herniation as a cause of back pain:*
  - major muscle weakness (strength three-fifths or less)
  - foot drop.

5 *Abdominal aortic aneurysm as a cause of back pain:*
  - abdominal pulsating mass
  - atherosclerotic vascular disease
  - pain at rest or nocturnal pain
  - age > 55 years.

6 *Inflammatory spinal disease as a cause of back pain:*
  - early morning stiffness
  - restricted spinal movements
  - peripheral joint involvement
  - iritis, skin rash (e.g. psoriasis), colitis, urethritis.

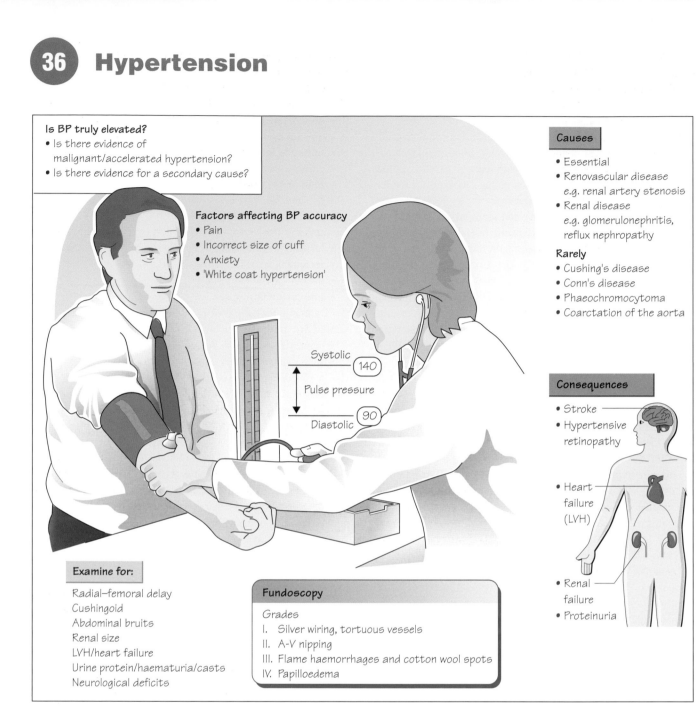

Is BP truly elevated?
- Is there evidence of malignant/accelerated hypertension?
- Is there evidence for a secondary cause?

Factors affecting BP accuracy
- Pain
- Incorrect size of cuff
- Anxiety
- 'White coat hypertension'

Systolic 140
Pulse pressure
Diastolic 90

Causes
- Essential
- Renovascular disease
  e.g. renal artery stenosis
- Renal disease
  e.g. glomerulonephritis, reflux nephropathy

Rarely
- Cushing's disease
- Conn's disease
- Phaeochromocytoma
- Coarctation of the aorta

Consequences
- Stroke
- Hypertensive retinopathy
- Heart failure (LVH)
- Renal failure
- Proteinuria

Examine for:
Radial–femoral delay
Cushingoid
Abdominal bruits
Renal size
LVH/heart failure
Urine protein/haematuria/casts
Neurological deficits

Fundoscopy
Grades
I. Silver wiring, tortuous vessels
II. A-V nipping
III. Flame haemorrhages and cotton wool spots
IV. Papilloedema

Hypertension is very common, usually clinically silent, potentially dangerous but treatable. Therefore, measurement of BP should be a routine procedure. The definition of BP above which hypertension is said to exist is difficult since it is distributed in the population as a normal distribution and increases with age. In a young adult BP of > 140/90 mmHg can be considered as hypertension and treatment is likely to be beneficial. In the presence of diabetes or renal disease, achieving levels of BP much lower than this has been shown to be of benefit. In an elderly person BP of ≥ 140/90 mmHg is common and may only warrant treatment in the presence of other cardiovascular risk factors. Some patients have elevated blood pressures in clinic ('white coat hypertension') and ambulatory 24-hour measurements and/or home measurements may be useful to define whether hypertension is really present.

History

Hypertension is usually asymptomatic. Rarely it can be accompanied by headaches, malaise or other symptoms of the causative diagnosis.

Find out how long a patient has been hypertensive (e.g. measurements at GP's, during pregnancy, in hospital notes, at medicals).

The consequences of hypertension are heart failure, renal failure, visual symptoms, stroke and ischaemic heart disease.

Rare causes of hypertension with specific symptoms are:
- Cushing's disease (weight gain, hirsutism, easy bruising).
- Phaeochromocytoma (paroxysmal symptoms: palpitations, collapse and flushing).
- Renal disease (microscopic haematuria/proteinuria and symptoms of renal failure).

Past medical history

- History of stroke, TIA, heart disease, renal disease?
- Other vascular risk factors?

Family history

There are very rare inherited specific causes of hypertension (e.g. Liddle's syndrome) but there is also a general genetic component to the development of hypertension.

Drugs

- What is the patient's current and/or previous medication? Does the patient have any intolerance to drugs?
- Ask about the patient's alcohol consumption.

Social history

- Ask about non-pharmacological methods (e.g. exercise, weight reduction, alcohol reduction, reduced sodium diet)?
- Ask about smoking and diet.

Direct questioning

- Headaches?
- Visual symptoms?

Examination

Blood pressure measurement using the auscultatory method

- Seat subject in calm, quiet environment with bared arm resting on support so that mid-point of upper arm is at level of heart.
- Ensure cuff is sufficiently large: the bladder should encircle > 80% of the upper arm.
- Place cuff so that mid-line of bladder is over the arterial pulsation of the brachial artery, with the lower edge of the cuff 2 cm above antecubital fossa where the head of the stethoscope is to be placed.
- Inflate the cuff and identify level of pressure at which brachial pulse disappears by palpation.
- Auscultate over the brachial artery and inflate cuff to 30 mmHg above the level previously determined by palpation.
- Deflate the bladder slowly whilst listening for the appearance (phase I) of the Korotkoff sounds, their muffling (phase IV) and their disappearance (phase V).

- Repeat several times, recording the systolic (phase I) and diastolic (phase V) pressures.
- Look for postural differences in BP.

(For the advantages and disadvantages of other methods of BP measurement see Pickering TG, Hall JE, Appel LJ *et al.* Recommendations for blood pressure measurement in humans and experimental animals. *Hypertension* 2005; **45**: 142–61.)

Further examination

Also examine for:

- pulse
- left ventricular hypertrophy (thrusting apex beat, displaced if secondary dilatation)
- fundoscopy
- radial femoral delay (coarctation)
- Cushingoid appearance
- abdominal bruits
- neurological deficits (TIA, CVA)
- any signs of heart failure
- check the urine dipstick for blood and protein.

First-line investigations

First-line investigations are ECG, creatinine and potassium. If in doubt about hypertension undertake 24-hour ambulatory measurement.

Assess the overall cardiovascular risk (age, gender, smoking history, renal disease, cholesterol and any known vascular disease) as this may influence the level of BP at which treatment of BP is beneficial.

Evidence

Abdominal bruits

In some studies, abdominal bruits are audible in up to 30% of healthy patients, have a large number of non-renovascular causes and are audible in up to 80% of patients with angiographically proven renal artery stenosis. They thus have a modest sensitivity and specificity for renal artery stenosis.

Turnbull JM. Is listening for abdominal bruits useful in the evaluation of hypertension? *JAMA* 1995; **274**: 1299–301.

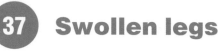

37 Swollen legs

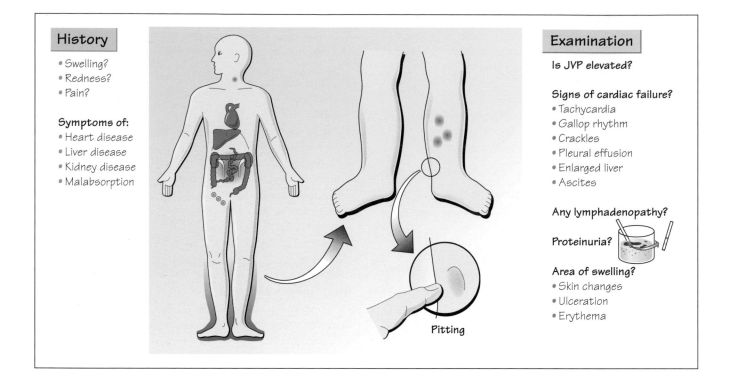

History
- Swelling?
- Redness?
- Pain?

Symptoms of:
- Heart disease
- Liver disease
- Kidney disease
- Malabsorption

Examination

Is JVP elevated?

Signs of cardiac failure?
- Tachycardia
- Gallop rhythm
- Crackles
- Pleural effusion
- Enlarged liver
- Ascites

Any lymphadenopathy?

Proteinuria?

Area of swelling?
- Skin changes
- Ulceration
- Erythema

Pitting

Swollen legs can be a manifestation of serious medical conditions including heart failure, DVTs and nephrotic syndrome. The symptoms in addition to the swelling may include pain.

History
- When was the leg swelling first noticed? Has it affected one or both legs?
- Is it painful? Has there been redness, exudates?
- Where does the swelling extend to? Is there also sacral oedema, ascites?
- Are there any associated symptoms (e.g. fever)?
- Are there any symptoms suggesting cardiac failure (e.g. chest pain, breathlessness or palpitations)?
- Are there any symptoms of liver disease (e.g. jaundice)?
- Are there any symptoms of renal disease (e.g. frothy urine [suggesting proteinuria])?
- Are there symptoms of malabsorption (e.g. weight loss, steatorrhoea)?
- Any prolonged immobility?

Past medical history
- Any previous leg swelling?
- Any previous DVTs, pulmonary emboli or varicose vein operations?
- Any history of cardiac, liver or renal disease?

Drugs
- Is the patient taking any diuretics or has the patient changed their medication recently?
- Is the patient taking any anticoagulants?

Family history
Any family history of oedema, thrombophilia (e.g. protein C, protein S deficiency or factor V Leiden)?

Examination
- Any oedema? Measure the legs. Is there pitting? How far up the leg does the swelling go?
- Is there redness, warmth, calf tenderness or dilated superficial veins?
- Any lymphadenopathy?
- Is the JVP elevated?
- Are there signs of cardiac failure (tachycardia, gallop rhythm, crackles, pleural effusion, enlarged liver, ascites)?
- Are there signs of liver disease or kidney disease?
- Any proteinuria?

38 Jaundice

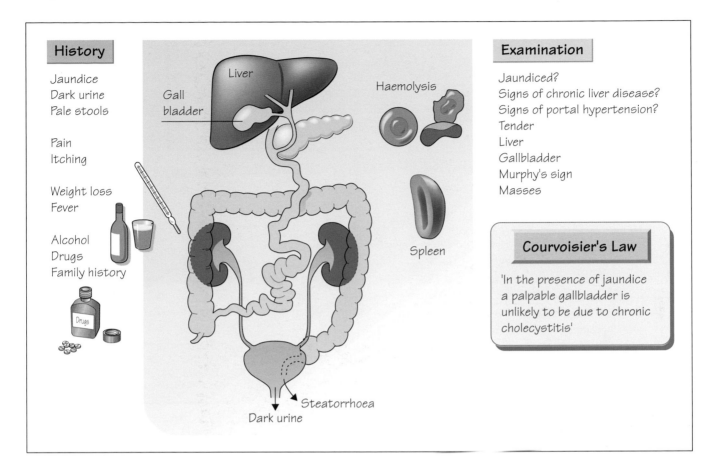

History

Jaundice
Dark urine
Pale stools

Pain
Itching

Weight loss
Fever

Alcohol
Drugs
Family history

Liver
Gall bladder

Haemolysis

Spleen

Steatorrhoea
Dark urine

Examination

Jaundiced?
Signs of chronic liver disease?
Signs of portal hypertension?
Tender
Liver
Gallbladder
Murphy's sign
Masses

Courvoisier's Law

'In the presence of jaundice a palpable gallbladder is unlikely to be due to chronic cholecystitis'

Jaundice may be a presenting symptom in many important conditions including advanced malignancy, gallstones, cirrhosis, hepatitis, haemolysis and carcinoma of the pancreas. The patient or others may notice the yellow coloration of the sclerae and skin, or features of associated conditions, such as malignancy or chronic liver disease that may result in presentation.

History

• When was the jaundice first noticed and by whom? What does the patient mean by jaundice? (Sometimes people think that jaundice means generally ill, off-colour or depressed.)
• Are there any other symptoms (abdominal pain, fever, weight loss, anorexia, steatorrhoea, dark urine, pruritus)?
• Any travel? Consider malaria or infectious hepatitis.
• Any features suggesting malignancy (e.g. weight loss, back pain), chronic liver disease (e.g. abdominal swelling due to ascites) or infective hepatitis?

Past medical history

Any history of:
• previous jaundice?
• known viral hepatitis?
• chronic liver disease or malignancy?
• blood transfusions?

• anaesthetics (especially halothane)?
• gallstones or previous cholecystectomy?

Drugs

Consider all medication, prescribed, illicit and alternative, as a potential cause of jaundice.

Alcohol

What is the patient's consumption of alcohol? Is the patient dependent on alcohol?

Family history

Consider inherited causes of jaundice (e.g. haemolytic anaemias, Gilbert's syndrome).

Examination

• Is the patient jaundiced? Look at sclerae.
• Are there signs of anaemia?
• Are there signs of weight loss, chronic liver disease?
• Any excoriations (suggesting pruritus)?
• Is there hepatomegaly, splenomegaly or both? Does the patient have a palpable gallbladder?
• Are there any abdominal masses or tenderness?
• Any features of portal hypertension?

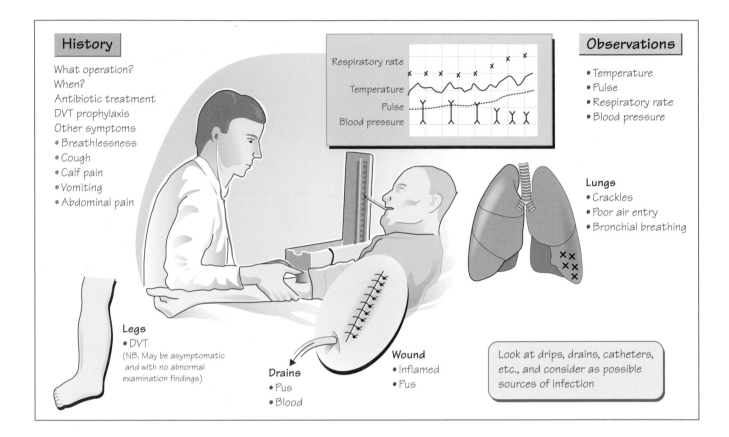

Fever is a common finding in the postoperative period and can point towards very important complications. Common causes include pulmonary atelectasis, chest infections, wound infections, pulmonary emboli, DVT and abscesses.

History
• When was the operation and what was the operation? Look at the operation and anaesthetic notes.
• Is the patient well or unwell?
• Does the patient have any symptoms (e.g. fever, rigors, cough, chest pain, haemoptysis, shortness of breath, calf pain, wound pain, wound discharge)?
• Are there any features suggesting an anastomotic breakdown (e.g. pain, ileus)?
• Is there a drain, drip, central line, etc., *in situ*?
• Has or is the patient receiving a blood transfusion?

Drugs
• Has the patient received any prophylactic or other antibiotics?

• Has the patient received any anticoagulation medication or TED stockings?
• Is the patient immunosuppressed?

Allergies
Does the patient have any allergies to medications?

Examination
• What is the patient's temperature? Look at the fever chart.
• Is there tachycardia, tachypnoea, cyanosis, respiratory distress?
• Examine the operative area carefully. Undress the wound. Is it inflamed, excessively tender or exuding pus?
• What is coming out of any drains?
• Examine drip sites for inflammation.
• Is there a subphrenic or pelvic abscess? Consider rectal examination.
• Are there any findings on examination of the chest to suggest atelectasis or consolidation?
• Are there any signs of DVT or pulmonary emboli?
• Any urinary abnormalities suggesting UTI?

40 Suspected meningitis

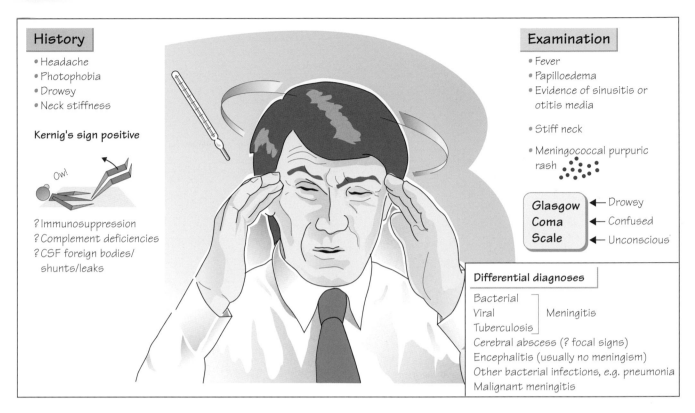

History
- Headache
- Photophobia
- Drowsy
- Neck stiffness

Kernig's sign positive

Ow!

? Immunosuppression
? Complement deficiencies
? CSF foreign bodies/
   shunts/leaks

Examination
- Fever
- Papilloedema
- Evidence of sinusitis or otitis media
- Stiff neck
- Meningococcal purpuric rash

Glasgow Coma Scale ← Drowsy
← Confused
← Unconscious

Differential diagnoses

Bacterial
Viral   Meningitis
Tuberculosis
Cerebral abscess (? focal signs)
Encephalitis (usually no meningism)
Other bacterial infections, e.g. pneumonia
Malignant meningitis

Bacterial meningitis may present with a combination of headache, neck stiffness, photophobia, confusion, drowsiness and fever. Viral meningitis, subarachnoid haemorrhage, cerebral abscess and encephalitis are important differential diagnoses. Give antibiotics urgently and admit the patient to hospital if there are features of meningitis. Consider the possibility of meningitis in close contacts.

History
- Does the patient have a headache? If so, when did the headache start? What is it like? Did it begin suddenly ('thunderclap') or gradually?
- Are there associated symptoms: photophobia, neck stiffness, nausea, vomiting, fever, drowsiness or confusion?
- Has the patient had any previous headaches?
- Are there any neurological symptoms: diplopia, focal weakness, sensory symptoms?
- Other systemic symptoms: nausea, vomiting, fever, rigors?

Past medical history
- Any history of previous meningitis, CSF leaks or shunts, recent severe head trauma, recent ear infection or sinusitis?
- Is the patient immunosuppressed?

Family and social history
- Any family history of meningitis, contact with patients with suspected meningitis or recent foreign travel?

Drugs
- Has the patient had recent antibiotics or any antibiotic allergies?

Examination
- Is the patient well or unwell? Alert, drowsy or unconscious?
- What is the patient's temperature?
- Check the pulse, BP and respiratory rate.
- Any rash, especially of meningococcal septicaemia, neck stiffness, photophobia or Kernig's sign?
- Are there any abnormalities on neurological examination?
- Fundi: normal papilloedema?
- Examine the throat, nose, ears and mouth.
- Perform a full general examination looking particularly for other septic foci.

Evidence

'The absence of all three of fever, neck stiffness and altered mental status virtually eliminates a diagnosis of meningitis.'
Attia J, Hatala R, Cook DJ & Wong JG. The rational clinical examination. Does this adult patient have acute meningitis? *JAMA* 1999; **282**: 175–81.

Anaemia

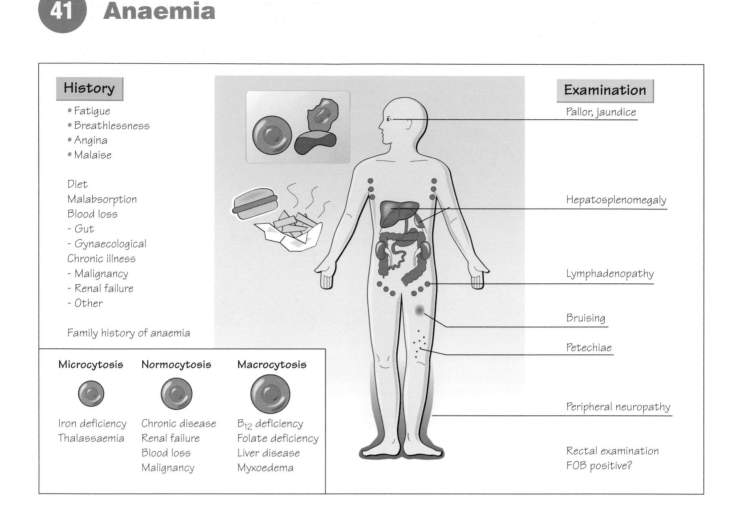

History

- Fatigue
- Breathlessness
- Angina
- Malaise

Diet
Malabsorption
Blood loss
- Gut
- Gynaecological
Chronic illness
- Malignancy
- Renal failure
- Other

Family history of anaemia

Microcytosis	Normocytosis	Macrocytosis
Iron deficiency	Chronic disease	B_{12} deficiency
Thalassaemia	Renal failure	Folate deficiency
	Blood loss	Liver disease
	Malignancy	Myxoedema

Examination

Pallor, jaundice

Hepatosplenomegaly

Lymphadenopathy

Bruising

Petechiae

Peripheral neuropathy

Rectal examination
FOB positive?

Anaemia may present with a variety of subtle symptoms. These can include fatigue, reduced exercise tolerance, shortness of breath and worsening angina. However, anaemia is often discovered incidentally when a blood count is undertaken routinely or during the course of investigation of another illness. The underlying cause of the anaemia, such as GI haemorrhage, may also bring the patient to medical attention. Anaemia is not a diagnosis and requires an explanation.

History

- What are the patient's symptoms? Fatigue, malaise, breathlessness, chest pain, none?
- Have these developed suddenly or gradually?
- Are there any clues to the cause of anaemia?
- Question dietary adequacy and iron content. Are there any symptoms consistent with malabsorption? Are there any features of GI blood loss (dark stools, blood per rectum, vomiting 'coffee grounds')?
- If the patient is female, is there excessive menstrual blood loss? Ask about frequency and duration of periods and the use of tampons and pads.
- Are there any other sources of blood loss?

Past medical history and functional enquiry

- Are there any previous suggestions of chronic renal disease?
- Any history of any chronic illness (e.g. rheumatoid arthritis or symptoms suggesting malignancy)?
- Are there any features of bone marrow failure (bruising, bleeding, unusual or recurrent infections)?
- Are there any features of vitamin deficiency such as peripheral neuropathy (with vitamin B_{12} deficiency/subacute combined degeneration of the cord [SACDOC])?
- Any reasons to suspect haemolysis (e.g. jaundice, known leaking prosthetic valve)?
- Any history of previous anaemia or investigations such as GI endoscopy?
- Any dysphagia (due to an oesophageal lesion producing anaemia or a web as a consequence of iron deficiency anaemia)?

Family history

Any family history of anaemia? Consider particularly sickle cell disease, thalassaemia and inherited haemolytic anaemias.

Travel

Ask about travel and consider the possibility of parasitic infections (e.g. hookworm and malaria).

Drugs

Certain drugs are associated with blood loss (e.g. NSAIDs producing gastric erosions or bone marrow suppression due to cytotoxic agents).

Examination

• Is the patient well or unwell? Is the patient breathless or shocked due to acute blood loss?

• Are there any signs of anaemia? Look for conjunctival and palmar pallor. (NB. Significant anaemia may be present without obvious clinical signs.)

• Is there koilonychia ('spoon'-shaped nails) or angular cheilitis as seen in long-standing iron deficiency?

• Any sign of jaundice (due to haemolytic anaemia)?

• Any circumoral freckling (Osler–Weber–Rendu syndrome)?

• Any telangiectasia (hereditary haemorrhagic telangiectasia)?

• Are there any signs of deficient or defective platelets (e.g. bruising, petechiae)?

• Any signs of abnormal white cells or features of infection?

• Are there features of malignancy? Any recent weight loss, masses, clubbing or lymphadenopathy?

• Is there hepatomegaly, splenomegaly or abdominal masses?

• Is the rectal examination normal? Any faecal occult blood (FOB)?

• Are there signs of peripheral neuropathy? (This suggests vitamin B$_{12}$ or folate deficiency)

Evidence

Pallor can suggest the presence of anaemia (although its absence does not rule out anaemia). Conjunctival pallor was assessed for its ability to predict the presence of severe anaemia (haemoglobin = 90 g/L). LR calculated for conjunctival pallor present, borderline and absent was: pallor present, LR 4.5 (1.80–10.99); pallor borderline, LR 1.80 (1.18–2.62); pallor absent, LR 0.61 (0.44–0.80).

Sheth TN, Choudhry NK, Bowes M & Detsky AS. The relation of conjunctival pallor to the presence of anaemia. *J Gen Intern Med* 1997; **12**: 102–6.

42 Lymphadenopathy

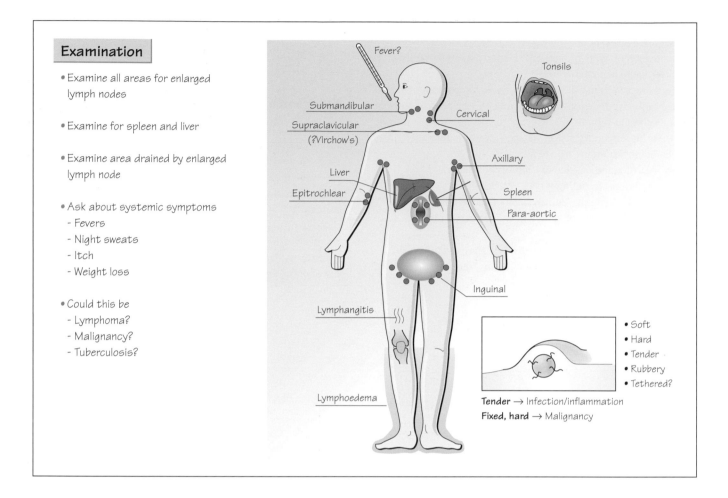

Examination

- Examine all areas for enlarged lymph nodes
- Examine for spleen and liver
- Examine area drained by enlarged lymph node
- Ask about systemic symptoms
  - Fevers
  - Night sweats
  - Itch
  - Weight loss
- Could this be
  - Lymphoma?
  - Malignancy?
  - Tuberculosis?

Fever?
Tonsils
Submandibular
Cervical
Supraclavicular (?Virchow's)
Axillary
Liver
Epitrochlear
Spleen
Para-aortic
Inguinal
Lymphangitis
Lymphoedema

- Soft
- Hard
- Tender
- Rubbery
- Tethered?

Tender → Infection/inflammation
Fixed, hard → Malignancy

Enlarged lymph nodes are common with self-limiting viral infections but can also be due to serious conditions such as malignancy or TB. It is important to consider pathology in the area drained by any enlarged lymph node.

History
- Which glands have been noticed as enlarged and for how long? Are they still increasing in size? Are they painful?
- Have there been any associated symptoms (e.g. weight loss, fevers, night sweats, pruritus, alcohol induced pain, cough, sore throat, rash)? (Weight loss, fevers, night sweats are the 'B' symptoms of lymphoma.)
- Any contact with glandular fever, TB? Any other infectious conditions?

Examination
- Is the patient well or unwell? Is the patient febrile?
- Examine the enlarged lymph nodes.
- Examine for lymphadenopathy elsewhere.
- Where are they enlarged? What do they drain? Examine carefully (e.g. very careful examination of breasts for axillary lymph nodes, full throat examination with laryngoscopy if abnormal cervical node enlargement).
- Are they painful, soft, rubbery, craggy, tethered?
- Is the overlying skin normal?
- Is the drained skin normal? Are there any lesions (e.g. cellulitis, abscess, melanoma)?
- Examine the mouth and throat (tonsils).
- Is spleen enlarged?
- Any lymphoedema?

Table 42.1 Common causes of lymphadenopathy.

Generalized	Local
Lymphoma	Bacterial infection
Glandular fever	Cancer
Other infections (e.g. other viral infections, brucellosis)	TB
SLE	
Drugs	
Sarcoid	

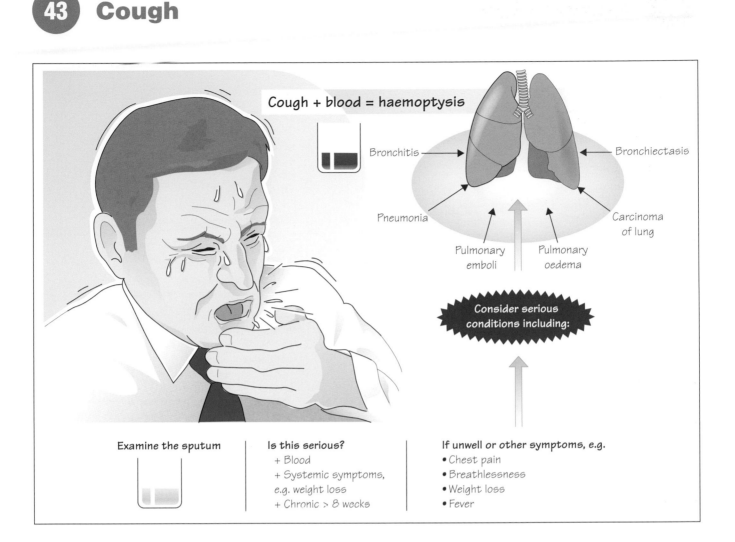

Cough + blood = haemoptysis

Bronchitis

Bronchiectasis

Pneumonia

Carcinoma of lung

Pulmonary emboli

Pulmonary oedema

Consider serious conditions including:

Examine the sputum

Is this serious?
+ Blood
+ Systemic symptoms, e.g. weight loss
+ Chronic > 8 weeks

If unwell or other symptoms, e.g.
• Chest pain
• Breathlessness
• Weight loss
• Fever

History

Cough is a very common symptom. It may be caused by mild, self-limiting illnesses, such as the common cold, or can be due to serious respiratory disease, such as carcinoma of the bronchus. It is essential to establish the duration of the cough, whether it is productive of sputum and whether there are symptoms suggestive of serious disease, such as haemoptysis, breathlessness, chest pain or weight loss.

Examination

• What is the colour, amount of sputum?
• Any blood (haemoptysis)?
• Is there evidence of serious acute illness?
• Is there fever, tachycardia, tachypnoea, chest pain or breathlessness?
• Is there a history of chronic respiratory disease?
• Are there features of sinusitis (e.g. maxillary toothache, purulent nasal secretions or facial pain)?

• Are there systemic features suggesting serious underlying illness (weight loss, fevers, anorexia)?
• Is the patient a smoker (current or ex-smoker)?
• Has the patient been exposed to particular infectious agents (e.g. pertussis, allergens or new medications [especially ACE inhibitors])?
• Carry out a full respiratory system examination.
• Are there any signs of consolidation, pulmonary oedema, clubbing or crackles?

Causes of haemoptysis

Causes of haemoptysis include:
• bronchitis
• pneumonia
• PE
• pulmonary oedema
• carcinoma of bronchus
• bronchiectasis
• pulmonary haemorrhage (e.g. Goodpasture's syndrome).

44 Confusion

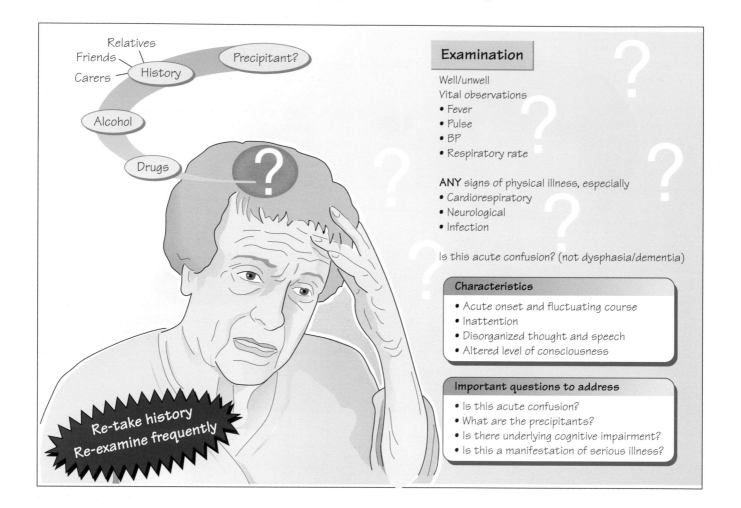

Examination

Well/unwell
Vital observations
• Fever
• Pulse
• BP
• Respiratory rate

ANY signs of physical illness, especially
• Cardiorespiratory
• Neurological
• Infection

Is this acute confusion? (not dysphasia/dementia)

Characteristics
• Acute onset and fluctuating course
• Inattention
• Disorganized thought and speech
• Altered level of consciousness

Important questions to address
• Is this acute confusion?
• What are the precipitants?
• Is there underlying cognitive impairment?
• Is this a manifestation of serious illness?

Relatives
Friends
Carers
History
Precipitant?
Alcohol
Drugs

Re-take history
Re-examine frequently

Confusion (or acute confusional states or delirium) is a common presentation of illness and is found in over 10% of patients aged over 65 years who are referred to hospital. It may be due to mild illnesses, such as UTI, or be an indicator of life-threatening conditions, such as myocardial infarction. The confusion often limits the quality of the history that can be obtained from the patient and so it is particularly important to obtain a history from relatives or any other witnesses. A very long history of confusion may point to dementia, but any deterioration in the patient requires an explanation.

Acute onset and fluctuating course are characteristic. Changes may be particularly apparent at night. There is usually a reduced ability to maintain attention to external stimuli: the patient is easily distractible and it is difficult to engage the patient in conversation. Thought may be disorganized and/or speech incoherent.

History
• When did the patient first become confused? How did it manifest?
• Any clear precipitants (e.g. change in medication, recent operation, hospitalization, alcohol withdrawal)?

• Any other symptoms (e.g. urinary frequency, fever, headache, cough, chest pain, other causes of pain)?
• Are there any other features (e.g. unable to walk or urinary incontinence)?
• Are there any features of psychiatric illness (e.g. depression)?
• What have relatives, friends or other carers noticed?
• Any recent falls, head injuries? (Consider subdural haematoma.)

Past medical history
• Any previous episodes of confusion?
• Any significant physical or psychiatric illnesses?

Drugs
• Gather a full drug history.
• Are there any recent changes in medication?

Alcohol
• Does the patient have a problem with alcohol dependence or withdrawal?

Family and social history

Establish the usual domestic arrangements, if there are any changes and the patient's functional abilities.

Functional enquiry

A full functional enquiry is vital and may reveal symptoms of an underlying physical condition, such as chest infection or subdural haematoma.

Examination

- Is the patient well or unwell?
- Are there any systemic features of illness (e.g. tachycardia, dehydration, fever, tachypnoea)?
- Could there be hypoglycaemia or hypoxia?
- Give a full clinical examination.
- Any cardiorespiratory disturbance (e.g. with cyanosis, respiratory distress or signs of cardiac failure)?
- Look carefully for any focal neurological signs.
- Examine the urine for signs of infection.
- Are they confused (rather than, for example, dysphasic)?
- Document with the Mini Mental Status Examination (see Chapter 110) and the Confusion assessment method section (below).
- If there are no clues in the history or examination pointing towards the cause of the confusion, investigations, such as ECG, arterial blood gases, chest X-ray, urine microscopy, dipstick and blood cultures are likely to be required.

The confusion assessment method

Key diagnostic features of the acute confusional state are:

1 Acute onset and fluctuating course.

2 Inattention.

3 Disorganized thinking—usually manifests as incoherent or disorganized speech.

4 Altered level of consciousness—ranges from vigilance (delirium tremens) to lethargy and coma.

Scoring the confusion assessment method

Consider the diagnosis of delirium if features 1 and 2 AND either feature 3 or 4 are present. This requires extra consideration in cases with suspected concurrent dementia or with prominent psychotic features.

1 *Acute onset?* Is there evidence of an acute change in mental status from the patient's baseline?

2 *Inattention:*

   A. Did the patient have difficulty focusing attention? (e.g. easily distractible or having difficulty keeping track of what was being said):

      (a) Not present at any time during interview

      (b) Present at some time during interview but in mild form

      (c) Present at some time during interview in marked form

      (d) Uncertain.

   B. If present or abnormal, did this behaviour fluctuate during the interview (i.e. tend to come and go or increase and decrease in severity):

      (a) Yes

      (b) No

      (c) Uncertain

      (d) Not applicable.

   C. If present or abnormal, describe this behaviour.

3 *Disorganized thinking.* Was the patient's thinking disorganized or incoherent? (e.g. rambling or irrelevant conversation, unclear or illogical flow of ideas, or unpredictable switching from subject to subject)

4 *Altered level of consciousness.* Overall, how would you rate the patient's level of consciousness:

   (a) Alert (normal)

   (b) Vigilant (hyperalert, overly sensitive to environmental stimuli, startled very easily)

   (c) Lethargic (drowsy, easily aroused)

   (d) Stupor (difficult to arouse)

   (e) Coma (unrousable)

   (f) Uncertain.

5 *Disorientation.* Was the patient disoriented at any time during the interview? (e.g. thinking that he or she was somewhere else, using the wrong bed or misjudging the time of day)

6 *Memory impairment.* Did the patient demonstrate any memory problems during the interview, such as an inability to remember events in the hospital or difficulty remembering instructions?

7 *Perceptual disturbances.* Did the patient have any evidence of perceptual disturbances (e.g. hallucinations, illusions or misinterpretations)?

8 *Psychomotor agitation.* At any time during the interview, did the patient have an unusually increased level of motor activity? (e.g. restlessness, picking at bedclothes, tapping fingers or making frequent sudden changes of position)

9 *Psychomotor retardation.* At any time during the interview, did the patient have an unusually decreased level of motor activity? (e.g. sluggishness, staring into space, staying in one position for a long time, or moving very slowly)

10 *Altered sleep–wake cycle.* Did the patient have evidence of disturbances of the sleep–wake cycle? (e.g. excessive daytime sleepiness with insomnia at night)

Evidence

Inouye SK, vanDyck CH, Alessi CA *et al*. Clarifying confusion: the confusion assessment method. *Ann Intern Med* 1990; **113**: 941–8.

Lump

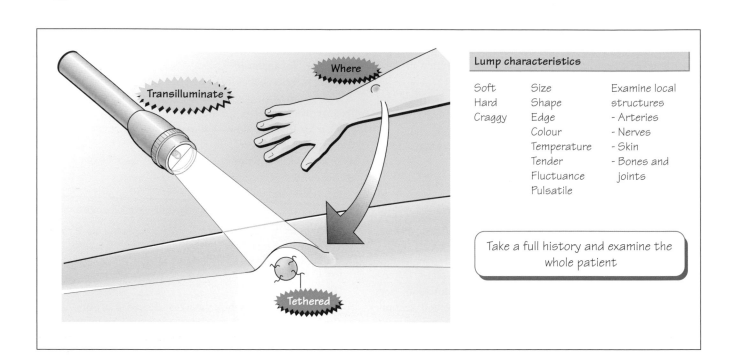

Lumps can be a manifestation of benign or malignant disease. A careful history and examination is vital in determining their likely nature.

History

• Where is the lump? How was it noticed (suddenly appeared, pain, itch, bleeding, change in pigmentation, etc.)?
• Is it enlarging? Is it producing local symptoms?
• Any other symptoms (e.g. weight loss, malaise or change in bowel habit)?

Past medical history

Any history of serious illnesses or other lumps?

Examination

• Where is the lump? Describe its location accurately. Is it associated with a particular organ (e.g. thyroid, breast)? Measure the size, document accurately and consider taking a photographic record.
• Are there multiple lumps?
• Any overlying skin change? (e.g. discoloration, erythema)
• What is the consistency of the lump: rubbery, soft, hard or craggy? Is it fluctuant? Is it hot or of normal temperature?

• Is the lump subcutaneous, deep, tender, pulsatile, pigmented?
• Is the lump mobile or fixed? Is it tethered to skin or underlying tissues? Does it move with, for example, swallowing?
• Is there a cough impulse? Does it transilluminate?
• Auscultate: is there a bruit?
• Is there associated lymphadenopathy?
• THEN examine the whole patient!

Evidence

Distinguishing a mole from a melanoma

• Use the seven-point checklist. Has there been a change in size, shape or colour? Has there been bleeding or crusting, sensory change? Diameter > 7 mm?
• Or use the ABCD checklist: **A**symmetry; irregular **B**order; **C**olour, variegation; **D**iameter, > 6 mm.
Both checklists had a high sensitivity and specificity in the diagnosis of melanoma.
Whited JD & Grichnik JM. Does this patient have a mole or a melanoma? *JAMA* 1998; **279**: 696–701.

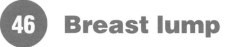

Breast lump

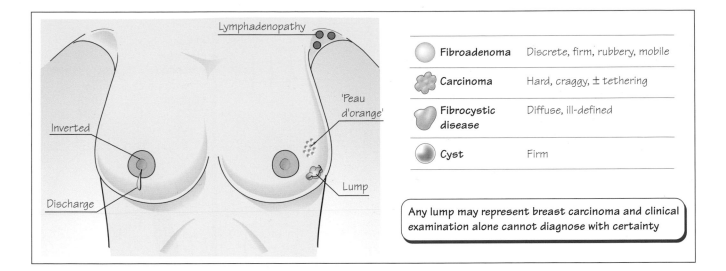

Fibroadenoma	Discrete, firm, rubbery, mobile
Carcinoma	Hard, craggy, ± tethering
Fibrocystic disease	Diffuse, ill-defined
Cyst	Firm

Any lump may represent breast carcinoma and clinical examination alone cannot diagnose with certainty

Breast lumps may be noticed by the patient, revealed during mammography or found during clinical examination. They have a variety of causes including carcinoma, abscesses and benign lumps.

History

• When was the lump first noticed? How? Has it changed in size or character since?
• Any variation with menstrual cycle? Any nipple discharge?
• Any pain?
• Are there any other symptoms? Lymphadenopathy, fever, other lumps, weight loss, back pain?

Past medical history

• Any previous breast lumps? If so, what treatment (e.g. mastectomies, local excision, radiotherapy, chemotherapy, breast reconstruction, other breast operations)?
• Any history of any other serious illnesses?
• What is the pregnancy history? Has the patient undergone lactation or menarche?

Drugs

Has the patient taken oestrogens or tamoxifen? Has the patient undergone chemotherapy?

Family history

Any family history of breast or ovarian cancer (e.g. *BRCA1/2* genetic predisposition)?

Examination

• Ensure (as always) that the patient is comfortable, warm, has privacy and the presence of a chaperone if appropriate and that you have clearly explained what you are going to do.
• *Inspect* the breasts. Are they symmetrical? Is there an obvious lump, any tethering of the skin? Is the overlying skin abnormal (e.g. *peau d'orange* appearance, puckering, ulceration)?
• Are the nipples normal, inverted, any discharge?
• *Palpate.* Palpate the breasts, gently initially and then more firmly using the pulps of the first three fingers. Use gentle circular motions and examine each quadrant of the breast and the axillary tail. Take time to examine carefully. It may be helpful to examine with the arm elevated above the head and with the patient sitting at 45°.
• Are there any lumps? Where? What size? What is their consistency: firm, soft rubbery, craggy, etc.?
• Is the lump tender? Examine the overlying skin for discoloration and tethering. Examine for tethering of the lump to deep structures.
• Examine for axillary and other lymphadenopathy.
• Are the arms normal or swollen?
• Look for possible metastatic spread and non-metastatic manifestations of malignancy features of infection.
  See Chapter 13.

47 Palpitations/arrhythmias

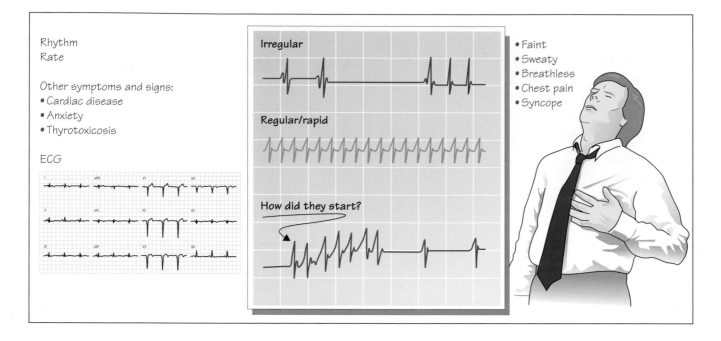

Rhythm
Rate

Other symptoms and signs:
• Cardiac disease
• Anxiety
• Thyrotoxicosis

ECG

Irregular

Regular/rapid

How did they start?

• Faint
• Sweaty
• Breathless
• Chest pain
• Syncope

Palpitations are an awareness of the heart beating. The symptoms arising from irregularity of the heart beat can vary from the slight and inconsequential (feeling a skipped beat due to a ventricular ectopic) to the major and life threatening (no cardiac output with unconsciousness due to ventricular fibrillation). It is important to analyse the symptoms carefully and assess the existence of underlying cardiac or systemic illness, such as coronary artery disease, anxiety or thyrotoxicosis. Bradyarrhythmias (slow heart beat) do not usually produce a sense of palpitations but produce dizziness, syncope, heart failure or fatigue.

History
• Describe the palpitations in detail? What do you mean by the term palpitation?
• What precipitated it (e.g. fright, chest pain)?
• How did it start (instantaneously is more common with tachyarrhythmias whilst an onset over minutes may occur with the awareness of sinus tachycardia)?
• How long did it last for? What terminated it (e.g. Valsalva, medication, spontaneous)?
• What were the accompanying symptoms: faintness, sweat, breathlessness, chest pain, thumping in the chest or neck, loss of consciousness? Any post-event polyuria (suggesting tachycardia producing atrial natriuretic factor release)?
• What was the rate of the palpitations? Was it regular or irregular (tap out)?
• Are there any other symptoms of cardiac disease (e.g. chest pain, exertional breathlessness, orthopnoea, PND)?
• Are there any symptoms of thyrotoxicosis (e.g. tremor, sweaty, goitre, eye signs)?

• Witness description and ECG during an attack are very helpful.

Past medical history
Any past history of collapses, presyncope, previous palpitations, ECG monitoring, 24-hour ECG tape results, cardiac disease or embolic events (e.g. stroke)?

Drugs
• Has the patient taken any anti-arrhythmics or any drugs with pro-arrhythmic effects? Any drugs that could cause electrolyte disturbance (e.g. loop diuretics and hyperkalaemia), anticoagulants?
• Ask about alcohol, caffeine intake and smoking.

Family history
Any family history of premature cardiac disease or arrhythmias?

Examination
• Is the patient well or unwell?
• Airway, Breathing, Circulation
• What is the BP? Are there signs of shock?
• Oxygen by mask, ECG monitoring and intravenous access if unwell
• Pulse: check rate, volume and rhythm
• Carry out a full cardiac examination
• Are there signs of heart failure?
• Are there signs of thyrotoxicosis?
• Carry out an ECG examination

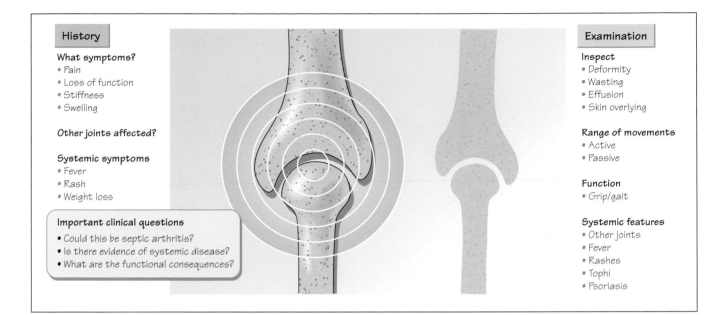

History

What symptoms?
- Pain
- Loss of function
- Stiffness
- Swelling

Other joints affected?

Systemic symptoms
- Fever
- Rash
- Weight loss

Important clinical questions
- Could this be septic arthritis?
- Is there evidence of systemic disease?
- What are the functional consequences?

Examination

Inspect
- Deformity
- Wasting
- Effusion
- Skin overlying

Range of movements
- Active
- Passive

Function
- Grip/gait

Systemic features
- Other joints
- Fever
- Rashes
- Tophi
- Psoriasis

Joint problems may arise due to trauma, infection or as a consequence of a systemic illness.

It is important to consider septic arthritis in any painful joint, particularly if there are systemic features of infection. Classically the joint is very tender with reduced range of movement and warmth, and a joint aspiration may be required to make the diagnosis and distinguish from conditions such as gout.

History

- What is the joint problem: pain, stiffness, swelling, deformity?
- What joint or joints are affected?
- How did the symptoms begin? Was there trauma or sudden or gradual onset?
- When are the symptoms worst? What exacerbates them? What alleviates them?
- Has there been any locking of the joint or giving way?
- Have there been any systemic features (e.g. rash, fever, rigors or weight loss)?
- What are the functional consequences (e.g. unable to walk, rise from a chair or write a letter)?

Past medical history

- Any previous joint problems: rheumatism or arthritis?
- Any joint replacement surgery?
- Any other serious illnesses?
- Any gout, arthritis, etc.?

Drugs

Any medications to treat, for example, NSAIDs, antibiotics, allopurinol, corticosteroids, etc.?

Family and social history

Any family history of arthritis or musculoskeletal problems?

Occupational history

What are the social consequences of the joint problem?

Examination

- Is the patient in pain or uncomfortable? Any abnormal posture?
- Is there evidence of systemic inflammation/infection? Fever, tachycardia, tachypnoea, hypotension?
- Any other signs of rheumatological disease (e.g. butterfly rash, gouty tophii, psoriasis, nodules)?
- Carry out a full general examination looking for systemic manifestations of rheumatological disease
- Inspect the affected joint(s): examine the unaffected joint first
- Is there swelling, erythema, deformity, muscle-wasting abnormalities of overlying skin?
- Palpate carefully. Is there tenderness, warmth, effusion or synovial thickening?
- Examine the active and passive movements of the joint
- Examine function (e.g. gait, grip)
- Examine other joints

Red eye

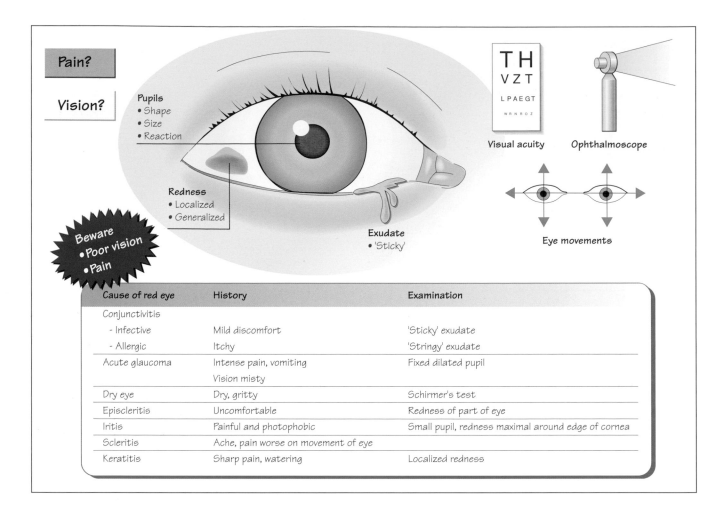

Cause of red eye	History	Examination
Conjunctivitis		
- Infective	Mild discomfort	'Sticky' exudate
- Allergic	Itchy	'Stringy' exudate
Acute glaucoma	Intense pain, vomiting	Fixed dilated pupil
	Vision misty	
Dry eye	Dry, gritty	Schirmer's test
Episcleritis	Uncomfortable	Redness of part of eye
Iritis	Painful and photophobic	Small pupil, redness maximal around edge of cornea
Scleritis	Ache, pain worse on movement of eye	
Keratitis	Sharp pain, watering	Localized redness

Red eye may be a manifestation of a benign self-limiting condition, such as viral conjunctivitis, or it may be due to a sight-threatening emergency such as acute glaucoma. Red eye is due to inflammation of the conjunctiva or episclera. A careful history and examination is essential to establish the correct diagnosis.

History

- How long has the eye(s) been red?
- Is there discomfort or irritation?
- Is it painful? Is it worse with eye movement? Is there a headache with it?
- Is vision impaired at all?
- Is the eye 'sticky'? Any exudate?
- Is the eye dry or gritty?
- Are there any systemic features (e.g. fever, malaise, vomiting, arthralgia or rashes)?
- Is there any eye itching or seasonal variation?
- Any photophobia?

Past medical history

- Any previous history of eye problems?

- Does the patient wear contact lenses?
- Any previous history of known illnesses (e.g. sarcoid, immunosuppression)?

Family history

Any family history of glaucoma?

Examination

- Are there any systemic findings (e.g. fever, arthritis)?
- Inspect the eyes:
  - Is the redness in one or both eyes?
  - Is it localized or generalized?
  - Are there exudates?
  - Is the visual acuity normal?
  - Are the pupils normal and responsive to light?
  - Are eye movements normal?
- Examine with an ophthalmoscope. A Schirmer's test and/or slit-lamp examination may also be required.

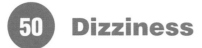

50 Dizziness

History

- What?
- When?
  - Precipitation
- Deafness
- Tinnitus

- Other symptoms?
  e.g. nausea, vomiting

Examination

Any signs of shock, hypotension?

Any cardiovascular abnormalities?

Any neurological abnormalities?
  Especially:
- Hearing
- Nystagmus
- Balance
- Cerebellar function

Feeling dizzy is a common symptom and can be caused by serious neurological or cardiovascular conditions. However, dizziness has a variety of benign causes and it encompasses a variety of different symptoms, and so it can be difficult to reach a precise diagnosis.

History

- What does the patient actually mean by the term dizzy? Does the patient mean unsteadiness, true vertigo (sensation of surroundings moving), feeling faint, headache, etc?
- Is the patient dizzy at present? What does it feel like? How long and how often is the patient dizzy?
- Are there any precipitants? Head movement/position, change in posture, exertion, etc?
- Any deafness, tinnitus?
- Are there any accompanying symptoms (e.g. nausea, vomiting, headache, palpitations, chest pain, etc.)?
- Are there any other symptoms (e.g. other neurological symptoms such as weakness or cardiovascular symptoms such as chest pain)?
- What alleviates the dizziness (e.g. sitting down)?

Past medical history

Any previous history of:
- Serious cardiac or neurological disease?
- Episodes or syncope?

Drugs

- Is the patient taking any drugs that might cause the symptom (e.g. diuretics producing postural hypotension)?
- Is the patient taking any treatment (e.g. vestibular 'sedatives')?

Examination

- Perform a full examination with particular emphasis on cardiovascular and neurological systems.
- Are there any signs of dehydration, shock, or anaemia?
- Check the pulse, BP and postural hypotension.
- Any heart murmurs?
- Are there any neurological signs? Examine particularly gait, hearing and for nystagmus.
- Examine the external auditory meatus.
- Test vestibular function and perform Hallpike's manoeuvre.
- Questions to address are:
  - Any evidence of cardiovascular disease?
  - Any evidence of vestibular, cerebellar or other neurological disease?

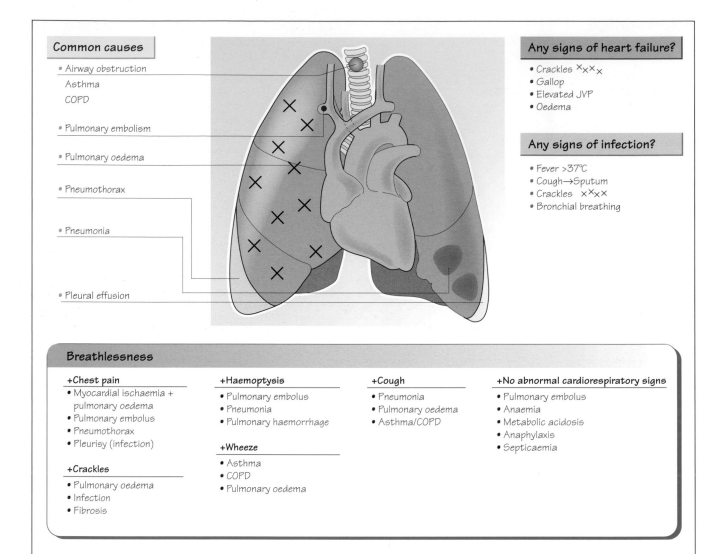

Common causes

- Airway obstruction
  Asthma
  COPD
- Pulmonary embolism
- Pulmonary oedema
- Pneumothorax
- Pneumonia
- Pleural effusion

Any signs of heart failure?

- Crackles ×××ₓ
- Gallop
- Elevated JVP
- Oedema

Any signs of infection?

- Fever >37℃
- Cough→Sputum
- Crackles ×××ₓ
- Bronchial breathing

Breathlessness

+Chest pain
- Myocardial ischaemia + pulmonary oedema
- Pulmonary embolus
- Pneumothorax
- Pleurisy (infection)

+Crackles
- Pulmonary oedema
- Infection
- Fibrosis

+Haemoptysis
- Pulmonary embolus
- Pneumonia
- Pulmonary haemorrhage

+Wheeze
- Asthma
- COPD
- Pulmonary oedema

+Cough
- Pneumonia
- Pulmonary oedema
- Asthma/COPD

+No abnormal cardiorespiratory signs
- Pulmonary embolus
- Anaemia
- Metabolic acidosis
- Anaphylaxis
- Septicaemia

Shortness of breath is a symptom that may be due to a very wide variety of diseases affecting the cardiovascular and respiratory symptoms. It may also be a manifestation of metabolic acidosis, anaemia, septicaemia or even anxiety.

History

- How long has the patient been breathless?
- How did it start: suddenly or gradually? What was the patient doing when it started: lying down, running, walking, etc?
- Is it getting worse?
- What brings it on? What alleviates it (e.g. posture, medication or oxygen)?
- Any orthopnoea or PND?
- Are there any accompanying symptoms (e.g. chest pain, cough, palpitations, haemoptysis and wheeze)?
- What is your exercise tolerance? What does the breathlessness stop you doing?

Past medical history

- Have there been any previous episodes?
- Any history of any cardiovascular or respiratory diseases (especially heart failure, asthma. COPD or pulmonary emboli)?
- Are there any potential causes of acidosis (e.g. diabetic ketoacidosis, renal failure)?
- Are there any allergies?
- Does the patient smoke?

Drugs

- What treatments has the patient taken? Any exposure to drugs with respiratory side-effects (e.g. amiodarone and pulmonary fibrosis)?
- Any use of home oxygen/nebulizers/inhalers?

Social history

- How has breathlessness interfered with any activities?

- What can't the patient do that the patient would like to do?
- Have there been any occupational exposures (e.g. pneumoconiosis)?

Examination

- Is the patient unwell and in need of resuscitation including intubation and artificial ventilation?
- Give oxygen by mask (use controlled oxygen flow if history of COPD and monitor arterial blood gases for hypercapnia)
- Is there tachypnoea, tachycardia, fever, cyanosis, anaemia or shock?
- Any use of accessory muscles, audible wheeze or stridor?
- Are there any signs of heart failure or fluid overload (e.g. crackles, gallop rhythm, elevated JVP, peripheral oedema)?
- Are there any signs that suggest infection? (e.g. fever, sputum, signs of consolidation)
- Are there any signs of pleural effusion? (dull to PN, reduced BS)
- Are there any signs of pneumothorax? (hyperresonant to PN, reduced BS)
- Are there any signs of pulmonary embolus? (raised JVP, pleural rub or signs of DVT)
- Signs of respiratory distress:
  - tachypnoea
  - use of accessory muscles
  - tachycardia
  - unable to speak in sentences because of breathlessness
  - anxiety
  - cyanosis
  - stridor
  - drowsy or confused.

Evidence

In breathless patients presenting to an emergency department, the features that increased the probability of it being due to heart failure were a past history of heart failure (LR = 5.8), the symptom of paroxysmal nocturnal dyspnoea (LR = 2.6), orthopnoea (LR = 2.2), breathlessness on exertion (LR = 1.3), a third heart sound (S3 gallop) (LR = 11), jugular venous distension (LR = 5.1), pulmonary crackles (LR = 2.8), leg oedema (LR = 2.3), the chest radiograph showing pulmonary venous congestion (LR = 12.0), and the electrocardiogram showing atrial fibrillation (LR = 3.8).

Wang CS, FitzGerald JM, Schulzer M, Mak E & Ayas NT. Does this dyspneic patient in the emergency department have congestive heart failure? *JAMA* 2005; **294**, 1944–56.

52 Dysuria and haematuria

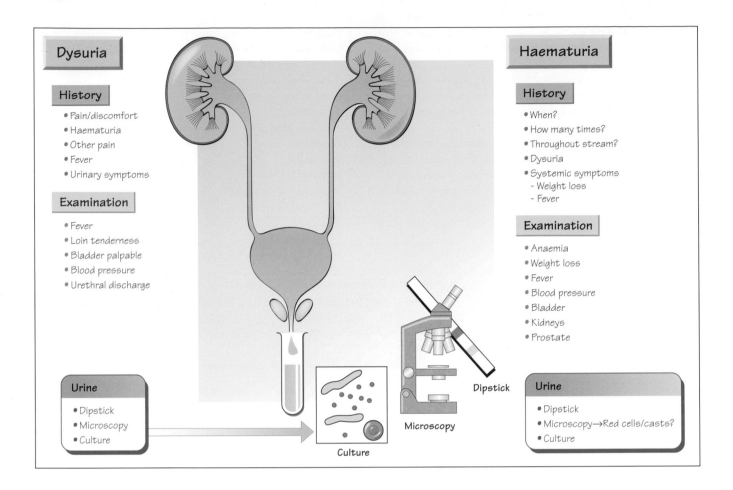

Dysuria
- History
  - Pain/discomfort
  - Haematuria
  - Other pain
  - Fever
  - Urinary symptoms
- Examination
  - Fever
  - Loin tenderness
  - Bladder palpable
  - Blood pressure
  - Urethral discharge
- Urine
  - Dipstick
  - Microscopy
  - Culture

Culture

Microscopy

Dipstick

Haematuria
- History
  - When?
  - How many times?
  - Throughout stream?
  - Dysuria
  - Systemic symptoms
    - Weight loss
    - Fever
- Examination
  - Anaemia
  - Weight loss
  - Fever
  - Blood pressure
  - Bladder
  - Kidneys
  - Prostate
- Urine
  - Dipstick
  - Microscopy→Red cells/casts?
  - Culture

Dysuria

Dysuria is the symptom of pain or discomfort when passing urine. The commonest cause by far is UTI but other conditions such as urinary calculi, urethritis, prostatitis and malignancy of the lower urinary tract can also produce dysuria.

History

• Ask the patient when is the pain or discomfort? Whilst or during attempting to urinate?
• Is there associated haematuria, penile or vaginal discharge, offensive smelling urine, cloudy urine or passage of 'grit' or calculi?
• Any loin pain? Suprapubic pain?
• Has the episode been associated with recent instrumentation, sexual intercourse or dehydration?
• Are there any other urinary symptoms (e.g. hesitancy, poor stream, terminal dribbling, incontinence)?
• Are there any systemic features such as weight loss, fever, rigors, sweats or confusion?
• Has a urine sample been sent for analysis?

Past medical history

Any previous episodes of dysuria, UTIs, urinary calculi, renal disease or diabetes mellitus?

Family history

Any family history of recurrent UTIs, particularly those associated with reflux nephropathy?

Drugs

• Is the patient taking any antibiotic treatment?
• Does the patient have any allergies to antibiotics?

Examination

• Is the patient well or unwell?
• Any fever?
• Any loin tenderness?
• Is the bladder palpable?
• BP elevated?
• Any penile or vaginal discharge?
• Consider rectal examination of prostate if prostatitis suspected
• Obtain mid-stream ('clean catch') urine sample. Tests: microscopy for cells and casts; dipstick for blood, protein, leucocytes, nitrites and culture.

Haematuria

Large amounts of blood may be detected in the urine by the patient, smaller amounts (e.g. in glomerulonephritis) can produce a 'smoky' appearance and even smaller quantities can be detected using dipsticks or microscopy. The presence of blood in the urine may be due to malignancy anywhere in the renal tract, calculi, infection, glomerulonephritis or other renal diseases and is common in women during menstruation. The presence of microscopic haematuria is common affecting up to 5% of the population in some surveys. Persistent microscopic haematuria usually warrants careful consideration of the possibility of underlying glomerulonephritis or malignancy. This will include a full history and examination with particular focus on any symptoms arising from the urinary tract, proteinuria and hypertension. Investigations such as ultrasound, renal biopsy and cystoscopy are often required to define the cause.

History

• Is there haematuria? If so, when and how many times?
• Where in the stream is it noticed: throughout or just terminally (suggesting lower tract disease)?
• Are there any associated features such as dysuria, fever, frequency, loin pain?
• Are there any other urinary symptoms such as hesitancy, poor stream, terminal dribbling, incontinence?
• Are there any systemic symptoms such as weight loss, itch, nausea, anorexia?
• Has haematuria been noticed previously (e.g. with dipstick during medicals)?

Past medical history

Any history of previous haematuria or of other diseases that affect the renal tract?

Drugs

• Is the patient taking any anticoagulants? (But haematuria still suggests an underlying abnormality.)
• Is the patient taking any anti-hypertensives?

Family history

Is there a family history of renal diseases (e.g. polycystic kidney disease)?

Examination

• Is the patient well or unwell?
• Are there any signs of weight loss, fever, anaemia or renal failure?
• Check BP and check for signs of hypertensive damage (e.g. retinopathy, left ventricular hypertrophy).
• Are there any abdominal masses, palpable bladder, kidneys or an enlarged prostate?
• Obtain a mid-stream ('clean catch') urine sample. Tests: microscopy for cells and casts; dipstick for blood, protein, leucocytes, nitrites and culture.

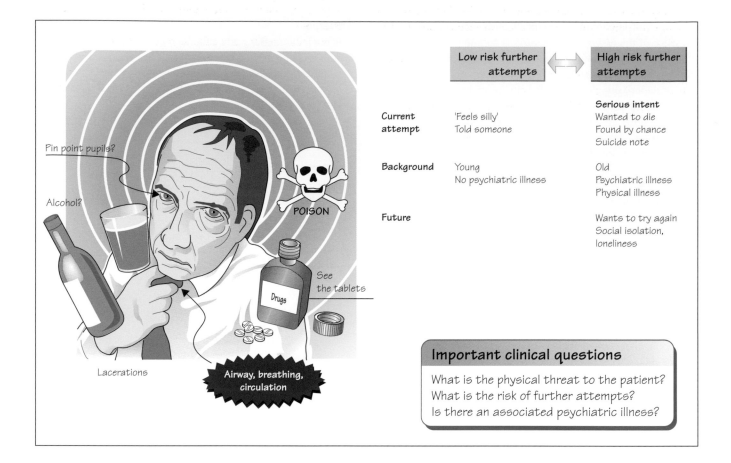

	Low risk further attempts	High risk further attempts
Current attempt	'Feels silly' Told someone	**Serious intent** Wanted to die Found by chance Suicide note
Background	Young No psychiatric illness	Old Psychiatric illness Physical illness
Future		Wants to try again Social isolation, loneliness

Pin point pupils?

Alcohol?

POISON

See the tablets

Drugs

Lacerations

Airway, breathing, circulation

Important clinical questions

What is the physical threat to the patient?
What is the risk of further attempts?
Is there an associated psychiatric illness?

Attempted suicide is a very common reason for hospital admission. It is important to establish the continuing medical threat from medications or toxins, to consider whether there is underlying psychiatric disease, to understand the personal and social background to the attempt, and to assess the risk of further attempts. The majority of attempts are not life threatening, use an overdose of medication (commonest drugs are paracetamol, aspirin, tricyclic antidepressants and opiates) and do not have a serious underlying psychiatric disorder.

History

• Gather history from patient, relatives, other witnesses and ambulance officers.
• When was the attempt made, where and with what? Consider the possibility of multiple drug overdose, the use of alcohol, carbon monoxide poisoning from exhaust fumes, self-harm by laceration, insulin overdose, etc.
• How was the patient found? Did they tell someone of the attempt? Did they phone an ambulance and, if not, who did?
• Was a suicide note found? Were empty tablet containers found?

• What other medications might the patient have had access to?
• What is the patient's age and sex? (Attempted suicide or parasuicide is more common in young women; successful suicide is more common in men.)
• What symptoms are there since the overdose (e.g. sleepiness, fits, vomiting)?
• What led to the suicide attempt?
• Did they want to die? Was it a 'cry for help'?
• How do they feel about it now: silly or disappointed that they failed?

Past medical history

• Have there been previous suicide attempts? If so, when, how and why?
• Any known psychiatric illnesses? If so, what treatment was the patient given?
• Any history of any other significant medical conditions?

Drugs

• What is the patient's normal medication?
• Do they take any illicit drugs?
• What other medications does the patient have access to?

Examination

- Examine the adequacy of the airway and ensure it is not obstructed.
- Assess and optimize breathing and circulation. Hypotension is a common finding with a wide variety of medications used in overdose.
- Assess the level of consciousness with Glasgow Coma Score.
- Check for vital observations.
- Check for signs of drug overdose:
  - pinpoint pupils and depressed respiration with opiates
  - smell of alcohol
  - cherry red skin colour with carbon monoxide poisoning
  - hyperventilation with aspirin poisoning
  - jaundice with late presenting (> 48 hours) paracetamol overdose
  - obvious lacerations or other signs of self harm.
- Perform a careful clinical examination.
- Look at the tablets, the tablet containers and prescriptions.
- Assess the patient's mental state looking particularly for depression, psychosis and risk of further attempts.

54 Immunosuppressed patients

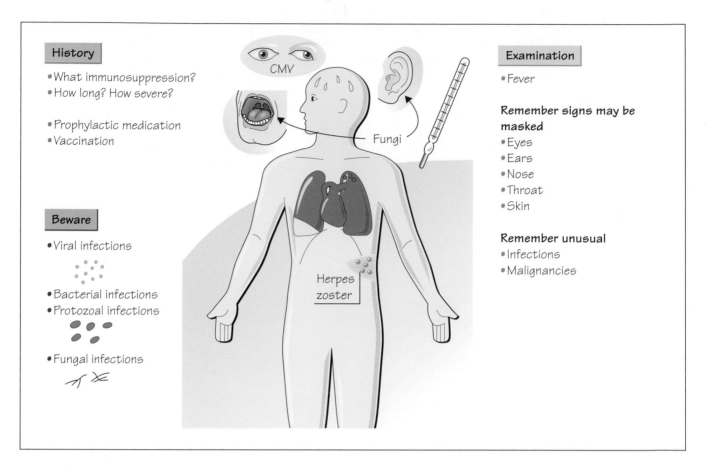

History
- What immunosuppression?
- How long? How severe?
- Prophylactic medication
- Vaccination

CMV

Fungi

Beware
- Viral infections
- Bacterial infections
- Protozoal infections
- Fungal infections

Herpes zoster

Examination
- Fever

Remember signs may be masked
- Eyes
- Ears
- Nose
- Throat
- Skin

Remember unusual
- Infections
- Malignancies

Patients who are immunosuppressed may present with masked or unusual symptoms. For example, corticosteroids may reduce the severity of signs of an intra-abdominal perforation, and an isolated fever in a neutropaenic patient is much more likely to represent a serious infection than in an otherwise healthy patient. Furthermore, patients who are immunosuppressed may be subject to unusual infectious and malignant diseases.

History
- Establish the cause of the immunosuppression: is it congenital (e.g. chronic granulomatous disease, acquired due to HIV infection, chemotherapy, splenectomy or a lymphoproliferative disorder)?
- What is the severity and duration of the immunosuppression (e.g. undetectable T-cell count or small dose of corticosteroid)?
- What is the presentation: fever, cough or other symptoms?
- Have there been previous infections or malignancies?
- Has there been prophylactic treatment or vaccination (e.g. septrin for *Pneumocystis carinii* pneumonia)?

Past medical history
- Any history of previous infections or malignancies?
- Ask about the history and cause of the immunosuppression.

Social history
Ask about foreign travel, pets and any possible contact with infectious disease.

Examination
- Is there fever?
- Undertake a full examination but particularly:
  - examine carefully the mouth, tongue, throat, ears, eyes and fundi
  - examine the skin for malignancy (e.g. Kaposi's sarcoma, warts, stigmata of infection)
  - consider that signs such as those of an acute abdomen may be 'masked', or that the fever may not be apparent
  - consider the reactivation of infections such as TB or herpes zoster.

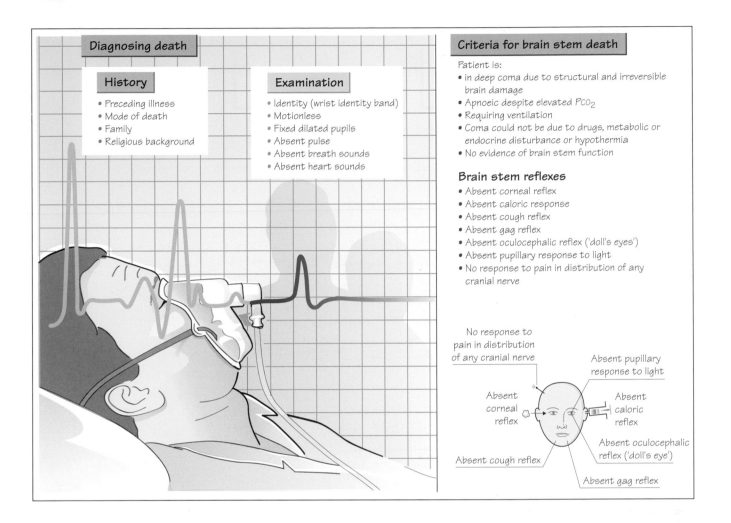

Diagnosing death

History
- Preceding illness
- Mode of death
- Family
- Religious background

Examination
- Identity (wrist identity band)
- Motionless
- Fixed dilated pupils
- Absent pulse
- Absent breath sounds
- Absent heart sounds

Criteria for brain stem death

Patient is:
- in deep coma due to structural and irreversible brain damage
- Apnoeic despite elevated P_{CO_2}
- Requiring ventilation
- Coma could not be due to drugs, metabolic or endocrine disturbance or hypothermia
- No evidence of brain stem function

Brain stem reflexes
- Absent corneal reflex
- Absent caloric response
- Absent cough reflex
- Absent gag reflex
- Absent oculocephalic reflex ('doll's eyes')
- Absent pupillary response to light
- No response to pain in distribution of any cranial nerve

No response to pain in distribution of any cranial nerve

Absent pupillary response to light

Absent corneal reflex

Absent caloric reflex

Absent oculocephalic reflex ('doll's eye')

Absent cough reflex

Absent gag reflex

The diagnosis of death is often obvious. The body is cool, motionless and pale.

In establishing the diagnosis of death an understanding of the recent history is important. For example, patients who are profoundly hypothermic may appear dead but in fact may be capable of resuscitation. It is also vital to establish with certainty the identity of the body.

History
- When did the patient die? When was the patient last seen alive?
- What happened in their final moments (e.g. cardiopulmonary resuscitation, agonal respirations but surrounded by relatives, etc.)?

Past medical history
What were the events and illnesses preceding death?

Family and social history
- What was the patient's social, family and religious background?

- What relatives are there? What do they know of the patient's death and any previous condition?

Examination
- The body is motionless.
- There is no palpable pulse.
- There are no audible heart sounds.
- There are no audible breath sounds.
- The pupils are fixed, dilated and unresponsive to light.

Brain stem death
Patients who have sustained a critical brain insult may have developed brain stem death, be incapable of recovery, but with artificial ventilation may still have intact peripheral spinal reflexes and cardiac function. In these circumstances brain stem death testing may be undertaken particularly if consideration is being given to organ donation.

The criteria for making the diagnosis of **brain stem death** are shown in the figure above and are usually performed by two senior clinicians at least 12 hours apart.

56 Shock

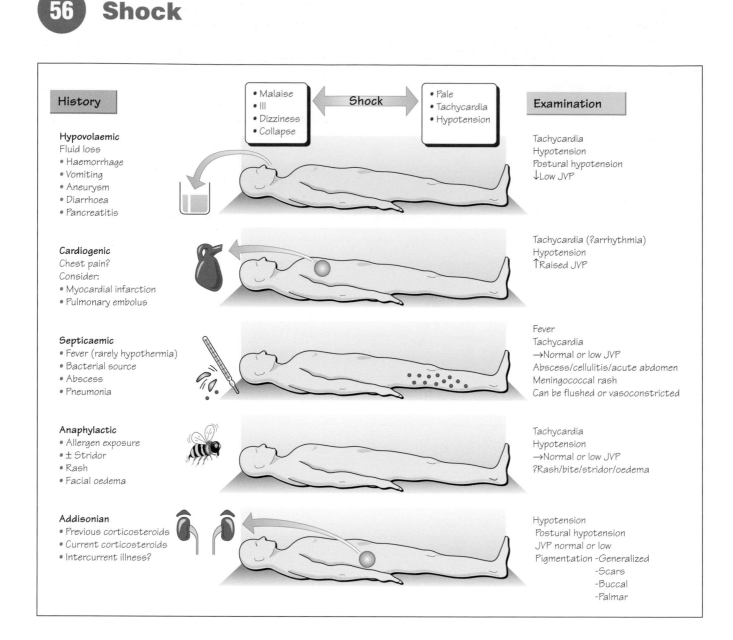

Shock is an important clinical presentation. It requires prompt recognition and accurate diagnosis of its cause. Shock is defined as insufficient perfusion of vital organs. It may manifest with non-specific malaise, dizziness, faintness or unconsciousness, or with symptoms of the underlying cause. The common aetiologies include hypovolaemia (e.g. due to GI haemorrhage), cardiogenic shock (due to myocardial infarction), pulmonary embolus, anaphylaxis, intra-abdominal catastrophes (e.g. bowel perforation, pancreatitis, ischaemic bowel) and septicaemia.

History

• When did the illness start? What were the symptoms?
• Has there been any chest pain, haemoptysis or breathlessness?
• Are there any symptoms suggesting volume depletion (e.g. vomiting, haematemesis, diarrhoea, melaena, polyuria)?

• Has there been any exposure to potential allergens (e.g. foods, drugs, venom)?
• Are there any symptoms suggesting septicaemia (e.g. fever, rigors, sweats, local infection [cough, chest pain, breathlessness, abscess, meningism, rash, inflamed joint])?
• Get additional history from relatives, especially if the patient is profoundly unwell and unable to give a clear history.

Past medical history

• Any previous episodes of shock?
• Any previous serious cardiac disease (e.g. myocardial infarction)?
• Any history of immunosuppression?
• Any known abdominal pathologies (e.g. aneurysm, previous pancreatitis)?

Drugs

• Is the patient taking or recently taken corticosteroids? (Consider the possibility of Addison's disease.)
• Is the patient taking any medication with anaphylactic potential?
• Is there the possibility of overdose with cardiodepressant drugs?

Allergies

Are there any known allergies?

Examination

• As for any ill patient, ensure preservation of the airway, adequate breathing and full examination. In particular, assess the *signs of shock*:
  • pulse: tachycardia or even bradycardia
  • BP: postural drop if not hypotensive
  • skin colour (pallor) and temperature
  • reduced urine output.
• The presence of shock requires urgent treatment (give oxygen, obtain venous access with large calibre lines, give intravenous fluids promptly whilst monitoring closely and obtain blood for cross-matching) and accurate diagnosis. Examine carefully for *volume status*:
  • check skin turgor
  • check the mucous membranes (dry?)
  • check the JVP: elevated or depressed? (may need measurement of CVP if there is any uncertainty)
  • check the pulse, BP (postural changes) and pulsus paradoxus (decrease in systolic pressure on inspiration).
• Examine for any potential sources of *volume loss* (e.g. ruptured aortic aneurysm, GI haemorrhage) (rectal examination for melaena?).
• Examine for signs of *major cardiac or respiratory disease* (e.g. murmurs [e.g. new VSD]), pleural rub (e.g. PE), Kussmaul's sign (rise in JVP on inspiration suggesting pericardial constriction/tamponade), cyanosis or raised respiratory rate.
• Examine carefully for signs or sources of *sepsis* and for *abdominal pathology* (e.g. pulmonary consolidation, joints, meningism, abscesses, rashes, abdominal tenderness, rebound guarding, ileus).
• Examine for signs consistent with *anaphylactic reaction*: rash, oral, laryngeal oedema and stridor.
• Examine for signs of *Addison's disease*: palmar, buccal pigmentation, signs of previous corticosteroid use.
• The assessment should proceed rapidly in concert with *therapy* that could include:
  • oxygen
  • intravenous access
  • intravenous fluids
  • intravenous antibiotics
• And *investigations* to include:
  • ECG (and ECG monitoring)
  • arterial blood gases (and/or pulse oximetry)
  • chest X-ray
  • blood cultures.

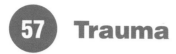 **Trauma**

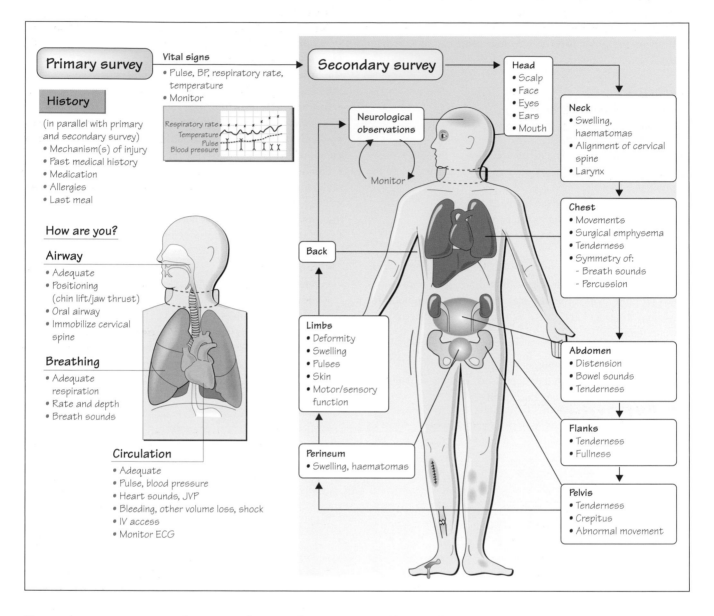

Trauma is a common reason for presentation to a doctor or to a hospital. The severity can obviously range from mild cuts and bruises to multiple life-threatening injuries of major organs. It is vital to undertake a systematic assessment of the patient to establish the nature and severities of the injuries and the threat that they pose. It is vital to obtain a full and accurate history from the patient and any other witnesses in order to indicate the likely severity of injuries and other possible hazards that they may have been exposed to. For example, a victim of a motor vehicle accident may have had a fit or myocardial infarction that caused them to crash or an assault victim may have a serious abdominal injury as well as the obvious facial contusions. It is also essential to obtain a full medical background: a minor head injury may have severe consequences in an anticoagulated patient who already has mild cognitive impairment.

Think carefully if the mechanism of injury and its consequences are compatible. Prolonged unconsciousness after a fall sustaining a small scalp laceration might be due to a primary subarachnoid haemorrhage, not due to the head injury itself. A simple trip that produces a fractured neck of femur may suggest underlying osteoporosis or other pathological fracture.

History

In serious injury, history will need to be undertaken at the same time as resuscitation and examination.
• When was the trauma? What happened?
• If in a motor vehicle accident, where was the patient sitting, were they wearing a seatbelt and what was the speed of the vehicles involved? What injuries did any other passengers sustain? What caused the accident? What happened immediately prior to the accident?

- Has there been exposure to other hazards (e.g. smoke, fumes)?
- What does the patient remember? Gather history from other witnesses, paramedics, police, etc.
- Determine the pre-hospital care that has been delivered and the time of the patient's last meal.

Past medical history

- Any history of any significant medical conditions?
- Any history of cardiorespiratory compromise or any other likely problems if anaesthesia is required?

Drugs

- Particularly consider anticoagulation and immunosuppression.
- Ask about the patient's recent alcohol and recreational drug intake.
- Has the patient got tetanus immunization?

Allergies

Does the patient have any allergies?

Family and social history

You may need to consider possibility of non-accidental injury.

Examination

If the history suggests the possibility of significant trauma then:

Primary survey (or ABCD)

Begin the primary survey as soon as you see the patient. A quick look can tell you a lot. Are they breathing? Do they look at you? Is the C-spine immobilized?

Airway

- Is the airway preserved? If not, correct with positioning (chin lift and jaw thrust), oral airway, suction and if necessary intubation (with in-line immobilization to protect the cervical spine).
- Ask, 'How are you?' If the patient responds in a clear voice, the airway is patent—at present. A clear voice, quiet respirations and a normal mental state rule out significant obstruction.
- Listen: snoring sounds suggest obstruction, while gurgles suggest secretions, vomit or blood in the airway. These sounds indicate the need to clear the airway, usually followed by intubation. Hoarseness or pain with speaking may indicate laryngeal injury, which can result in airway obstruction. Agitation can be due to hypoxia. Altered conscious level may be due to carbon dioxide retention.
- Assess future risk to the airway by looking for foreign bodies or loose teeth, and test for a gag reflex if unconscious.

Breathing

- Is the patient breathing adequately? If not administer 100% oxygen and mouth-to-mouth resuscitation or other ventilation.
- If the patient's respirations are not obvious to you, put your ear to the patient's mouth. While watching the chest for movement, listen and feel for the motion of air on your cheek. Assess the rate of respirations and their depth: listen to the chest for breath sounds.

Circulation

- Is it adequate? What is the pulse and BP? Is there obvious volume loss, active bleeding? Obtain venous access, give fluids, start external cardiac massage if no output. Monitor the patient's circulation with ECG and frequent measurements of pulse and BP. Stop any active, external bleeding by applying pressure directly over the wound.
- If shock is present give fluids and consider underlying causes, such as hypovolaemia, pericardial tamponade or tension pneumothorax.
- Hypovolaemia or shock may produce apprehension, drowsiness and even unresponsiveness. The peripheries may be pale, cold and bluish or mottled.
- Examine for peripheral pulses. If a radial pulse can be felt, the systolic BP is probably above 80 mmHg.
- Examine pulse rate and rhythm, BP, heart sounds and JVP.
- Immobilize the head and neck, and maintain the cervical spine in a neutral position. Assume a cervical spine injury is present until proven otherwise.

Disability (conscious level) (or disorders of the CNS)

- What is the conscious level? Use the Glasgow Coma Score to document (see Chapter 33).
- Examine pupil size, equality and reactivity.

Secondary survey

- Ensure the patient is fully undressed.
- Obtain complete vital signs. BP, pulse rate, respiratory rate, and temperature. Seek further history.
- Inspect the *head* for lacerations, haematomas, and tenderness. Test the facial bones for crepitus or instability. Check the eyes for foreign bodies and direct injuries. Look at the eardrums for rupture or blood.
- Examine the *neck* for swelling, haematomas, and misalignment of the posterior spinous processes.
- Palpate the larynx for crepitus, tenderness and stability.
- Re-examine the *chest* for chest wall motion, crepitus (surgical emphysema), tenderness, symmetry of breath sounds and percussion.
- Examine the *heart* for position of the apex beat, level of JVP, murmurs and muffled heart tones.
- Examine the *abdomen* for distension, bowel sounds, and tenderness.
- Palpate the *flanks* for tenderness and fullness, and compress the *pelvis* to elicit tenderness or crepitus.
- Examine for integrity of the pubic symphysis and evaluate the scrotum and perineum for haematomas and swelling. Do a rectal exam, and check the urethral meatus for blood.
- Inspect and palpate *arms and legs* for deformity, swelling, and skin injuries. Check all peripheral pulses. Test motor function and skin sensation, if the patient's level of consciousness allows.
- Log-roll the patient so the *back* can be examined.
- Digital rectal examination.

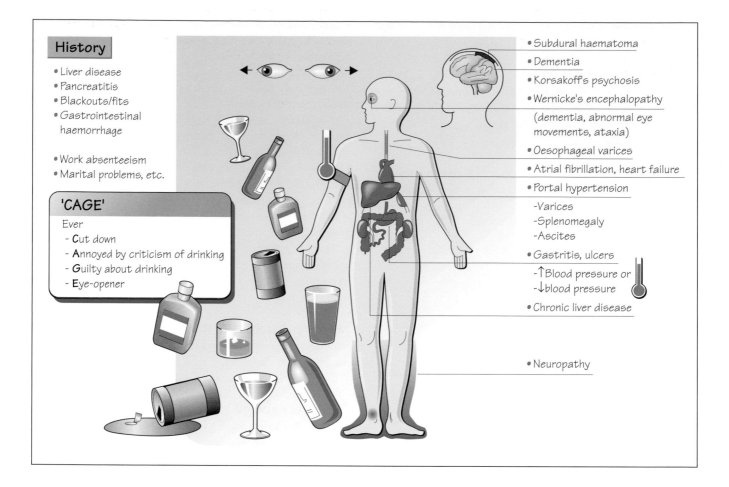

History

- Liver disease
- Pancreatitis
- Blackouts/fits
- Gastrointestinal haemorrhage

- Work absenteeism
- Marital problems, etc.

'CAGE'

Ever
- **C**ut down
- **A**nnoyed by criticism of drinking
- **G**uilty about drinking
- **E**ye-opener

- Subdural haematoma
- Dementia
- Korsakoff's psychosis
- Wernicke's encephalopathy (dementia, abnormal eye movements, ataxia)
- Oesophageal varices
- Atrial fibrillation, heart failure
- Portal hypertension
  - Varices
  - Splenomegaly
  - Ascites
- Gastritis, ulcers
  - ↑Blood pressure or
  - ↓blood pressure
- Chronic liver disease

- Neuropathy

The excess consumption of alcohol can produce many clinical presentations. Acute intoxication or drunkenness is a common finding in some patients with trauma, in road accidents or with head injuries. Chronically, alcohol excess may present with liver failure, neuropathy, cardiac disease, cognitive impairment and the social problems of dependency.

History

- How much does the patient drink? What do they drink and how often?
- How many units of alcohol does the patient drink in a week?

CAGE questionnaire

- Have you ever felt you should **C**ut down on your drinking?
- Have people **A**nnoyed you by criticising your drinking?
- Have you ever felt bad or **G**uilty about your drinking?
- Have you ever had a drink first thing in the morning to steady your nerves or get rid of a hangover (**E**ye-opener)?

Past medical history and functional enquiry

- Establish the history and current situation regarding liver dis-

ease, pancreatitis, gastritis, GI haemorrhage, jaundice, abdominal pain or swelling.
- Assess the history and current situation regarding hypertension, arrhythmias or cardiomyopathy.
- Establish the history and current situation regarding neuropathy, memory difficulties, cognitive impairment, psychosis or hallucinations.
- Establish the history and current situation regarding blackouts or fits and anxiety.
- Consider fetal alcohol syndrome.
- Establish the history and current situation regarding sexual dysfunction.
- Assess the history and current situation regarding gout.
- Establish the history and current situation regarding cancer of the mouth, oesophagus and liver.
- Establish the history and current situation regarding TB.

Social history

- Have there been any requests for medical certificates?
- Does the patient have any marital problems, and has there been any domestic violence?
- Has there been any absenteeism at work?

- Does the patient have any financial difficulties?
- Have there been any prosecutions for violent behaviour or driving offences?

Examination

- Is the patient orientated? Is the patient well or unwell? Is the patient intoxicated?
- Is the patient smelling of alcohol?
- Check for hypertension, atrial fibrillation and other tachycardias.
- Any signs of cardiac failure?

- Any signs of chronic liver disease?
- Is there abdominal pain/tenderness? Consider pancreatitis, acute alcoholic hepatitis, gastritis or peptic ulceration.
- Any peripheral neuropathy?
- Any confusion, confabulation (Korsakoff's psychosis)?
- Any abnormalities of eye movements, dementia, unsteadiness (Wernicke's syndrome)?
- Any focal deficits or reduced conscious level? Consider subdural haematoma.
- Any epileptiform convulsions?

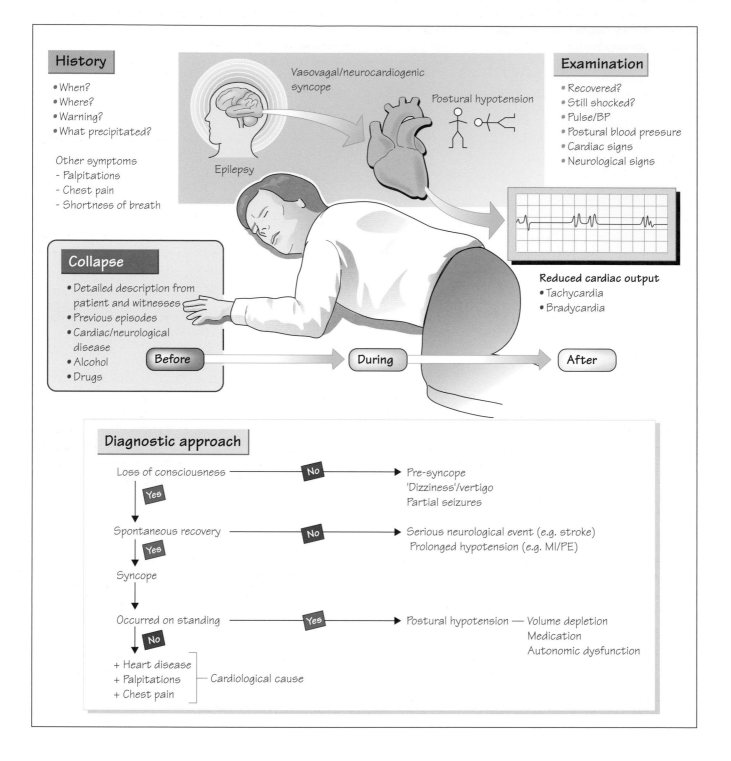

History

- When?
- Where?
- Warning?
- What precipitated?

Other symptoms
- Palpitations
- Chest pain
- Shortness of breath

Collapse

- Detailed description from patient and witnesses
- Previous episodes
- Cardiac/neurological disease
- Alcohol
- Drugs

Before → During → After

Vasovagal/neurocardiogenic syncope

Epilepsy

Postural hypotension

Examination

- Recovered?
- Still shocked?
- Pulse/BP
- Postural blood pressure
- Cardiac signs
- Neurological signs

Reduced cardiac output
- Tachycardia
- Bradycardia

Diagnostic approach

Loss of consciousness — **No** → Pre-syncope
'Dizziness'/vertigo
Partial seizures

↓ **Yes**

Spontaneous recovery — **No** → Serious neurological event (e.g. stroke)
Prolonged hypotension (e.g. MI/PE)

↓ **Yes**

Syncope

↓

Occurred on standing — **Yes** → Postural hypotension — Volume depletion
Medication
Autonomic dysfunction

↓ **No**

+ Heart disease
+ Palpitations — Cardiological cause
+ Chest pain

Collapses, falls, funny turns and faints, etc. are very common reasons for presentation to doctors and can be manifestations of serious underlying cardiac or neurological dysfunctions. Common causes include bradycardias, tachycardias, vasovagal attacks, postural hypotension and epilepsy, although often a clear cause is not identified.

History

In taking a history from a patient who has collapsed, it is vital to determine whether there was loss of consciousness or not. A detailed description of the collapse should be obtained from the patient and any available witnesses.

• When and where did the patient collapse? What was the patient doing? How did he/she feel immediately prior to the episode? Was there any warning or prodrome? Did it follow standing, vigorous coughing, nausea? How long did the patient take to recover? Was the patient unconscious? For how long was he/she unconscious? Are there any symptoms suggesting blood loss? A good memory of events during the episode suggests that consciousness was not lost. Significant injury suggests an absence of warning and often loss of consciousness.

• Were there other symptoms (e.g. nausea, sweating, palpitations, chest pain, breathlessness, etc.)?

• Were there any convulsive movements? Any tongue biting, urinary incontinence?

• The detailed observations of witnesses should be sought of events prior to, during and after the collapse. What colour was the patient before during and after the attack? Was the patient pale, flushed, blue, sweating? Was the patient's pulse palpable during attacks?

Syncope can be defined as a sudden, brief loss of consciousness associated with loss of postural tone and spontaneous recovery. This should be distinguished from episodes without loss of consciousness or postural tone, which are often described as dizziness or pre-syncope, or episodes in which the patient describes a sensation of movement of themselves or their surroundings, which is termed vertigo.

Any previous episodes should be similarly analysed in detail.

Past medical history

• Any history of cardiovascular disease, neurological disease?
• Does the patient have a pacemaker?
• Any history of epilepsy?

Drugs

• Is the patient taking any drugs (particularly those that might produce hypotension)?
• Establish the patient's alcohol history.

Functional enquiry

It is particularly important to determine the presence of cardiovascular disease and so a full functional enquiry seeking symptoms such as palpitations, chest pain, breathlessness, etc., must be undertaken.

Family history

A family history of sudden death might suggest the presence of long QT syndrome or an inherited cardiomyopathy.

Examination

• Does the patient look well or unwell?
• Has the patient made a complete recovery?
• Any continuing shock, hypotension or neurological deficit?
• A full examination should be undertaken with particular attention being paid to the pulse, BP, including postural measurements, presence of cardiac murmurs and any neurological signs. Look for signs of trauma sustained during the collapse including tongue biting.

Table 59.1 Differential diagnosis of collapse.

	Seizure	Vasovagal syncope	Cardiac cause
Precipitant	None (stroboscopic lights)	Pain, exercise Micturition, stress Prolonged standing	None?
Premonitory symptoms	Aura? None	Sweating Nausea	None Chest pain Palpitations
During event	Rhythmic movements Urinary incontinence Tongue biting	Rarely movements Pale	Pale Rarely movements
After event	Disorientation Injury? Unconscious > 5 min Aching muscles	Rarely injured	Flushed Injury?

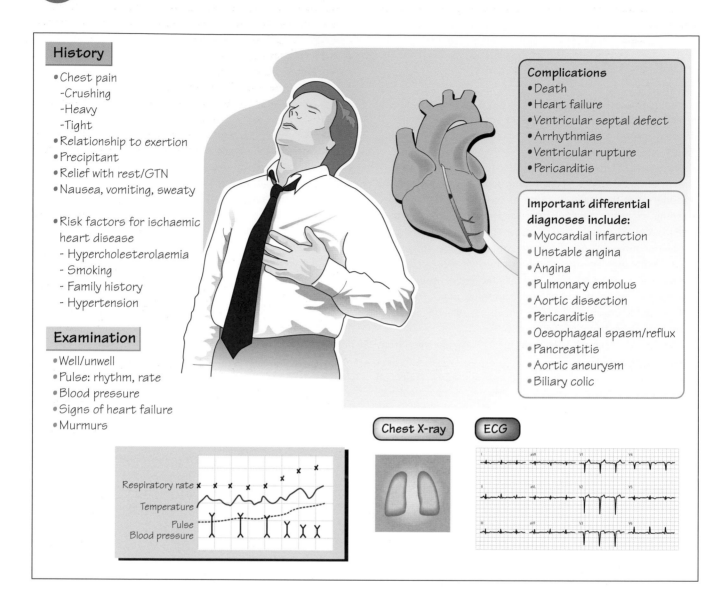

History

- Chest pain
  - Crushing
  - Heavy
  - Tight
- Relationship to exertion
- Precipitant
- Relief with rest/GTN
- Nausea, vomiting, sweaty

- Risk factors for ischaemic heart disease
  - Hypercholesterolaemia
  - Smoking
  - Family history
  - Hypertension

Examination

- Well/unwell
- Pulse: rhythm, rate
- Blood pressure
- Signs of heart failure
- Murmurs

Complications
- Death
- Heart failure
- Ventricular septal defect
- Arrhythmias
- Ventricular rupture
- Pericarditis

Important differential diagnoses include:
- Myocardial infarction
- Unstable angina
- Angina
- Pulmonary embolus
- Aortic dissection
- Pericarditis
- Oesophageal spasm/reflux
- Pancreatitis
- Aortic aneurysm
- Biliary colic

Chest X-ray

ECG

Respiratory rate
Temperature
Pulse
Blood pressure

Myocardial infarction and angina are usually due to coronary atherosclerosis. They are very common: myocardial infarction has an incidence of 0.5% per year whilst angina has a prevalence of over 15% in people over 65 years of age. Angina may be described as stable in which attacks of chest pain are usually short-lived (< 15 minutes), provoked by exertion and alleviated by rest and/or GTN. Unstable angina is longer lasting chest pain on minimal or no exertion. It may be impossible to distinguish from myocardial infarction on clinical grounds alone and may be termed acute coronary syndrome. Myocardial infarction usually produces severe pain or tightness that lasts > 15 minutes and may be accompanied by nausea, sweating and vomiting.

History

• *Angina* is classically a central tight, chest pain or discomfort:

- induced by exertion or more rarely emotion
- radiates to the jaw and to the arms
- relieved by rest and by GTN tablets or spray
- sometimes experienced as exertional breathlessness.

• *Myocardial infarction* produces a more severe, longer lasting pain or tightness:

- radiates to the arms or jaw
- accompanied by nausea, vomiting, sweating and anxiety
- complicated by heart failure, shock and arrhythmias
- rarely presents without chest pain (particularly in the elderly or diabetic) as, e.g. new onset arrhythmia or worsening heart failure or even postoperative confusion.

• Ask in detail about the chest pains and other symptoms. Consider the possibility of other causes of chest pain, such as pulmonary emboli, aortic dissection and oesophageal reflux.

- Consider possible contraindications to thrombolysis (e.g. active bleeding, bleeding tendency, known peptic ulcer, recent stroke, recent operation, severe hypertension, previous allergic reaction).

Past medical history

- Any angina, myocardial infarction or any other cardiac disease?
- Any angioplasties, coronary artery bypass grafts, previous thrombolysis?
- Any diabetes mellitus?

Drugs

- Is the patient taking nitrates, aspirin, beta-blockers, ACE inhibitors or GTN tablets/spray?
- Is the patient taking any treatments for hypertension or hypercholesterolaemia?

Allergies

- Any allergies to streptokinase, aspirin or any other medication?

Family history

- Any family history of IHD or sudden death?
- Any family history of other causes of chest pain (e.g. aortic dissection)?

Social history

What is the patient's occupation and does angina interfere with their life or work?

Examination

- Does the patient need immediate resuscitation?
- Ensure airway and breathing. Give oxygen. Obtain intravenous access, ECG monitor and 12-lead ECG.
- Does the patient look unwell?
- Is the patient in pain, distressed, comfortable, vomiting, anxious, sweaty, pale, cyanosed or tachypnoiec?
- Is the patient well perfused or with cool peripheries?
- Any stigmata of hypercholesterolaemia or smoking?
- Is there anaemia or cyanosis or surgical scars (e.g. from CABG)?
- *Pulse*: check the rate, rhythm, volume and character. Are the peripheral pulses present and equal?
- *BP*: are both arms equal?
- *JVP*: is it elevated?
- *Chest movements*: is there symmetrical expansion?
- *Apex* beat?
- Is the pain reproduced/exaggerated by chest wall pressure?
- *Auscultation*: lung fields clear? Any added sounds—crackles, rub or wheeze? Check heart sounds for murmurs, pericardial rub and gallop.
- Examine for peripheral *oedema*, ankles and sacrum.
- *Abdomen*: any tenderness, guarding, rebound, bowel sounds, organomegaly, aneurysm?

- Any *urine* output?
- *CNS*: any weakness, focal deficits?
- An *ECG* is vital in the diagnosis of myocardial infarction.
- Examine carefully for the possible consequences of myocardial infarction:
  - arrhythmias
  - cardiogenic shock
  - heart failure (especially pulmonary oedema)
  - valvular dysfunction (especially mitral regurgitation) and, rarely, ventriculoseptal defect.
- If the patient has chest pain and shock or is unwell, consider myocardial infarction, unstable angina, pneumothorax (?tension), pulmonary embolus and aortic dissection.

Evidence

In patients undergoing coronary angiography for chest pain, patients who had normal coronary angiograms were compared with patients with significant stenoses on coronary angiography. The consistent reproduction of pain by exercise and the duration of pain for > 5 minutes was much more common in the patients with abnormal coronary angiography (Cooke *et al.* 1997).

There is an increased probability of myocardial infarction if:
- chest pain is radiating to both arms simultaneously (LR, 7.1)
- there is radiation of pain to the right arm or shoulder (LR, 4.7)
- there is radiation of pain to the left arm (LR, 2.3)
- the patient is sweating (LR, 2.0)
- the patient has nausea or is vomiting (LR, 1.9)
- the patient has a history of myocardial infarction (LR, 1.5–3.0)
- the pain is worse than previous angina or similar to previous myocardial infarction (LR, 1.9).

There is a decreased probability of myocardial infarction if:
- the patient has pleuritic chest pain (LR, 0.2)
- the chest pain is produced by palpation (LR, 0.3)
- there is sharp or stabbing pain (LR, 0.3)
- there is positional chest pain (LR, 0.3).

Cooke RA, Smeeton N & Chambers JB. Comparative study of chest pain characteristics in patients with normal and abnormal coronary angiograms. *Heart* 1997; **78**: 142–6.

Panju AA, Hemmelgarn BR, Guyatt GH & Simel DL. The rational clinical examination. Is this patient having a myocardial infarction? *JAMA* 1998; **280**: 1256–63.

Swap CJ & Nagurney JT. Value and limitations of chest pain history in the evaluation of patients with suspected acute coronary syndromes. *JAMA* 2005; **294**: 2623–9.

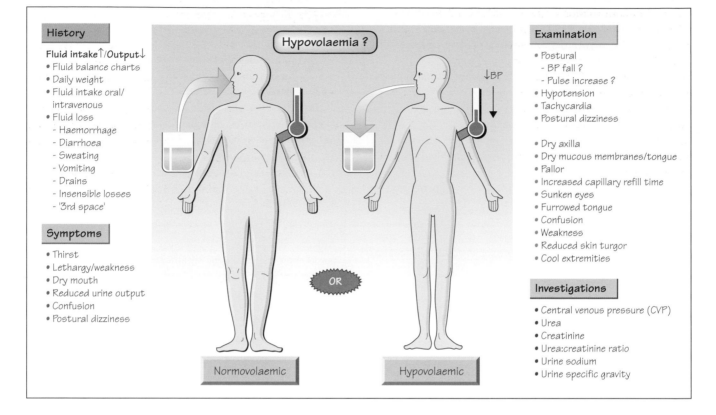

History

Fluid intake↑/Output↓
- Fluid balance charts
- Daily weight
- Fluid intake oral/ intravenous
- Fluid loss
  - Haemorrhage
  - Diarrhoea
  - Sweating
  - Vomiting
  - Drains
  - Insensible losses
  - '3rd space'

Symptoms

- Thirst
- Lethargy/weakness
- Dry mouth
- Reduced urine output
- Confusion
- Postural dizziness

Hypovolaemia ?

Normovolaemic

OR

Hypovolaemic

↓BP

Examination

- Postural
  - BP fall ?
  - Pulse increase ?
- Hypotension
- Tachycardia
- Postural dizziness

- Dry axilla
- Dry mucous membranes/tongue
- Pallor
- Increased capillary refill time
- Sunken eyes
- Furrowed tongue
- Confusion
- Weakness
- Reduced skin turgor
- Cool extremities

Investigations

- Central venous pressure (CVP)
- Urea
- Creatinine
- Urea:creatinine ratio
- Urine sodium
- Urine specific gravity

The determination of fluid status is vital in the management of many patients. Establishing whether there is hypovolaemia is particularly critical in the bleeding patient, in dehydration, during anaesthesia, in shock, in renal failure, following trauma or postoperatively. As ever, the history provides critical information and there are many useful clinical signs, of which BP, pulse rate and postural change in BP are particularly important and informative. A distinction is often made between patients with salt and water deficiency and those in whom there is simply dehydration. In dehydration, hypovolaemia with signs of circulatory instability may not occur until very severe, whilst volume depletion in which there is sodium and water loss can more rapidly produce dangerous hypovolaemia and circulatory instability, requiring prompt treatment with intravenous saline. In practice, the distinction may be difficult and more important is the recognition and treatment of hypovolaemia.

In otherwise healthy individuals, substantial blood loss or degrees of fluid depletion can be tolerated without very marked findings on clinical examination and subsequent losses can lead to catastrophic shock.

History

• Take a full history of any fluid gains and losses.
• Obtain information from the patient, relatives, nurses, fluid balance charts, prescription charts, anaesthetic records and daily weights.

• The symptoms of hypovolaemia can include:
  • general lethargy and weakness
  • postural dizziness
  • thirst
  • dry mouth
  • reduced urine output
  • feeling cold
  • shivering
  • shortness of breath and altered mental status if profound.

Examination

• Of central importance are:
  • the level of BP
  • the presence of a fall in BP on standing or sitting upright
  • tachycardia (or more rarely a bradycardia with very severe hypovolaemia)
  • postural changes in pulse rate.
• Careful documentation of weight change can be invaluable in determining fluid gains or losses.
• Other signs that should be sought are:
  • the level of JVP
  • pallor
  • the adequacy of peripheral perfusion
  • the dryness of mucous membranes
  • the presence of pulmonary and peripheral oedema.

- Investigations may be helpful, including: urea, creatinine, urea/creatinine ratio, sodium, haemoglobin, urine sodium, urine osmolarity, chest X-ray, pulse oximetry, CVP and PCWP by Swan–Ganz catheter.
- **If doubt about volume status, consider CVP monitoring.**
- Vital additional information can be gained from the measurement of CVP by insertion of a central venous line, or determination of pulmonary artery capillary wedge pressure (by the insertion of a Swan–Ganz catheter). However, because of the difficulties and risks in those patients with collapsed veins, central venous line insertion should not be attempted in those patients with hypovolaemia until resuscitation with fluid has taken place.
- **If hypovolaemia is present, treat promptly with intravenous fluids.**

Evidence

Normal response to standing upright:
- increase in heart rate by 10 b.p.m.
- slight fall in systolic BP (3 mmHg)
- slight rise in diastolic BP (5 mmHg).

However, a fall in systolic BP > 10 mmHg is found in 10% of normovolaemic individuals. In addition, severe postural dizziness or rise in pulse > 30 b.p.m. on standing has specificity of 96% for hypovolaemia.

In elderly patients, signs of confusion, non-fluent speech, weakness, dry mucous membranes, dry tongue, furrowed tongue, sunken eyes, dry axilla and delayed capillary refill are associated with severe dehydration.

McGee S, Abernethy WB IIIrd & Simel DL. Is this patient hypovolemic? *JAMA* 1999; **281**: 1022–9.

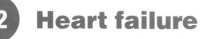

62 Heart failure

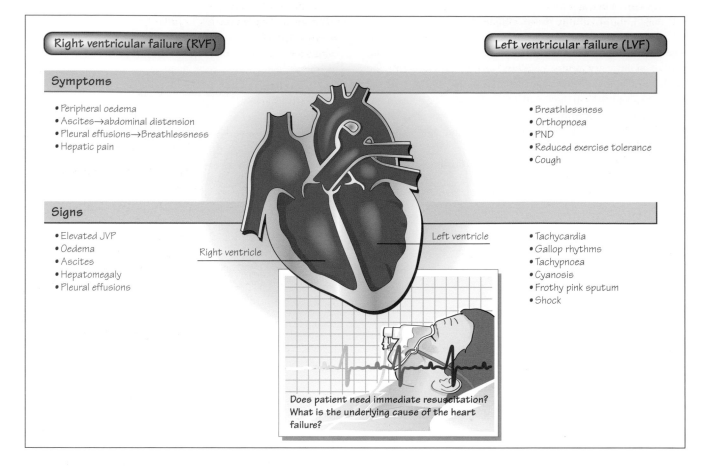

Right ventricular failure (RVF)

Symptoms

- Peripheral oedema
- Ascites→abdominal distension
- Pleural effusions→Breathlessness
- Hepatic pain

Signs

- Elevated JVP
- Oedema
- Ascites
- Hepatomegaly
- Pleural effusions

Right ventricle

Left ventricle

Left ventricular failure (LVF)

- Breathlessness
- Orthopnoea
- PND
- Reduced exercise tolerance
- Cough

- Tachycardia
- Gallop rhythms
- Tachypnoea
- Cyanosis
- Frothy pink sputum
- Shock

Does patient need immediate resuscitation? What is the underlying cause of the heart failure?

History

- The symptoms of heart failure are conventionally divided into left ventricular failure (LVF), right ventricular failure (RVF) or both (congestive cardiac or biventricular failure).
- **Heart failure is not a diagnosis and the underlying cause(s) should always be sought.** It is a very common reason for hospital admission accounting for 5% of admissions to medical wards.
- *Left ventricular failure:*
  - breathlessness
  - orthopnoea
  - paroxysmal nocturnal dyspnoea ('Do you have problems with your breathing at night?', 'Tell me more [ask directly about number of pillows]?')
  - less commonly wheeze, cough, frothy pink sputum
  - reduced exercise tolerance.
- *Right ventricular failure:*
  - peripheral oedema especially ankles, legs, sacrum
  - ascites
  - rarely jaundice, hepatic pain, nausea and reduced appetite (due to bowel oedema)
  - pleural effusions.
- *Acute heart failure* may present with sudden and severe shortness of breath, cyanosis and distress.

- *Chronic heart failure* can be associated with reduced exercise tolerance, peripheral oedema, lethargy, malaise and weight loss ('cardiac cachexia').

Past medical history

- Any chest pain? (Any recent myocardial infarction?)
- Any cardiac disease (especially myocardial infarction, angina, murmurs, arrhythmias or known valvular heart disease)?
- Any risk factors for atherosclerosis?
- Any respiratory or renal disease?
- Any cardiomyopathy?

Drugs

- What medication is the patient taking? Have there been any recent changes to the patient's medication: loop diuretics, spironolactone, NSAIDs, ACE inhibitors, beta-blockers, negative inotropes, digoxin?
- Is the patient taking any drugs that can produce cardiomyopathy (doxorubicin, cocaine)?
- Does the patient smoke?
- What is the patient's alcohol intake? (Consider the possibility of alcoholic cardiomyopathy.)

Functional enquiry

- Ask about exercise tolerance (e.g. flights of stairs, distance walking on the flat).
- Assess salt and water intake.
- Consider the possibility of renal failure.

Examination

The examination should aim to establish the presence of heart failure and its likely aetiology.

Causes

- **Causes of heart failure include:**
  - IHD (65%)
  - hypertensive heart disease (10%)
  - valvular heart disease, murmurs (10%)
  - cardiomyopathy (10%)
  - myocarditis (2%)
  - pericardial effusion/constriction (1%).
- **Exacerbating factors of heart failure include:**
  - anaemia
  - NSAIDs
  - renal impairment
  - arrhythmias.
- **Also remember non-cardiac causes of pulmonary oedema/ heart failure:**
  - high output states (e.g. thyrotoxicosis)
  - fluid overload (e.g. intravenous fluids, renal failure)
  - anaemia
  - phaeochromocytoma
  - allergic reactions (e.g. contrast)
  - ARDS
  - heroin.

Consequences

- Is the patient unwell, breathless, in pain, anxious, in need of immediate resuscitation?
- *The signs of left ventricular failure are:*
  - cold and clammy skin
  - tachycardia
  - gallop rhythm
  - tachypnoea, cyanosed, frothy pink sputum, wheeze
  - displaced apex beat
  - pulsus alternans (very rare)
  - hypotension or hypertension
  - cardiogenic shock.
- *The signs of right ventricular failure are:*
  - elevated JVP
  - peripheral oedema
  - ascites
  - hepatomegaly
  - pleural effusions.

Evidence

Jugular venous distension (which = 85–100% probability of increased filling pressure) is very helpful. Dyspnoea, orthopnoea, tachycardia, decreased systolic or pulse pressure, third heart sound, crackles, abdominojugular reflux and oedema are somewhat helpful (Badgett *et al.* 1997).

ECG and chest X-rays can add considerably to the specificity of detection of left ventricular dysfunction and should be considered essential in the assessment of any patient with suspected heart failure.

New York Heart Association grading of chronic heart failure severity

I Unlimited exercise tolerance.
II Symptoms on extra exertion (e.g. using stairs).
III Symptoms on mild exercise (e.g. walking).
IV Symptoms on minimal exertion or at rest.

Common errors

- Patients with severe LVF may be hypertensive (due to intense vasoconstriction and fluid overload).
- The wheezy, breathless patient may have LVF (not new onset asthma).
- Always define the underlying cause or exacerbation of the heart failure as it may be correctable (e.g. anaemia, valvular heart disease, tachyarrhythmia, etc.).

Badgett RG, Lucey CR & Mulrow CD. Can the clinical examination diagnose left-sided heart failure in adults? *JAMA* 1997; **277**: 1712–9.

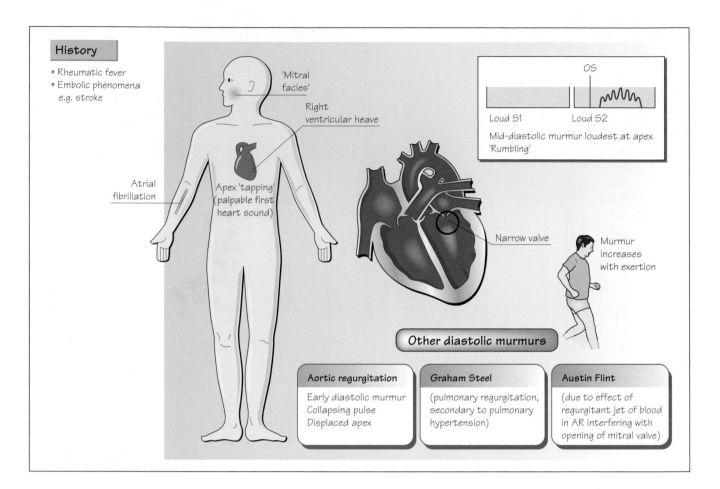

History
- Rheumatic fever
- Embolic phenomena e.g. stroke

'Mitral facies'

Right ventricular heave

Atrial fibrillation

Apex 'tapping' (palpable first heart sound)

OS

Loud S1

Loud S2

Mid-diastolic murmur loudest at apex 'Rumbling'

Narrow valve

Murmur increases with exertion

Other diastolic murmurs

Aortic regurgitation	Graham Steel	Austin Flint
Early diastolic murmur Collapsing pulse Displaced apex	(pulmonary regurgitation, secondary to pulmonary hypertension)	(due to effect of regurgitant jet of blood in AR interfering with opening of mitral valve)

Mitral stenosis is the narrowing of the mitral valve. It should be particularly looked for in patients with a history of rheumatic fever, new onset atrial fibrillation and unexplained pulmonary hypertension.

History
- Mitral stenosis may present with slowly progressive breathlessness, reduced exercise tolerance, cough, haemoptysis, recurrent bronchitis, ankle swelling and palpitations.
- There may have been embolic episodes (e.g. stroke/TIA).
- Rarely there are symptoms of endocarditis.

Past medical history
- Any rheumatic fever?
- Previous medical examinations: any murmurs noted?

Examination
- Examine for mitral facies.
- Examine for atrial fibrillation.
- Is there a tapping apex (palpable first heart sound)?
- Is there a loud first heart sound?
- Is there a loud pulmonary second sound?
- Is there an opening snap?
- Auscultate for a mid-diastolic murmur, low-pitched rumble (best heard at apex and in left lateral position).
- Is murmur more easily audible with exertion?
- The patient may have a parasternal heave from pulmonary hypertension and right ventricular hypertrophy.

64 Mitral regurgitation

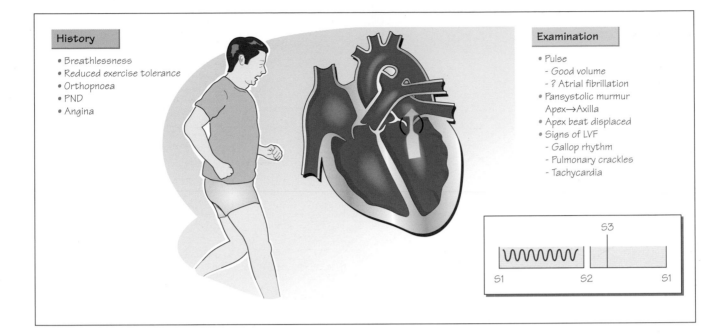

History
- Breathlessness
- Reduced exercise tolerance
- Orthopnoea
- PND
- Angina

Examination
- Pulse
  - Good volume
  - ? Atrial fibrillation
- Pansystolic murmur
  Apex→Axilla
- Apex beat displaced
- Signs of LVF
  - Gallop rhythm
  - Pulmonary crackles
  - Tachycardia

Mitral regurgitation is the abnormal regurgitation of blood through an incompetent mitral valve. It is usually discovered incidentally but it may be found during the examination of a patient with worsening heart failure. It can be due to progressive left ventricular dilatation, rheumatic fever, as a consequence of mitral valve prolapse or it can present acutely following chordal rupture due to ischaemia.

History
- Mitral regurgitation may present with increasing breathlessness, reduced exercise tolerance, orthopnoea, PND or angina.
- Any symptoms of infective endocarditis?

Past medical history
- Any IHD?
- Any rheumatic fever?
- Any known mitral valve prolapse?

Examination
- Any signs of infective endocarditis?

- The pulse usually has good volume; there may be atrial fibrillation.
- Any signs of left ventricular failure (gallop rhythm, pulmonary crackles, tachycardia)?
- Is the apex beat displaced?
- The pansystolic murmur is usually loudest at apex with radiation to axilla.

Mitral valve prolapse
- The patient may have a mid-systolic click and/or a systolic murmur:
  - 50% have click
  - 40% have late systolic murmur
  - 15% have pansystolic murmur
  - 20% have neither click nor murmur
  - 7% have severe incompetence.
- It is very common (up to 5% of the population).
- Murmur is increased with exercise or with the Valsalva manoeuvre.

65 Aortic stenosis

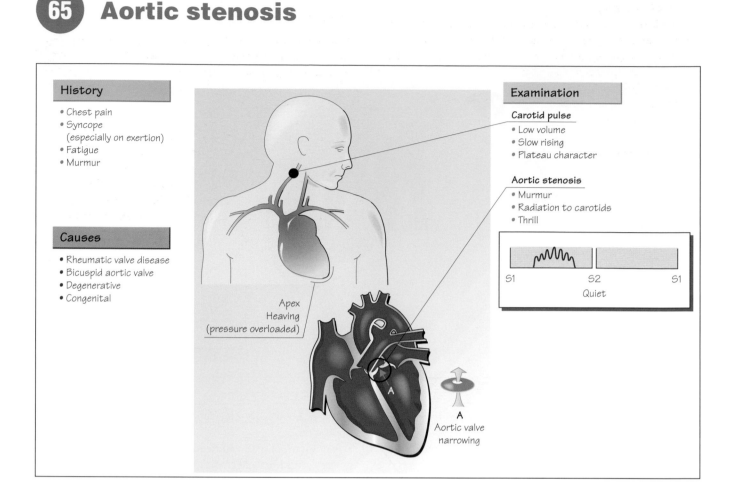

History

- Chest pain
- Syncope (especially on exertion)
- Fatigue
- Murmur

Causes

- Rheumatic valve disease
- Bicuspid aortic valve
- Degenerative
- Congenital

Apex
Heaving
(pressure overloaded)

A
Aortic valve
narrowing

Examination

Carotid pulse

- Low volume
- Slow rising
- Plateau character

Aortic stenosis

- Murmur
- Radiation to carotids
- Thrill

S1   S2   S1
Quiet

Aortic stenosis is narrowing of the aortic valve. It is most commonly due to progressive calcification of a degenerative or bicuspid valve. Look specifically for aortic stenosis in any patient with angina, shortness of breath or syncope.

History

Aortic stenosis may present with angina, breathlessness, syncope (including exertional syncope), sudden death or as an incidentally discovered murmur. There may be a gradual worsening of symptoms.

Past medical history

- Was the murmur previously audible? (Consider bicuspid aortic valve with progressive calcification.)
- Any history of rheumatic fever?

Functional enquiry

- Does the patient have shortness of breath?
- Does the patient have reduced exercise tolerance?
- Does the patient have chest pain?
- Did the patient have any collapse, especially exercise-induced collapse?
- Does the patient have a fever?

Family history

Any family history of valvular disease?

Examination

- *Pulse*: check for low volume, slow rising.
- *BP*: check for narrow pulse pressure.
- *Apex*: check for heaving.
- Check thrill.
- *Auscultation*: check for harsh ejection systolic murmur radiating to carotids and aortic area.
- Is the aortic second sound soft or absent?
- Check for fever, stigmata of infective endocarditis.
- NB. Particularly in the elderly patient, signs may be lacking.
- Murmur can decrease in intensity as aortic stenosis becomes more severe and left ventricular performance declines.
- Determine the severity of aortic stenosis.
  In mild aortic stenosis:
  - pulse character normal
  - normal BP
  - murmur is not loud and radiates minimally to neck
  - normal second heart sound
  - no thrill.
  Distinguish from mitral regurgitation:

- apex is thrusting
- first heart sound is soft and there may be a third heart sound
- murmur is pansystolic and radiates to axilla.

Distinguish from hypertrophic obstructive cardiomyopathy:
- pulse may be jerky in character
- apex may have double impulse
- loud fourth heart sound
- ejection systolic murmur which does not radiate to neck but increases in intensity with Valsalva manoeuvre and during squatting to standing.

Evidence

Absence of murmur over right clavicle helps to rule out aortic stenosis (LR, 0.1; 95% CI, 0.01–0.44). If any three of the following four findings are present, then LR of moderate to severe aortic stenosis = 40 (95% CI, 6.6–240]):

1 Slow carotid artery upstroke.
2 Reduced carotid artery volume.
3 Maximal murmur intensity at second right intercostal space.
4 Reduced intensity of second heart sound.

Etchells E, Bell C & Robb K. Does this patient have an abnormal systolic murmur? *JAMA* 1997; **277**: 564–71.

Etchells E, Glenns V, Shadowitz S, Bell C & Siu S. A bedside clinical prediction rule for detecting moderate or severe aortic stenosis. *J Gen Intern Med* 1998; **13**: 699–704.

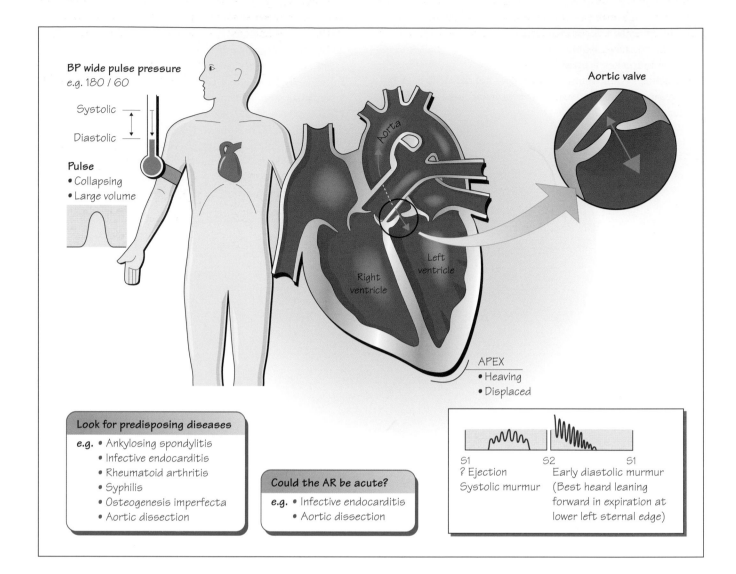

Aortic regurgitation is the disorder of the aortic valve in which an incompetent valve allows the regurgitation of blood back into the left ventricle. This may be due to incompetence of the valve leaflets themselves or dilatation of the aortic root. It should be specifically examined for in any patient with a low diastolic BP, a wide pulse pressure or who has symptoms that could represent endocarditis (e.g. fever, embolic phenomena).

History

• Aortic regurgitation may produce symptoms of breathlessness, reduced exercise tolerance, palpitations or other symptoms of cardiac failure. There may be a very gradual deterioration in symptoms. Acute aortic regurgitation, caused, for example, by infective endocarditis, may present with acute onset of breathlessness and shock.

• Are there any symptoms of infective endocarditis or aortic dissection?

Past medical history

Any history of:
• rheumatic fever?
• rheumatoid arthritis?
• ankylosing spondylitis?
• syphilis?
• osteogenesis imperfecta?
• Behçet's syndrome?
• known heart murmur (perhaps congenital bicuspid valve)?

Examination

• Are there any signs of endocarditis or aortic dissection? Are there any signs of tertiary syphilis, ankylosing spondylitis, rheumatoid arthritis or Marfan's syndrome?
• Is there a fever?
• Is there a collapsing pulse with large volume?
• Is there wide pulse pressure (> 50 mmHg) and low diastolic BP?

- Heaving apex: hyperdynamic and displaced?
- Is there an early diastolic murmur? (This is best heard at left sternal edge with patient leaning forward and with breath held at end of expiration.) (The patient may also have an ejection systolic murmur [without any coexistent aortic stenosis] due to high blood flow across valve.)
- Other eponymous signs (mostly only useful for showing off once the diagnosis has been made):
  - Corrigan's pulse ('water hammer' pulse) and sign (visible, vigorous arterial pulsations in neck)
- Quincke's sign (visible nail bed pulsation)
- De Musset's sign (head bobbing in time with the heart beat)
- Duroziez's sign (compression over the femoral artery with the stethoscope diaphragm produces a diastolic murmur)
- Hill's sign (BP higher [> 20 mmHg] in lower than higher extremities when horizontal)
- Austin–Flint murmur (diastolic murmur due to effect of regurgitant jet of blood interfering with opening of mitral valve).

Evidence

- If no aortic regurgitation murmur is heard (by a cardiologist), LR for moderate to severe aortic regurgitation is 0.1.
- If a typical aortic regurgitation murmur is heard, LR for moderate or greater aortic regurgitation is 4.0–8.3.

Choudhry NK & Etchells EE. The rational clinical examination. Does this patient have aortic regurgitation? *JAMA* 1999; **281**: 2231–8.

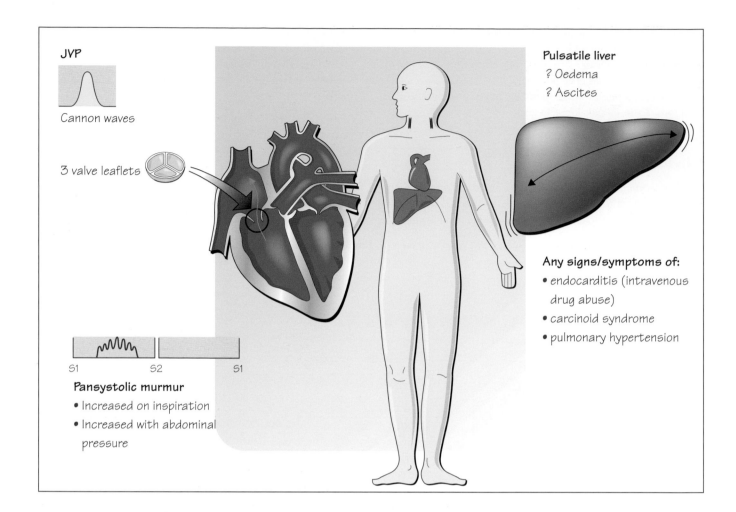

Tricuspid regurgitation is regurgitation of blood through an incompetent tricuspid valve.

History
The patient may present with symptoms of right-sided heart failure, such as oedema, abdominal swelling due to ascites, uncomfortable hepatic congestion or a pulsatile abdominal mass (liver).

Past medical history
Most commonly tricuspid regurgitation is due to right heart failure and dilatation (itself due to left heart failure). It is rarely caused by:
- endocarditis (intravenous drug abuse?)
- carcinoid syndrome (e.g. flushing)
- pulmonary hypertension
- congenital (Ebstein's anomaly)
- slimming drugs.

Examination
- Is there a fever?
- Are there splinter haemorrhages and other signs of infective endocarditis?
- Is the JVP elevated with prominent V waves?
- Is there a parasternal right ventricular heave?
- Is there a pansystolic murmur at left sternal edge increased on inspiration or with abdominal pressure (hepatojugular reflux)?
- Is there an enlarged, pulsatile liver?
- Is there oedema or ascites?

68 Pulmonary stenosis

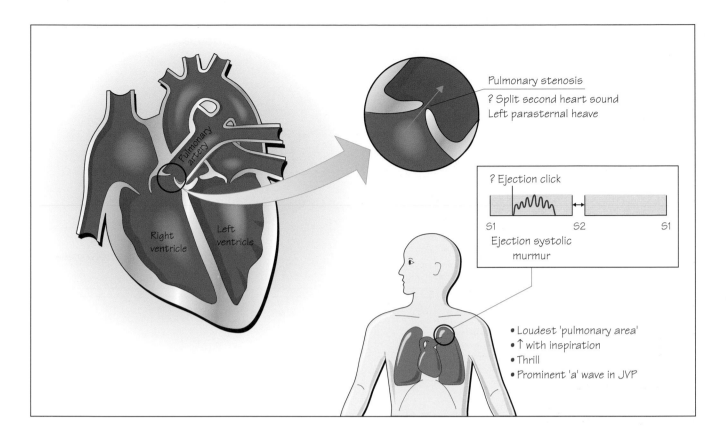

Pulmonary stenosis is a rare condition of the narrowing of the pulmonary valve, which may be congenital (< 10% of cases of congenital heart disease) and associated with Turner's syndrome, Noonan's syndrome, William's syndrome or tetralogy of Fallot, or acquired due to rheumatic fever. It may present with breathlessness or other symptoms of cardiac failure.

History
• Any known murmur?
• Any symptoms of cardiac failure?

Examination
• Is there left parasternal heave?
• Is the ejection systolic murmur (+ thrill?) loudest over pulmonary area, and is it louder during inspiration (may be an ejection click)?
• The second sound may be split.

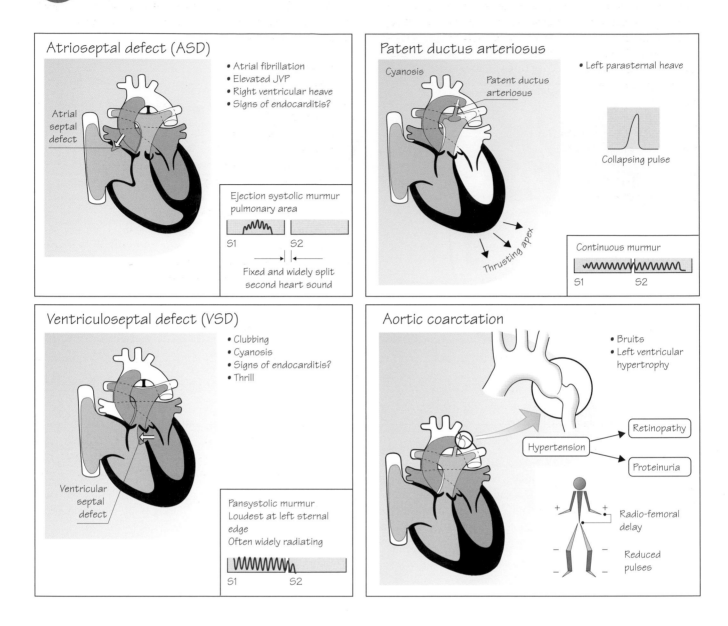

Atrioseptal defect (ASD)

Atrial septal defect

- Atrial fibrillation
- Elevated JVP
- Right ventricular heave
- Signs of endocarditis?

Ejection systolic murmur pulmonary area

S1   S2

Fixed and widely split second heart sound

Patent ductus arteriosus

Cyanosis

Patent ductus arteriosus

Thrusting apex

- Left parasternal heave

Collapsing pulse

Continuous murmur

S1   S2

Ventriculoseptal defect (VSD)

Ventricular septal defect

- Clubbing
- Cyanosis
- Signs of endocarditis?
- Thrill

Pansystolic murmur
Loudest at left sternal edge
Often widely radiating

S1   S2

Aortic coarctation

- Bruits
- Left ventricular hypertrophy

Hypertension

Retinopathy

Proteinuria

Radio-femoral delay

Reduced pulses

Atrioseptal defect
History

A murmur may be discovered incidentally, or the chronic left-to-right shunt may lead to right ventricular strain with the gradual development of symptoms of predominantly right-sided heart failure with peripheral oedema, breathlessness or palpitations. Atrioseptal defect accounts for one-third of congenital cardiac defects.

Vary rarely, there may be a history of symptoms of endocarditis.

Past medical history

Any previously heard murmur?

Family history

Any family history of congenital heart defects?

Examination

Is there:
- atrial fibrillation?
- an elevated JVP?
- a right ventricular heave?
- a widely split second heart sound?
- an ejection systolic murmur (pulmonary area)?
- peripheral oedema?
- hepatomegaly?
- signs of endocarditis?

Ventriculoseptal defect
History
This defect may be congenital or acquired (usually caused by ischaemic septal rupture following myocardial infarction). Again, a murmur may be heard incidentally or progressive symptoms of heart failure, breathlessness or palpitations may develop. It is the commonest congenital heart defect.

Vary rarely, there may be a history of symptoms of endocarditis.

Past medical history
Any previously heard murmur?

Family history
Any family history of congenital heart defects?

Examination
• Is the systolic murmur loudest at left sternal edge but widely radiating? The murmur is often very loud.
• Any signs of heart failure?
• If this is Eisenmenger's syndrome (reversal of shunt due to pulmonary hypertension), examine for cyanosis and clubbing. The murmur is quieter.
• Are there signs of endocarditis?
• Acute VSD following myocardial infarction may present with shock, hypotension, cyanosis, a loud new murmur and right-sided failure. Differential diagnosis includes acute mitral regurgitation due to chordal rupture in which there is usually pronounced orthopnoea and pulmonary oedema.

Aortic coarctation
This congenital condition of aortic narrowing may present with hypertension or be recognized due to impaired pulses in the legs.

History
The young adult might (very rarely) have symptoms of claudication, known hypertension or stroke. There is often associated aortic valve disease. Look specifically for a coarctation in any young patient with hypertension.

Examination
• Are there reduced leg pulses or radial femoral delay?
• Is there hypertension in the upper limbs and reduced BP in lower limbs?
• Is there left ventricular hypertrophy?
• Are there any widespread bruits over chest due to collaterals?
• Any evidence of end-organ damage from hypertension (e.g. proteinuria, hypertensive retinopathy)?

Patent ductus arteriosus
This usually presents during infancy. It does occasionally become noticed during adulthood but the clinical signs may be subtle. It can present with breathlessness or cyanosis. It constitutes 10% of cases of congenital heart disease.

History
• Is there a known murmur?
• Is there breathlessness?
• Patent ductus arteriosus can develop into Eisenmenger's syndrome or infective endocarditis.

Examination
• Is there cyanosis?
• Is the pulse collapsing in character?
• Is the apex thrusting in character with left parasternal heave?
• Is there a continuous 'machinery' murmur, widespread but loudest in the pulmonary area.
• Consider the possibility of other cardiac defects.

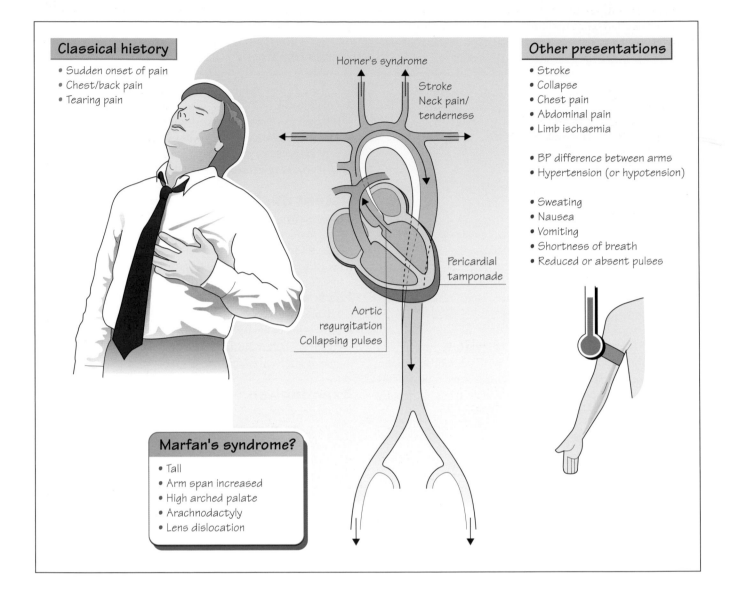

Classical history
- Sudden onset of pain
- Chest/back pain
- Tearing pain

Marfan's syndrome?
- Tall
- Arm span increased
- High arched palate
- Arachnodactyly
- Lens dislocation

Horner's syndrome

Stroke
Neck pain/
tenderness

Pericardial
tamponade

Aortic
regurgitation
Collapsing pulses

Other presentations
- Stroke
- Collapse
- Chest pain
- Abdominal pain
- Limb ischaemia

- BP difference between arms
- Hypertension (or hypotension)

- Sweating
- Nausea
- Vomiting
- Shortness of breath
- Reduced or absent pulses

Aortic dissection is a split in the wall of the aorta. Blood can enter this split and lead to vessel occlusion, aortic regurgitation and blood in the pericardial space. It is relatively rare with an incidence of 3/100 000 per year, but unrecognized or untreated it has a very high mortality rate. Consider the possibility of aortic dissection in any patient with chest pain or collapse.

History
The **classical** description of the pain of aortic dissection is of a sudden (instantaneous), severe, tearing pain located in the back (often interscapular region). However, other presentations occur: aortic dissection may present with sudden death, collapse, stroke, central anterior chest pain (mimicking acute myocardial infarction), abdominal or leg pain.

Accompanying symptoms may include nausea, sweating, vomiting and shortness of breath. The dissection can spread to involve other arteries such as the carotids (producing neck pain and tenderness or stroke), radial or femoral arteries (producing acute limb ischaemia), spinal arteries (producing paraparesis) or can extend proximally producing pericardial tamponade or acute aortic regurgitation.

Past medical history
There may be a history of previous aortic dissection, of hypertension or of conditions such as Marfan's syndrome.

Family history
Any family history of Marfan's syndrome?

Examination

- Is the patient well or unwell? Is the patient in pain or shocked?
- Check the pulse. Is the pulse equal in both arms? Are there absent peripheral pulses? Any collapsing character (actually rare in acute aortic regurgitation)?
- Check the BP, is it elevated? Are there any differences between the arms?
- Is there tenderness of carotids or of other blood vessels?
- Is there an early diastolic murmur of aortic regurgitation?
- Consider Horner's syndrome.
- Are there any neurological signs (e.g. hemiplegia, paraplegia)?
- Are there any signs of Marfan's syndrome (tall, increased arm span, high arched palate, lens dislocation)?

Evidence

Frequency of symptoms and signs (Hagan *et al.* 2000)

- Severe pain of abrupt onset (85%)
- Chest pain (73%)
- Back pain (53%)
- Syncope (9%)
- History of hypertension (70%)
- Marfan's syndrome (5%)
- Hypertension (49%)
- Murmur of aortic regurgitation (32%)
- Pulse deficit (15%)
- Stroke (5%)

The importance of history (Rosman *et al.* 1998)

A high quality history can contribute substantially to the accuracy of diagnosis of aortic dissection with questions addressing quality of pain, its radiation and sudden intensity at onset increasing the accuracy of diagnosis.

Inter-arm BP difference in normal patients (Singer & Hollander 1996)

Fifty-three per cent of 610 ambulant patients seen at an emergency department had inter-arm BP differences (BP measured by automated BP monitor) of > 10 mmHg and 19% had difference of > 19 mmHg.

Hagan PG, Nienaber CA, Isselbacher EM *et al.* The International Registry of Acute Aortic Dissection (IRAD): new insights into an old disease. *JAMA* 2000; **283**: 897–903.

Rosman HS, Patel S, Borzak S, Paone G & Retter K. Quality of history taking in patients with aortic dissection. *Chest* 1998; **114**: 793–5.

Singer AJ & Hollander JE. Blood pressure. Assessment of interarm differences. *Arch Intern Med* 1996; **156**: 2005–8.

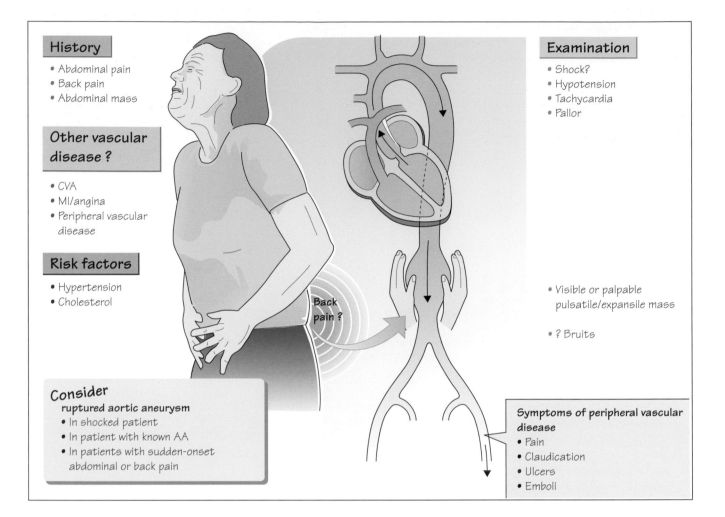

History
- Abdominal pain
- Back pain
- Abdominal mass

Other vascular disease ?
- CVA
- MI/angina
- Peripheral vascular disease

Risk factors
- Hypertension
- Cholesterol

Back pain ?

Consider
ruptured aortic aneurysm
- In shocked patient
- In patient with known AA
- In patients with sudden-onset abdominal or back pain

Examination
- Shock?
- Hypotension
- Tachycardia
- Pallor

- Visible or palpable pulsatile/expansile mass

- ? Bruits

Symptoms of peripheral vascular disease
- Pain
- Claudication
- Ulcers
- Emboli

An abdominal aortic aneurysm is an abnormal dilatation of the abdominal aorta and may present acutely with sudden onset of abdominal or back pain, with collapse or syncope or with loin pain. It may be found incidentally as a pulsatile abdominal mass, as a more gradual presentation with back pain or during investigation of peripheral vascular disease. It has a prevalence of 1–2% in people over 50 years of age and a 3–4% prevalence in people over 75 years of age. Risk factors other than age include smoking, a family history of abdominal aortic aneurysm and other atherosclerotic disease.

A ruptured or leaking aortic aneurysm should be considered in any patient presenting with the sudden onset of back pain, abdominal pain, shock or collapse. Unusually, it can mimic renal colic and other causes of the acute abdomen, such as pancreatitis and perforated peptic ulcer. The incidence of ruptured aortic aneurysm rises with age and is 20/100 000 in people aged 60–64 years, rising to 180/100 000 in people aged 80–84 years. The risk of rupture increases with aneurysm size and over 5 years the risk is: < 4.5 cm = 9%; 4.5–7.0 cm = 35%; > 7 cm = 75%.

History
- Abdominal aortic aneurysms are usually asymptomatic.
- They may present with pain, collapse, as an abdominal mass or with symptoms due to leg ischaemia.
- How did the pain start, gradually or suddenly? Where was it and was there any radiation to back, loin or legs?
- Was there any claudication? Any rest pain, embolic phenomenon, ulcers?

Past medical history
- Any known aneurysm?
- Any history of any other vascular disease (e.g. myocardial infarction, angina, peripheral vascular disease, renovascular disease)?
- Any hypertension?
- Any hypercholesterolaemia?
- Does/did the patient smoke?

Family history
Is there a family history of aneurysms?

Examination

- Is the patient well or unwell? Is the patient shocked, pale and distressed?
- *Examine the pulse*: tachycardia, thready?
- *Measure BP*: hypertension/hypotension?
- *Inspect the abdomen*: distension, pulsatile mass?
- *Palpate the abdomen*: tenderness, palpable, expansile, pulsatile mass?
- *Auscultate the abdomen*: abdominal bruits, femoral bruits? (NB. In ruptured aneurysm or hypotension, pulsatile mass may not be present.)
- Examine the peripheral pulses, especially the femoral pulses.
- **If any patient has abdominal or back pain together with signs of shock, consider a ruptured aortic aneurysm.**

Evidence

- Abdominal palpation for the presence of a widened aorta produced a LR of 15.6 for abdominal aortic aneurysms of > 4 cm.
- Abdominal palpation had a high sensitivity for aneurysms > 5 cm in patients without large girth (< 100 cm).

Fink HA, Lederle FA, Roth CS *et al*. The accuracy of physical examination to detect abdominal aortic aneurysm. *Arch Intern Med* 2000; **160**: 833–6.

Lederle FA & Simel DL. The rational clinical examination. Does this patient have abdominal aortic aneurysm? *JAMA* 1999; **281**: 77–82.

Infective endocarditis

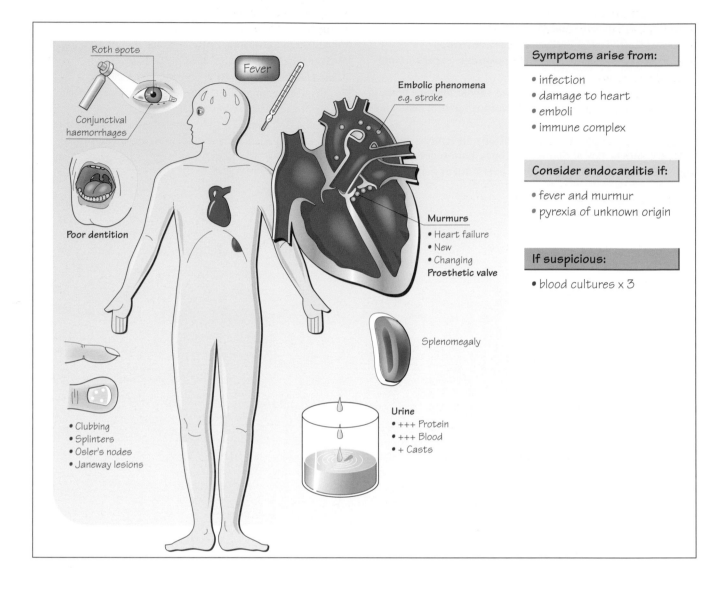

Symptoms arise from:

- infection
- damage to heart
- emboli
- immune complex

Consider endocarditis if:

- fever and murmur
- pyrexia of unknown origin

If suspicious:

- blood cultures x 3

Roth spots

Conjunctival haemorrhages

Fever

Poor dentition

Embolic phenomena e.g. stroke

Murmurs
- Heart failure
- New
- Changing
Prosthetic valve

Splenomegaly

Urine
- +++ Protein
- +++ Blood
- + Casts

- Clubbing
- Splinters
- Osler's nodes
- Janeway lesions

History

Patients with endocarditis can present with a wide variety of symptoms due to:
- the infection (fever, malaise, night sweats, anorexia, weight loss, rigors, mycotic aneurysms)
- damage to the heart (symptoms of heart failure, palpitations, collapse)
- embolic phenomenon (stroke, arterial embolus)
- immune complex phenomenon (rash, symptoms due to renal failure)
- other symptoms (dyspnoea, cough, myalgia, athralgia, back pain).

The presentation may be chronic with symptoms over weeks, months or acute with rapid deterioration (e.g. with *Staphylococcus aureus* endocarditis affecting the aortic valve). The prevalence of community-acquired endocarditis is 5/100 000 per year but rises to 150–2000/100 000 per year in intravenous drug abusers.

The signs of endocarditis should be sought in any patient with unexplained fever, new murmur, malaise, emboli or renal failure, particularly if there is a known valvular abnormality or prosthetic valve. However, up to a half of patients have no previously known cardiac disorder.

Past medical history

- Any known cardiac structural abnormality (e.g. known murmur or VSD)?
- Does the patient have a prosthetic valve?
- Any recent procedure that may have allowed bacteraemia (e.g. dental work)?

Drugs

- Any intravenous drug abuse?
- Any recent antibiotic treatment?

Allergies

Does the patient have any allergies to antibiotics?

Examination

- Is the patient well or unwell?
- Is there dentition or any other sources of infection?
- Is there a tunnelled central line for long-term antibiotics?
- Is the patient anaemic?
- Check the patient's temperature, pulse, BP (and pulse pressure).
- Are there splinter haemorrhages?
- Are there petechiae?
- Any murmurs? (If so, new or altered?)
- Any signs of cardiac failure?
- Any neurological signs?
- Any haematuria/proteinuria/casts?
- Very rarely there may be clubbing, Janeway lesions (non-tender erythematous, haemorrhagic or pustular lesions, often on the palms or soles), Osler nodes (tender, subcutaneous nodules, often in the pulp of the digits or the thenar eminence), Roth spots (white-centred retinal haemorrhages) or splenomegaly.

Evidence

Frequency of symptoms and signs (Watanakunakorn & Burkert 1993)

In native valve endocarditis (excluding intravenous drug abusers):

- **Symptoms (frequency):**
  - fever (66%)
  - malaise (40%)
  - arthralgia/myalgia (16%)
  - confusion (22%)
  - severe back pain (9%)
- **Signs (frequency):**
  - temperature > 37.7° (86%)
  - cardiac murmur (81%)
  - petechiae/embolic lesions (45%)
  - Osler nodes/Janeway lesions/Roth spots (10%)
  - congestive cardiac failure (52%)
  - microscopic haematuria (65%)

NB. In intravenous drug abusers with endocarditis, pleuritic chest pain occurs in 30%.

Modified Duke criteria for the diagnosis of infective endocarditis (Li *et al.* 2000)

Major criteria

- Microbiological isolation of typical organism or persistently positive blood cultures.
- Evidence of endocardial involvement (new valvular regurgitation or positive echocardiogram).

Minor criteria

- Predisposition to cardiac abnormalities:
  (a) *High risk*: previous endocarditis, aortic valve disease, rheumatic heart disease, prosthetic valve, aortic coarctation, complex cyanotic congenital heart disease.
  (b) *Moderate risk*: mitral valve prolapse with regurgitation, mitral stenosis, tricuspid valve disease, pulmonary stenosis, hypertrophic obstructive cardiomyopathy.
  (c) *Low risk*: atrioseptal defect, IHD, coronary artery bypass grafts, mitral valve prolapse (no regurgitation or intravenous drug use).
- Immunological: positive rheumatoid factor, glomerulonephritis, Osler nodes or Roth spots.
- Fever: temperature > 38°C.
- Vascular phenomena (major arterial emboli, septic pulmonary infarcts, mycotic aneurysm, intracranial haemorrhage, conjunctival haemorrhages and Janeway lesions).
- Microbiological findings: positive blood cultures or serological evidence of typical infection.

To meet the criteria requires the presence of two major, one major and three minor or five minor criteria. However, the diagnosis is excluded if there is a firm alternative diagnosis explaining evidence of infective endocarditis.

Li JS, Sexton DJ & Mick N. Proposed modifications to the Duke criteria for the diagnosis of infective endocarditis. *Clin Infect Dis* 2000; **30**: 633–8.

Watanakunakorn C & Burkert T. Infective endocarditis at a large community teaching hospital, 1980–90. A review of 210 episodes. *Medicine (Baltimore)* 1993; **72**: 90–102.

Pulmonary embolism and deep vein thrombosis

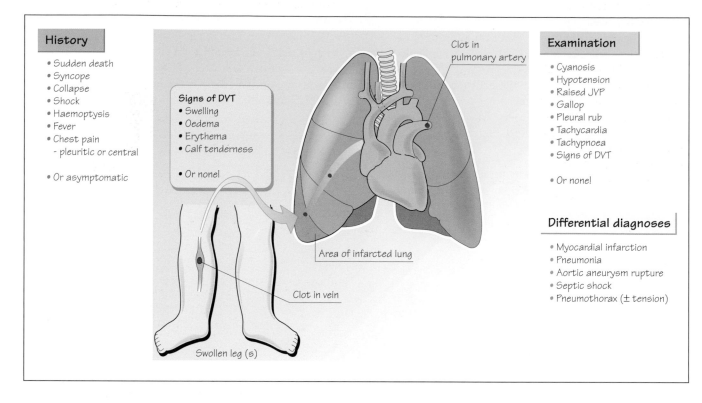

History
- Sudden death
- Syncope
- Collapse
- Shock
- Haemoptysis
- Fever
- Chest pain
  - pleuritic or central

- Or asymptomatic

Signs of DVT
- Swelling
- Oedema
- Erythema
- Calf tenderness

- Or none!

Clot in pulmonary artery

Area of infarcted lung

Clot in vein

Swollen leg (s)

Examination
- Cyanosis
- Hypotension
- Raised JVP
- Gallop
- Pleural rub
- Tachycardia
- Tachypnoea
- Signs of DVT

- Or none!

Differential diagnoses
- Myocardial infarction
- Pneumonia
- Aortic aneurysm rupture
- Septic shock
- Pneumothorax (± tension)

Pulmonary embolism

PE is an embolus (usually thromboembolic) to the lungs.

History

PE may present in a variety of different ways and the presentation depends upon the size of the emboli and the extent of pulmonary vascular obstruction:
- sudden death
- syncope
- shock
- haemoptysis
- breathlessness
- chest pain
- palpitations
- fever (even PUO).

A classical presentation would be with the sudden onset of pleuritic chest pain accompanied by breathlessness and haemoptysis or alternatively a sudden collapse in a postoperative patient shortly after straining at stool. Other patients may present simply with breathlessness, with pleuritic pain or with haemoptysis, but have little abnormality visible on chest X-ray.

PE occurs in over 1% of hospital inpatients and significant pulmonary emboli are found unexpectedly in the postmortems of over 10% of patients who die in hospital. A high index of suspicion is thus required. PE should be considered in any patient with chest pain, collapse, breathlessness, pleuritic pain, haemoptysis or shock.

Particular groups of patients are at greater risk, including immobile patients, postoperative patients, pregnant patients and patients with malignancy.

Past medical history

There may be a history of DVT, previous PE, recent surgery, prolonged travel or known malignant disease.

Family history

There may be a family history of PE or DVT, perhaps in association with an inherited tendency to increased thrombosis (e.g. factor V Leiden, protein C or protein S deficiency).

Drugs

Is the patient taking any anticoagulants, aspirin or using the oral contraceptive pill or oestrogen hormone replacement therapy?

Functional enquiry

Ask about any symptoms that might point to underlying malignancy.

Examination

- Is the patient well or unwell? Do they need urgent resuscitation including supplemental oxygen?
- Are they in pain, distressed, breathless, cyanosed, shocked?
- Is there:
  - blood stained sputum?
  - tachycardia?
  - hypotension?

- elevated JVP?
- right ventricular heave?
- pleural rub?
- peripheral oedema?
- signs of DVT?

(NB. Most patients with a PE will have few or none of these signs.)

- Examine for any features suggesting malignancy (e.g. abdominal mass) and consider the possibility of a pelvic mass obstructing venous return (perform rectal ± vaginal examinations).
- **The diagnosis of PE should be considered in any patient in whom there is a sudden collapse or cardiorespiratory deterioration.**
- **A significant PE may produce no signs and a high index of suspicion is thus required in patients with sudden breathlessness, collapse, haemoptysis or chest pain.**

Deep vein thrombosis
History
- DVT may present with leg (or very rarely arm):
  - swelling
  - pain
  - oedema
  - tenderness
  - redness
- or the patient may be asymptomatic.

Examination
- Is there swelling of calf (measure at fixed distance below tibial tuberosity)?
- Any oedema?
- Any redness?
- Tenderness of the leg?
- Superficial venous dilatation?
- The risk factors are as for PE.
- It often is not possible with the history and examination to conclude whether a red swollen leg is due to DVT or, for example, due to cellulitis. Investigations such as venography or ultrasound are often required.

Prediction rules

Clinical prediction rules (Tables 73.1 & 73.2) have been developed to predict pre-test probabilities and can be combined with tests such as D-dimers and CT scanning.

Table 73.1 Clinical prediction rule for deep vein thrombosis (DVT). High probability if score 3 or more, moderate if 1 or 2 and low if score is 0 or less.*

	Score
Active cancer (treatment or within 6 months or palliative)	1
Paralysis, paresis or recent plaster immobilization of legs	1
Major surgery or recently bedridden for > 3 days in last 4 weeks	1
Localized tenderness along the distribution of the deep venous system	1
Entire leg swelling	1
Calf swelling by > 3 cm when compared with the asymptomatic leg (measured 10 cm below the tibial tuberosity)	1
Pitting oedema (greater in the symptomatic leg)	1
Collateral superficial veins (nonvaricose)	1
Alternative diagnosis as likely or greater than that of DVT	−2

*From Anand SS, Wells PS, Hunt D *et al*. Does this patient have deep vein thrombosis? *JAMA* 1998; **279**: 1094–9.

Table 73.2 Clinical prediction rule for pulmonary embolism (PE). Low probability if score <2.0; moderate probability if score 2.0–6.0; high probability if score is >6.0.*

Clinical signs and symptoms of DVT (minimum of leg swelling and pain with palpation of the deep veins)	3.0 points
PE as or more likely than an alternative diagnosis	3.0 points
Heart rate greater than 100	1.5 points
Immobilization or surgery in the previous 4 weeks	1.5 points
Previous DVT/PE	1.5 points
Hemoptysis	1.0 points
Malignancy (on treatment, treated in the last 6 months or palliative)	1.0 points

*From Wells PS. Advances in the diagnosis of venous thromboembolism. *J Thromb Thrombolysis* 2006; **21**(1): 31–40.

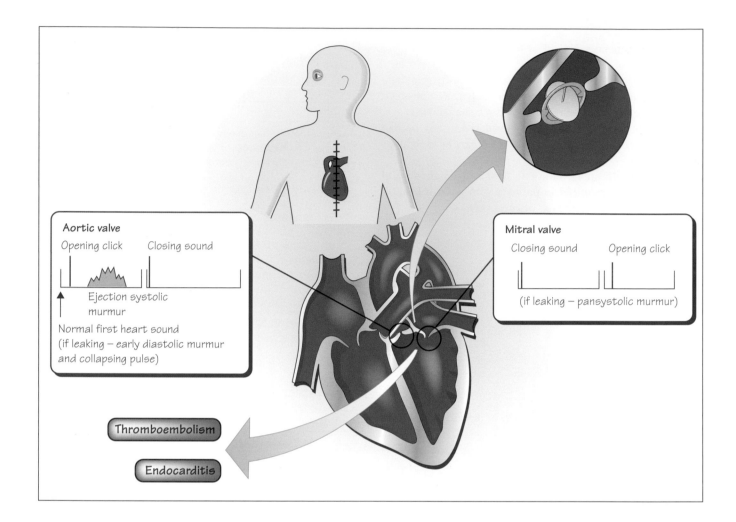

Cardiac valves are most commonly replaced when the native valve is severely stenosed or incompetent. The aortic and mitral valves are the commonest valves requiring replacement. The prosthetic valves may be mechanical (ball-cage [Starr–Edwards], tilting disc [Bjork–Shiley] or double tiliting disc [St. Jude]), cadaveric homografts or porcine heterografts. Anticoagulation is commonly required to prevent thromboembolism. The prosthetic valves may become infected causing endocarditis.

History
- Why was the valve replaced?
- What was the initial cause of the valvular pathology?
- What were the symptoms leading to valve replacement?
- Any symptoms suggestive of endocarditis or thromboembolism?
- Any symptoms suggestive of valvular leak (e.g. of heart failure)?

Drugs
Is the patient being treated with anticoagulants?

Examination
- Is there a thoracotomy scar?
- Any stigmata of endocarditis?
- Any signs of thromboembolism?
- Carry out a full cardiac examination looking for signs of cardiac failure.
- Metallic prosthetic sounds are often very loud and produce a loud closing sound at the same time as the native heart sound and may additionally produce a softer opening snap.

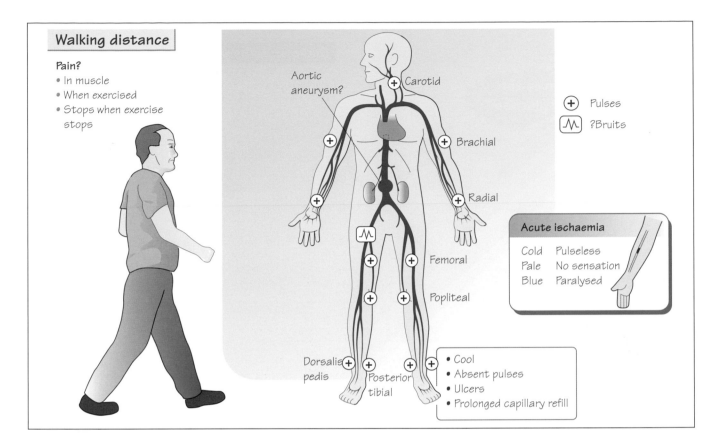

Walking distance

Pain?
- In muscle
- When exercised
- Stops when exercise stops

Aortic aneurysm?

Carotid

Brachial

Radial

Femoral

Popliteal

Dorsalis pedis

Posterior tibial

⊕ Pulses

〰 ?Bruits

Acute ischaemia

Cold   Pulseless
Pale   No sensation
Blue   Paralysed

- Cool
- Absent pulses
- Ulcers
- Prolonged capillary refill

Peripheral vascular disease usually presents in the legs with pain on walking but, if more severe, can cause rest pain and eventually skin ulceration and gangrene.

History
- Peripheral vascular disease classically produces calf pain on walking and is relieved by rest. How far can the patient walk before pain? Does is it improve with rest?
- Peripheral vascular disease can also produce buttock claudication, cauda equina claudication (pain on exercise in distribution of sacral nerve roots) and impotence.
- Ask if there is rest pain that may be improved by hanging the leg over the edge of bed. Ask about skin ulcers.
- Consider vascular disease elsewhere (e.g. aortic aneurysm, coronary, carotid and renovascular disease). (Patients with peripheral vascular disease have a threefold increased incidence of stroke and myocardial infarction).
- In acute ischaemia there is the sudden onset of a painful, cold limb which on examination is pale, pulseless, perishingly cold, painful, paraesthetic and paralysed.
- Consider emboli and examine for embolic source.

Past medical history
- Any previous symptoms, reconstructive vascular surgery, angioplasties, amputations, hypercholesterolaemia, other vascular disease, diabetes mellitus or hypertension?

- Has the patient taken any treatments such as aspirin or anticoagulants?
- Does the patient smoke?

Examination
- Look carefully at the legs and arms. Are there colour changes, ulcers, temperature changes, loss of hair?
- Is there prolonged capillary refill, venous guttering or postural colour change?
- Examine the peripheral vascular tree for pulses, auscultate for bruits (especially carotid and femoral) and examine for aortic and popliteal aneurysms. Consider coronary, carotid and renovascular disease. Consider measurement of the ankle-brachial pressure index.

Evidence

In patients with leg symptoms, the most useful findings in diagnosing peripheral vascular disease are the presence of cool skin (LR, 5.9), the presence of at least one bruit (LR, 5.6) or any palpable pulse abnormality (LR, 4.7). The absence of any bruits (iliac, femoral, or popliteal) (LR, 0.39) or pulse abnormality (LR, 0.38; 95% CI, 0.23–0.64) reduces the likelihood of peripheral vascular disease.

Khan NA, Rahim SA, Anand SS, Simel DL & Panju A.
   Does the clinical examination predict lower extremity peripheral arterial disease? *JAMA* 2006; **295**: 536–46.

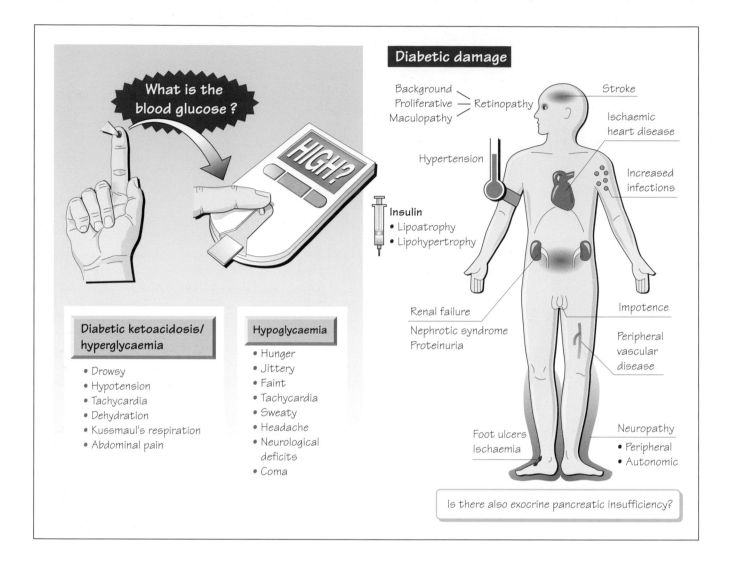

Diabetes mellitus is characterized by elevated blood glucose and is due to decreased secretion or effectiveness of insulin. It is common and Type 1 diabetes mellitus (formerly insulin-dependent diabetes mellitus, IDDM) has a prevalence of 0.5%, whilst Type 2 diabetes mellitus (formerly non-insulin dependent diabetes mellitus, NIDDM) has a prevalence approaching 2%.

History

Diabetes mellitus may initially present acutely with diabetic ketoacidosis; hyperglycaemic coma; with the osmotic diuretic effects of hyperglycaemia (polyuria, polydipsia, nocturia); the adverse end-organ effects of diabetes (IHD, retinopathy, peripheral vascular disease, peripheral neuropathy); or the complications of increased susceptibility to infection (e.g. UTI, candidal thrush). Alternatively, it may be discovered incidentally during blood or urine testing.

Diabetic ketoacidosis

This can occur as the first presentation of diabetes mellitus, or it can occur in those patients with known diabetes mellitus. There may be a gradual onset of symptoms with thirst and polyuria. Other symptoms include breathlessness, abdominal pain, drowsiness, confusion or even coma. On examination there may be evidence of acidosis (rapid, Kussmaul respiration [deep and sighing]), of dehydration (with hypotension, tachycardia and postural fall in BP) or of pre-existing diabetic damage (e.g. retinopathy, neuropathy). There may be symptoms or signs of a precipitating illness, such as bacterial infection with fever, rigors, etc. Similar presentations can occur with non-ketotic hyperglycaemia but without signs of acidosis. Acidosis can also occur in diabetic patients due to lactic acidosis; rarely this is associated with the use of metformin.

Hypoglycaemia

Hypoglycaemia occurs commonly in diabetics due to insulin or hypoglycaemic administration or during times of inadequate caloric intake. It can also occur in alcoholics, with tumours secreting glucagon, with malnutrition and, rarely, in sepsis.

The symptoms of hypoglycaemia are a feeling of hunger, jitteriness, faint feeling, tachycardia, sweating and a range of neurological symptoms from headache to neurological deficits to coma. The prompt recognition of hypoglycaemia is essential so that treatment (intravenous glucose) can be administered and irreversible neurological damage avoided. In any diabetic patient who is unwell and in any comatose or drowsy patient prompt bedside determination of blood glucose must be performed. If no facilities for blood glucose measurement exist, glucose should be administered to avoid the neurological damage from potential hypoglycaemia. Some diabetics will be very familiar with the symptoms of hypoglycaemia and be able to correct it by eating. However, hypoglycaemia may occur without premonitory symptoms in some patients, particularly at night or if on beta-blockers.

Past medical history
• Any history of known diabetes mellitus? If so, what was the mode of presentation and what was the treatment? What was the monitoring of control: frequency of urine testing, blood testing, HbA_1C, record books, awareness of hypoglycaemia? Ask about previous complications.
• Previous admissions for hypoglycaemia/hyperglycaemia?
• Vascular disease: cardiac ischaemia (myocardial infarction, angina, CCF), peripheral vascular disease (claudication, rest pain, ulcers, foot care, impotence) peripheral neuropathy, autonomic neuropathy (symptoms of gastroparesis—vomiting, bloating, diarrhoea)?
• Retinopathy, visual acuity, laser treatments?
• Hypercholesterolaemia, hypertriglyceridaemia?
• Renal dysfunction (proteinuria, microalbuminuria)?
• Hypertension—treatments?
• Diet/weight/exercise?

Drugs
• Is the patient taking any treatment for diabetes: diet alone, oral hypoglycaemics or insulin?

• Ask about drugs that can be diabetogenic (e.g. corticosteroids, cyclosporin).
• Ask about the patient's smoking and alcohol use/history.
• Does the patient have any allergies?

Family and social history
• Any family history of diabetes mellitus?
• Any interference of diabetes with life?
• Who actually draws up the insulin/tests blood sugar, etc. (spouse/patient/nurse)?

Examination
• Is the patient acutely unwell?
• What is the blood glucose? TEST IT!
• Any smell of ketones? Are there any signs of tachypnoea or Kussmaul's respiration (deep, sighing)?
• Any evidence of dehydration due to hyperglycaemia (tachycardia, hypotension, postural hypotension, dry mucous membranes, reduced skin turgor, etc.)?
• Is the patient drowsy, confused or comatose?
• What is the patient's temperature?
• Check the cardiovascular system: BP? Are there signs of cardiac failure?
• Check peripheral vasculature for: pulses present, bruits?
• Check feet for: ulcers, cellulitis, neuropathy (sensation to light touch), pin prick, monofilament, vibration sense, joint position sense, reflexes and autonomic neuropathy (postural BP, response to Valsalva).
• Check eyes for visual acuity and pupillary responses.
• Perform fundoscopy for: dot + blot haemorrhages, proliferative retinopathy, maculopathy.
• Check for any hypertensive changes.
• Check urine for: proteinuria, glucose, ketones.
• Look for and treat dangerous acute complications of diabetes mellitus (e.g. hypoglycaemia, diabetic ketoacidosis).
• Consider infective or other precipitant to deterioration.
• Examine for end-organ diabetic damage.

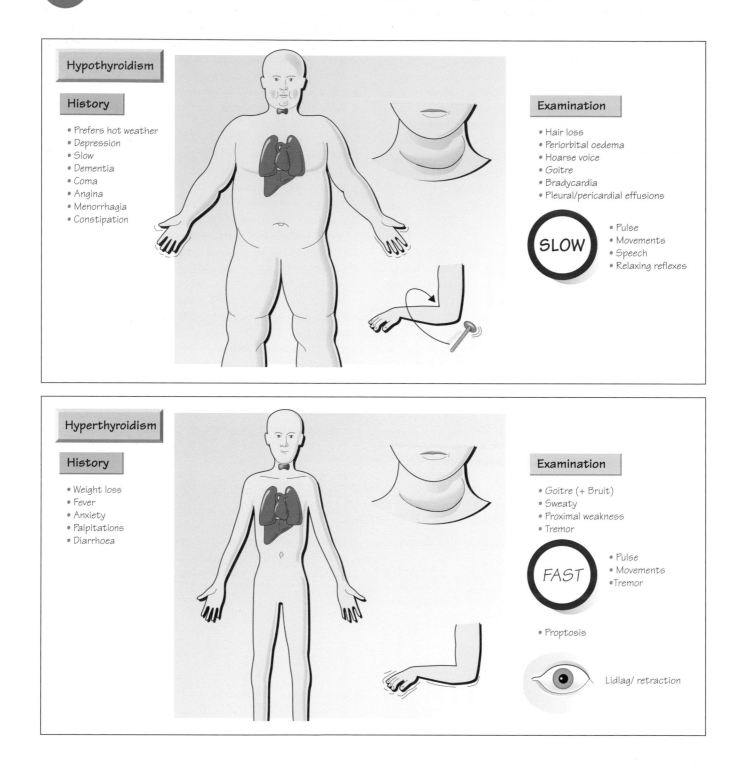

Hypothyroidism

History

- Prefers hot weather
- Depression
- Slow
- Dementia
- Coma
- Angina
- Menorrhagia
- Constipation

Examination

- Hair loss
- Periorbital oedema
- Hoarse voice
- Goitre
- Bradycardia
- Pleural/pericardial effusions

SLOW
- Pulse
- Movements
- Speech
- Relaxing reflexes

Hyperthyroidism

History

- Weight loss
- Fever
- Anxiety
- Palpitations
- Diarrhoea

Examination

- Goitre (+ Bruit)
- Sweaty
- Proximal weakness
- Tremor

FAST
- Pulse
- Movements
- Tremor

- Proptosis

Lidlag/ retraction

Hypothyroidism

Hypothyroidism, the deficiency of thyroid hormones, is common (1% of hospitalized patients) and can present with a variety of subtle and non-specific symptoms. These include tiredness, mental and physical slowness, cold intolerance, weight gain, constipation, carpal tunnel syndrome, menorrhagia, dementia and hypothermia. Very rarely severe hypothyroidism may present with coma. However, the classical signs described below may not be present, particularly in the elderly.

Past medical history

- Any known history of hypothyroidism? If so, ask about thyroxine replacement therapy, dose and duration?
- Any history of IHD?

- Any history of hypercholesterolaemia?
- Any previous radioiodine treatment (for thyrotoxicosis)?
- Any history of other endocrine/autoimmune conditions?

Drugs

Is the patient receiving thyroxine or amiodarone?

Family history

Any family history of thyroid disease?

Examination

- Is there a goitre?
- Does the patient have:
  - slow speech?
  - coarse hair?
  - lethargic movements?
  - facial oedema?
  - bradycardia?
  - hoarse voice?
  - carpal tunnel syndrome?
  - anaemia?
  - hair loss (scalp and eyebrows)?
  - a 'peaches and cream' complexion?
  - pericardial/pleural effusions?
  - peripheral oedema?
  - slow relaxing reflexes?

Hyperthyroidism

Thyrotoxicosis, an excess of thyroid hormones, is common affecting 0.5% of hospital inpatients. It can produce a variety of symptoms including anxiety, tremor, weight loss, palpitations, eye changes and goitre. However, as in hypothyroidism, patients with thyrotoxicosis may not present with clear symptoms or signs and a high index of suspicion is required, particularly in the elderly.

Past medical history

- Any history of previously known thyrotoxicosis? If so, what treatments were used, including radioactive iodine and drugs such as carbimazole, propylthiouracil and beta-blockers?
- Any history of other autoimmune diseases?

Family history

Any family history of thyroid disease?

Examination

- Does the patient have:
  - tachycardia, atrial fibrillation?
  - hyperkinetic movements, agitation?
  - fine tremor?
  - warm sweaty palms?
  - a goitre?
  - proximal weakness?
  - heart failure?
- Check eye signs: proptosis, lid retraction, lid lag?

Evidence

Clinical symptoms and signs are useful in the diagnosis of hypothyroidism but a high index of suspicion is required because hypothyroidism may exist with minimal symptoms and no classical signs.

Table 77.1 Symptoms and signs in hypothyroidism.

Symptom or sign	Frequency of sign in hypothyroid patient (%)	Frequency of sign in normal controls (%)
Cold intolerance	64	38
Reduced sweating	54	14
Weight gain	54	23
Paraesthesia	52	18
Constipation	48	15
Slow-relaxing ankle reflexes	77	7
Dry skin	76	34
Coarse skin	60	19
Periorbital puffiness	60	4
Cold skin	50	20
Slow movements	36	1
Hoarseness	34	13
Impaired hearing	22	3

Zulewski H, Muller B, Exer P, Miserez AR, Staub JJ. Estimation of tissue hypothyroidism by a new clinical score: evaluation of patients with various grades of hypothyroidism and controls. *J Clin Endocrinol Metab* 1997; **82**: 771–6.

Table 77.2 Symptoms and signs in thyrotoxicosis.

Symptom or sign	Frequency in patients with thyrotoxicosis (%)	Frequency in controls (%)
Dyspnoea	81	40
Palpitations	75	26
Tiredness	80	31
Preference for cold	73	41
Excess sweating	68	31
Nervousness	59	21
Increased appetite	32	2
Weight loss	52	2
Hot hands	76	44
Diarrhoea	8	0
Finger tremor	66	26
Pulse over 90	68	19
Average pulse	100	78
Atrial fibrillation	19	0
Goitre	87	11
Exophthalmos	34	2
Lid lag	62	16
Hyperkinesis	39	9
Sweating hands	72	22

Wayne EJ. The diagnosis of thyrotoxicosis. *Br Med J* 1954; **1**: 411.

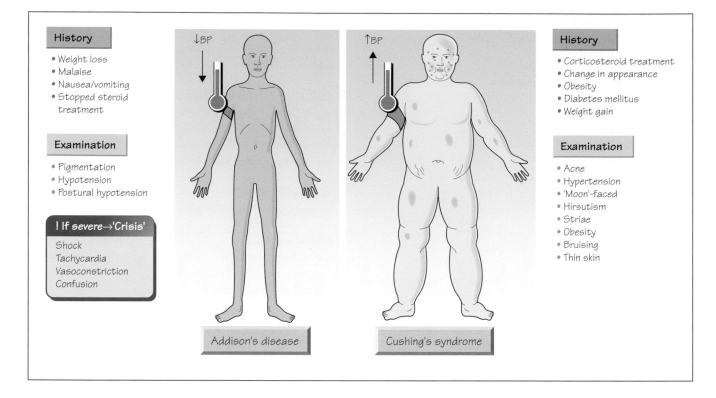

Addison's disease

Cushing's syndrome

Addison's disease

Addison's disease is the deficiency of mineralocorticoid hormones. It has a prevalence of 10/100 000.

History

Addison's disease may present with fatigue, faintness, nausea, vomiting, depression, postural dizziness, myalgia, cold intolerance, weight loss or, if severe, with more profound illness with shock (Addisonian crisis).

Past medical history

- Any history of:
  - corticosteroid therapy? (If so was it suddenly stopped?)
  - malignancy (adrenal metastases)?
  - tuberculosis?
  - other autoimmune conditions (e.g. vitiligo, hypothyroidism)?
- Any evidence of pituitary disease (hypopituitarism)?

Examination

- Is the patient unwell and pale?
- Does the patient have:
  - hypotension, postural hypotension?
  - pigmentation, especially buccal, skin creases, scars?

Cushing's syndrome

Cushing's syndrome arises from an excess of glucocorticoids. It is very common due to the therapeutic administration of corticosteroids.

History

Cushing's syndrome may present with hirsutism, weight gain, change in body/face shape, easy bruising or be noticed incidentally.

Past medical history

Any history of corticosteroid usage?

Examination

Does the patient have:
- thin skin?
- multiple ecchymoses?
- a 'buffalo' hump?
- a 'moon' face?
- centripetal obesity?
- hypertension?
- glycosuria?

79 Hypopituitarism

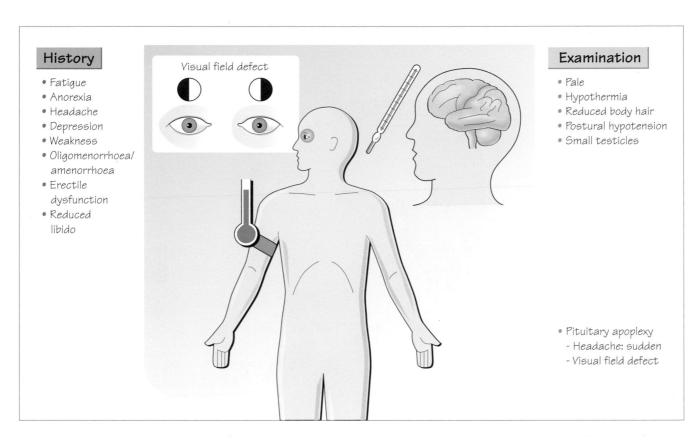

History
- Fatigue
- Anorexia
- Headache
- Depression
- Weakness
- Oligomenorrhoea/ amenorrhoea
- Erectile dysfunction
- Reduced libido

Visual field defect

Examination
- Pale
- Hypothermia
- Reduced body hair
- Postural hypotension
- Small testicles

- Pituitary apoplexy
  - Headache: sudden
  - Visual field defect

This is deficiency of thyroid, adrenal, gonadal and growth hormones due to pituitary disease. Thus in any patient with such hormonal deficiency the possibility of other deficiencies should be entertained. Rarely it may develop acutely with pituitary apoplexy in which there is haemorrhagic infarction of a pituitary tumour, usually accompanied by sudden severe headache and often with visual field defects. Hypopituitarism has a prevalence of 30/100 000.

History
Does the patient have:
- fatigue?
- anorexia?
- reduced libido?
- menstrual disturbances?
- headache?
- depression?
- weakness?
- symptoms of hypothyroidism?

Past medical history
- Any history of a known pituitary adenoma?
- Any irradiation treatment to the pituitary?
- Any severe postpartum haemorrhage (Sheehan's syndrome)?

Drugs
Has the patient taken any hormone replacement therapy: thyroxine, hydrocortisone, testosterone, oestrogen or growth hormone?

Examination
Does the patient have:
- pale (classically 'alabaster' skin)?
- reduced body hair?
- soft skin with fine wrinkles?
- hypothermia?
- hypotension (postural)?
- visual field defect?
- atrophic breasts?
- small testicles?

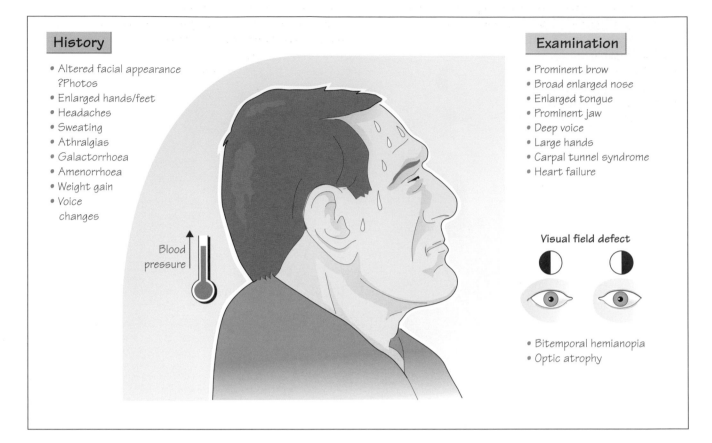

Acromegaly is the syndrome of excess growth hormone secretion, usually from a pituitary tumour. Acromegaly may present with the effects of excess growth hormone, such as a change in facial appearance or an increase in foot or hand size. The changes occur gradually and may be noticed by friends and family or when seeking medical attention for another complaint, such as hypertension or hyperglycaemia. Acromegaly has a prevalence of 6/100 000.

The pituitary tumour can encroach upon the optic nerves and produce visual symptoms, such as visual blurring or signs such as bitemporal hemianopia. There is also an increased incidence of heart failure, hypertension and hyperglycaemia.

History

• Does the patient have an altered facial appearance (ask to see previous photographs)?
• Does the patient have enlarged feet (ask about change in shoe size/fitting) and hands (rings no longer fit)?
• Any visual blurring, reduced peripheral vision?
• Are there any symptoms of hyperglycaemia, such as polyuria and polydipsia?

• Does the patient have:
  • headaches?
  • fatigue?
  • weight gain?
  • galactorrhoea?
  • menstrual irregularity?
  • erectile impotence?
  • increased sweating?
  • carpal tunnel syndrome?
  • arthralgias?

Past medical history

• Any history of known acromegaly?
• Has the patient taken any treatments with radiotherapy, drugs, surgery?
• Any associated hypopituitarism?

Drugs

• Is the patient taking somatostatin or dopaminergic agonists?
• Is the patient taking endocrine replacement (e.g. thyroxine, corticosteroids)?

Examination

- Does the patient have:
  - prominent facial features?
  - a broad, enlarged nose, prominent brow (supraorbital ridge), protruding (prognathic) jaw and an enlarged tongue?
  - interdental separation?
  - thick, greasy skin?
  - mild hirsutism?
  - a deep voice?
  - large hands ('spade-like')?
  - large feet?
- Are there signs of carpal tunnel syndrome?
- Are there signs of arthritis?
- Does the patient have hypertension?
- Are there signs of heart failure?
- Does the patient have bitemporal hemianopia (may have upper bitemporal quadrantonopia or it may only affect one eye)?
- Does the patient have optic atrophy?
- Dipstick urine for glycosuria.

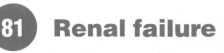

81 Renal failure

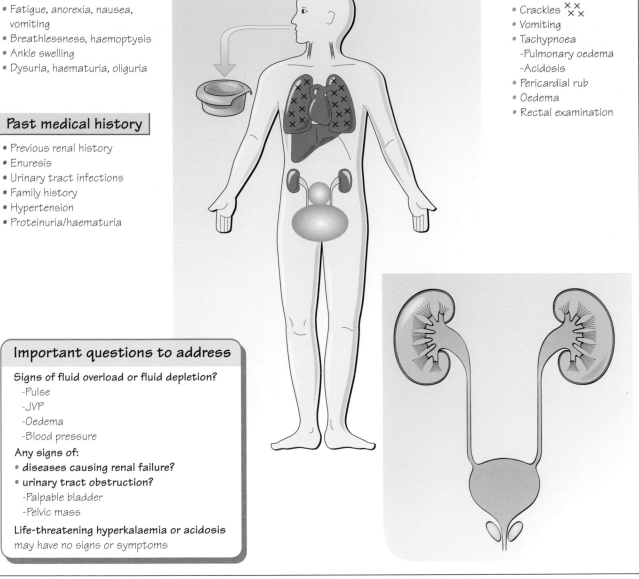

History

- Fatigue, anorexia, nausea, vomiting
- Breathlessness, haemoptysis
- Ankle swelling
- Dysuria, haematuria, oliguria

Past medical history

- Previous renal history
- Enuresis
- Urinary tract infections
- Family history
- Hypertension
- Proteinuria/haematuria

Examination

- Crackles ×× ××
- Vomiting
- Tachypnoea
  - Pulmonary oedema
  - Acidosis
- Pericardial rub
- Oedema
- Rectal examination

Important questions to address

Signs of fluid overload or fluid depletion?
- Pulse
- JVP
- Oedema
- Blood pressure

Any signs of:
- diseases causing renal failure?
- urinary tract obstruction?
  - Palpable bladder
  - Pelvic mass

Life-threatening hyperkalaemia or acidosis
may have no signs or symptoms

In the assessment of the patient with renal failure it is important to try to establish the likely cause of the renal failure, its duration and whether life-threatening complications have developed, such as pulmonary oedema.

Renal failure may be discovered incidentally when renal function is estimated with measurement of urea or creatinine, with hypertension or with symptoms of renal failure. Dramatic presentations of acute renal failure can occur with profound acidosis, pulmonary oedema or encephalopathy.

History

- Does the patient have any symptoms of renal failure (e.g. nausea, vomiting, breathlessness [due to acidosis or pulmonary oedema]) or peripheral oedema? Any itching, hiccoughs, peripheral neuropathy, fatigue, malaise, reduced urine output, polyuria or nocturia haematuria?
- Any enuresis in childhood?
- Any associated symptoms: haemoptysis, rash, back pain, fever, weight loss, or neuropathy?

• Is the patient undergoing treatment for renal failure (e.g. haemodialysis, peritoneal dialysis, renal transplant)?

Past medical history
• Any previously known renal disease?
• Any previous hypertension or proteinuria?
• Any complications of renal disease: hypertension, renal bone disease or cardiac disease?
• Any procedures to enable dialysis (e.g. arteriovenous fistula formation, peritoneal dialysis catheter [Tenckhoff])?

Drugs
Ask about:
• any drugs that might cause renal disease (e.g. NSAIDs, angiotensin-converting enzyme inhibitors or antibiotics)
• any specific treatments for renal failure (e.g. erythropoietin)
• any drugs that could accumulate and cause toxicity in renal failure (e.g. digoxin).

Family history
Any family history of renal disease (e.g. polycystic kidney disease, reflux nephropathy)?

Social history
Any interference with life by symptoms or by treatments such as dialysis?

Examination
• Is the patient unwell? Life-threatening complications of renal failure include pulmonary oedema, acidosis and hyperkalaemia.
• Are they breathless? Is there a Kussmaul pattern of respiration (deep and sighing due to acidosis)?
• Is there cyanosis?
• Is there evidence of fluid overload? Crackles in the lungs, gallop rhythm, elevated JVP, peripheral oedema, hypertension?
• Is there fluid depletion or shock? Hypotension, postural fall in BP, tachycardia, cool peripheries, peripheral vasoconstriction?
• Any signs of specific diseases causing renal failure (e.g. polycystic kidneys, vasculitic rash, sites of sepsis, pancreatitis, renal arterial bruit)?
• Any evidence of effects of renal dysfunction (e.g. anaemia, metabolic flap, acidosis, drowsy, bleeding tendency)?
• Or any evidence of severe hypertension (e.g. left ventricular hypertrophy, hypertensive retinopathy)?
• Examine carefully for any signs of obstruction. Palpable bladder, enlarged prostate, pelvic mass?
• Examine the urine with dipstick for blood, protein, glucose, leucocytes and microscopy for cells and casts.

Polycystic kidney disease

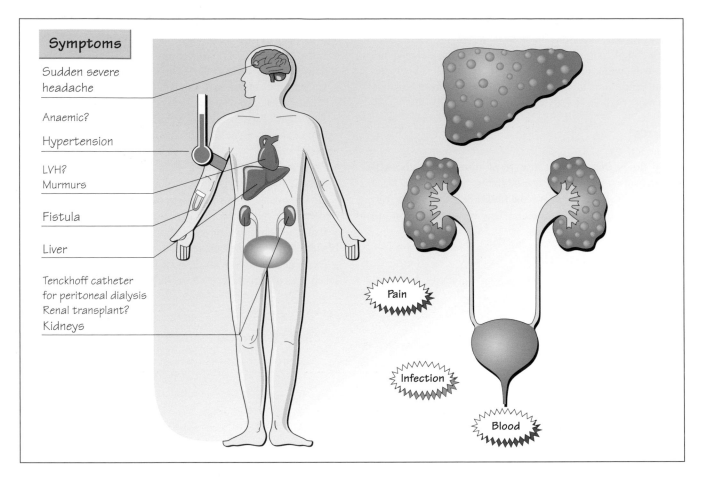

Symptoms

Sudden severe headache

Anaemic?

Hypertension

LVH?
Murmurs

Fistula

Liver

Tenckhoff catheter for peritoneal dialysis
Renal transplant?
Kidneys

Pain

Infection

Blood

Polycystic kidney disease is inherited in an autosomal dominant manner in which gradually enlarging renal cysts are associated with progressive renal impairment. It may present with chronic renal failure or be found during screening of relatives of patients with the disease. More unusually it can present with an abdominal mass, with hypertension or with rupture of an associated intracranial Berry aneurysm causing a subarachnoid haemorrhage. The renal failure most commonly manifests in middle age and might present with vomiting, nausea, anorexia, itching, fatigue, polyuria, etc. The cysts can bleed producing haematuria, become infected or be painful. There is an increased incidence of cardiac disease including valvular abnormalities, herniae and diverticular disease. It has a prevalence of 0.1%.

History
• Local symptoms: pain (flank, abdominal, back), gross haematuria, UTIs?
• Symptoms of renal failure?
• Requirement for dialysis/transplant?
• Symptoms of subarachnoid haemorrhage (sudden severe headache)?

Past medical history
Does the patient show signs of hypertension, cardiac disease or subarachnoid haemorrhage?

Drugs
Is the patient taking anti-hypertensives or medication required following the development of renal failure (e.g. erythropoietin, phosphate binders)?

Family history
An accurate family history is required.

Examination
• Signs of chronic renal failure (anaemia, fluid overload)?
• Examine for dialysis access: fistula, central line, transplant and Tenckhoff catheter.
• Examine for hypertension and check for end-organ damage (e.g. retinopathy, left ventricular hypertrophy).
• Are there bilateral palpable kidneys? (Classically ballottable, irregular and bilateral [though may be difficult to palpate or only palpable unilaterally].)
• Is there an enlarged cystic liver? (Liver failure is rare.)
• Examine for mitral valve prolapse, aortic regurgitation and mitral regurgitation.

83 Nephrotic syndrome

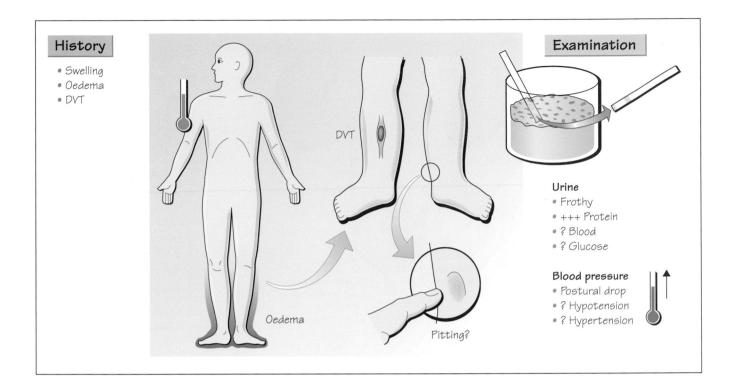

History
- Swelling
- Oedema
- DVT

DVT

Oedema

Pitting?

Examination

Urine
- Frothy
- +++ Protein
- ? Blood
- ? Glucose

Blood pressure
- Postural drop
- ? Hypotension
- ? Hypertension

Nephrotic syndrome is defined as proteinuria > 4.5 g/day with hypoalbuminaemia and peripheral oedema. It presents with oedema usually of the legs but sometimes progressing to involve the trunk and, rarely, oedema can be noticeable in the face. The proteinuria can cause the urine to be frothy. There is an increased incidence of thromboembolism.

History
- Is there history of oedema? If so, where?
- Has the patient passed frothy urine?
- Are there any symptoms suggesting PE or DVT?

Past medical history
Any history of:
- known renal disease (especially glomerulonephritis)?
- previous renal biopsy?
- previous episodes of oedema and response to treatment?
- previous proteinuria?
- other associated diseases such as SLE?

Drugs
- Is the patient using diuretics?
- Does the patient take any immunosuppressive medication (e.g. corticosteroids, cyclophosphamide, cyclosporin)?
- Is the patient using NSAIDs (can cause nephrotic syndrome)?
- Is the patient anticoagulatcd?

Examination
- Does the patient have oedema or pitting?
- Check the patient's BP.
- What is the patient's fluid status? Overloaded/elevated JVP? Hypovolaemic (hypotension and postural drop)?
- Undertake urine dipstick/microscopy.
- Check the patient's weight (most accurate indicator of fluid loss/gain).

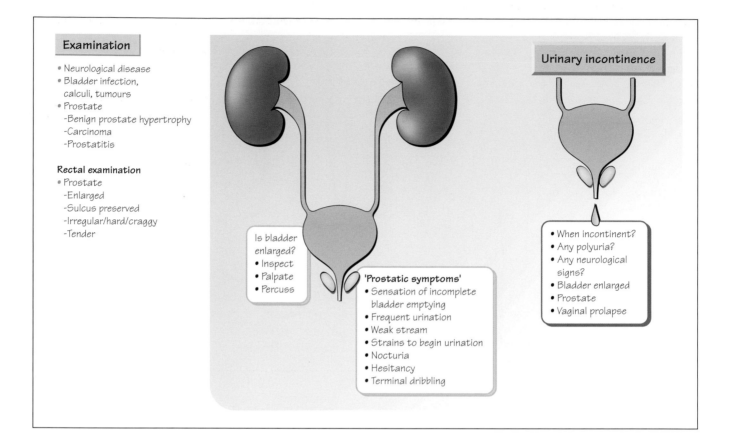

84 Urinary symptoms

Examination

- Neurological disease
- Bladder infection, calculi, tumours
- Prostate
  -Benign prostate hypertrophy
  -Carcinoma
  -Prostatitis

Rectal examination
- Prostate
  -Enlarged
  -Sulcus preserved
  -Irregular/hard/craggy
  -Tender

Is bladder enlarged?
- Inspect
- Palpate
- Percuss

'Prostatic symptoms'
- Sensation of incomplete bladder emptying
- Frequent urination
- Weak stream
- Strains to begin urination
- Nocturia
- Hesitancy
- Terminal dribbling

Urinary incontinence
- When incontinent?
- Any polyuria?
- Any neurological signs?
- Bladder enlarged
- Prostate
- Vaginal prolapse

Urinary retention

The commonest cause of urinary retention is benign prostatic hypertrophy in men. Other causes include UTI, neurological disease or prostatic malignancy. It is important to establish whether there are other symptoms from the urinary tract, whether there is renal failure and if malignant disease could be responsible.

History

- When did the patient last pass urine?
- Does the patient feel the desire to pass urine?
- Is there pain or discomfort?
- Any recent haematuria?
- Any recent dysuria?
- Any strangury (painful desire but inability to pass urine)?
- Are there normally any difficulties with urinary stream? Does the patient have any hesitancy? Does the patient have a good urinary stream or terminal dribbling?
- Are there any symptoms suggestive of neurological disease (e.g. numbness or weakness of limbs)?
- Any faecal incontinence?

Past medical history

- Are there any previous episodes of urinary retention?
- Ask about previous operations, especially transurethral resection of prostate (TURP) or open prostatectomy.

- Any history of UTI?
- Any history of renal calculi?
- Any history of neurological diseases?

Drugs

- Is the patient taking any drugs that can promote urinary retention (e.g. tricyclic antidepressants)?
- Is the patient taking any treatments for UTI, prostatic hyperplasia/malignancy?

Examination

- Is the patient well or unwell? Fluid overloaded/in pain?
- Are there systemic features of infection (fever, tachycardia, loin tenderness)?
- Is the bladder enlarged? (Examine by palpation and percussion.)
- Is the prostate enlarged on rectal examination?
- Is the sulcus preserved? Is it hard and craggy (consider carcinoma of the prostate)? Is it tender (consider prostatitis)?
- If appropriate, are there any abnormalities on vaginal examination?
- Are there any abnormal neurological signs?
- Examine carefully for peripheral sensation including sacral area and the presence of tendon reflexes.

Urinary incontinence

Urinary incontinence in men is usually caused by prostatic enlargement. In women the commonest cause is pelvic floor weakness following childbirth, followed by detrusor instability. Other causes include immobility, dementia, stroke and in the context of any serious illness.

History

• When is the patient incontinent?
• Is it precipitated by coughing, straining, laughing (stress incontinence)?
• Is there excessive urine production (polyuria)?
• Is there immobility preventing the patient from getting to the toilet or diminished awareness due to sedation or confusion?

Past medical history

Ask about:
• childbirth, pregnancies and operations (e.g. hysterectomies, TURPs)

• neurological conditions (e.g. dementia, stroke)
• specific surgical procedures for incontinence.

Drugs

• Is the patient taking diuretics, treatments for detrusor instability or desmopressin?
• Is the patient taking hypnotics or anti-cholinergics?

Examination

• Look carefully for any signs of neurological disease.
• Is the bladder enlarged? Could this be retention with 'overflow'?
• Examine for vaginal prolapse, urethrocoele.
• Examine prostate with rectal examination.
• Is the patient constipated?

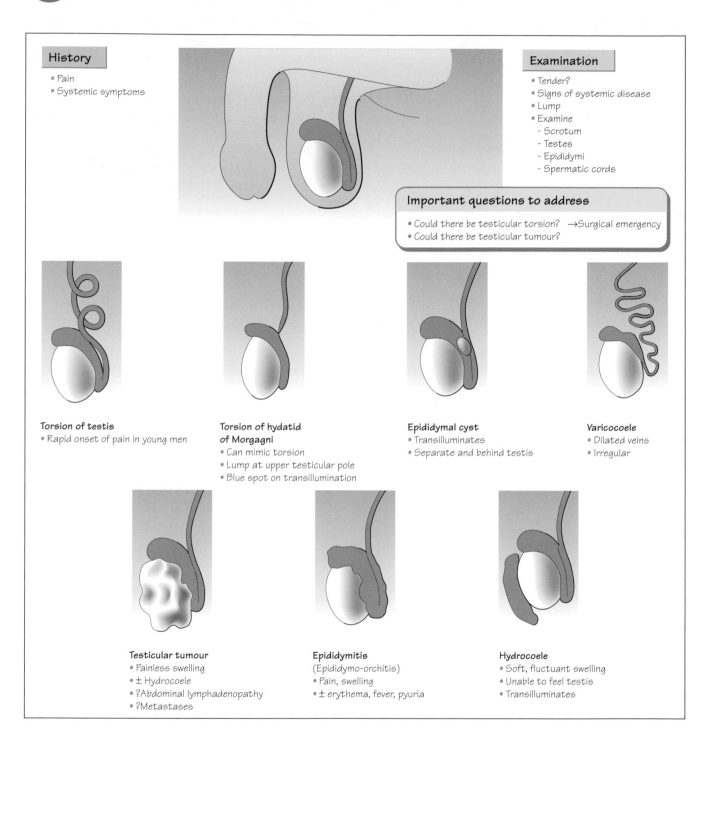

History
- Pain
- Systemic symptoms

Examination
- Tender?
- Signs of systemic disease
- Lump
- Examine
  - Scrotum
  - Testes
  - Epididymi
  - Spermatic cords

Important questions to address
- Could there be testicular torsion? →Surgical emergency
- Could there be testicular tumour?

Torsion of testis
- Rapid onset of pain in young men

Torsion of hydatid of Morgagni
- Can mimic torsion
- Lump at upper testicular pole
- Blue spot on transillumination

Epididymal cyst
- Transilluminates
- Separate and behind testis

Varicocoele
- Dilated veins
- Irregular

Testicular tumour
- Painless swelling
- ± Hydrocoele
- ?Abdominal lymphadenopathy
- ?Metastases

Epididymitis
(Epididymo-orchitis)
- Pain, swelling
- ± erythema, fever, pyuria

Hydrocoele
- Soft, fluctuant swelling
- Unable to feel testis
- Transilluminates

Testicular lumps may present with discomfort, pain or the lump may be noticed by the patient. Testicular lumps may represent benign pathology, such as a hydrocoele, or be due to a highly malignant but treatable teratoma or seminoma.

History

• How was the lump first noticed? Is it enlarging? Has there been pain or discomfort?
• Are there any other genitourinary symptoms (e.g. dysuria)?
• Are there any systemic symptoms (e.g. fever, weight loss, rigors) or symptoms of metastatic disease (e.g. back pain, haemoptysis)?
• Has there been bowel disturbance (e.g. with strangulated hernia)?

Past medical history

Any history of previous testicular lumps, herniae?

Examination

• Is the patient uncomfortable and in pain?
• Are there features of infection or metastatic disease?
• Examine for fever, anaemia, lymphadenopathy, hepatomegaly and jaundice.
• Examine the scrotum: any obvious swelling, change in skin colour?
• Palpate the testes: are they symmetrical, is there a lump, is there generalized or local swelling, are they of similar consistency? Is there localized tenderness, warmth? Identify the epididymis and spermatic cord. Any cough impulse?
• Is there transillumination of any swelling?
• Also examine the penis, the urine for pyuria, and consider digital rectal examination of the prostate.

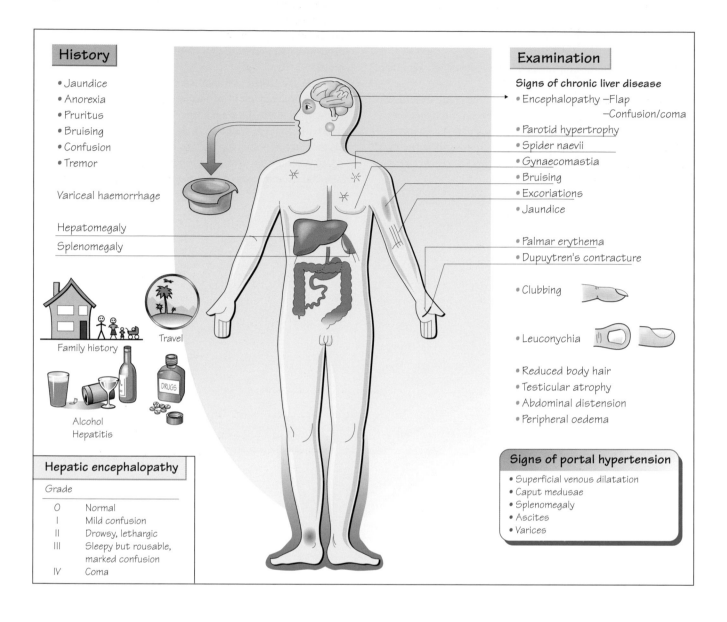

History

- Jaundice
- Anorexia
- Pruritus
- Bruising
- Confusion
- Tremor

Variceal haemorrhage

Hepatomegaly
Splenomegaly

Family history
Travel

Alcohol
Hepatitis

Examination

Signs of chronic liver disease

- Encephalopathy —Flap
  —Confusion/coma
- Parotid hypertrophy
- Spider naevii
- Gynaecomastia
- Bruising
- Excoriations
- Jaundice

- Palmar erythema
- Dupuytren's contracture

- Clubbing

- Leuconychia

- Reduced body hair
- Testicular atrophy
- Abdominal distension
- Peripheral oedema

Hepatic encephalopathy

Grade	
0	Normal
I	Mild confusion
II	Drowsy, lethargic
III	Sleepy but rousable, marked confusion
IV	Coma

Signs of portal hypertension

- Superficial venous dilatation
- Caput medusae
- Splenomegaly
- Ascites
- Varices

Chronic liver disease may present with features of impaired synthetic function such as oedema, bruising or jaundice; with features of portal hypertension such as ascites, abdominal pain or variceal haemorrhage; or with general malaise, pruritus, fatigue and anorexia. Alternatively the underlying aetiology, such as excess alcohol consumption, may bring the problem to light or it may be discovered incidentally during routine blood testing.

Important causes include alcohol-induced liver disease, viral hepatitis, autoimmune liver disease, primary biliary cirrhosis, haemochromatosis, primary sclerosing cholangiitis and Wilson's disease. Chronic liver disease has a prevalence of 100/100 000.

History

- Is there jaundice, bruising, abdominal distension, anorexia, pruritus, peripheral oedema, confusion or tremor?

- When were symptoms first noted? Has there been any deterioration and, if so, why? Has there been any change in medication or evidence of infection?
- Have friends or relatives noticed any changes?
- Is the patient's urine dark? Are the patient's stools pale?

Past medical history

- Has the patient ever been jaundiced?
- Any history of haematemesis or melaena?
- Any history of previous hepatitis? If so, how acquired (e.g. blood transfusion, intravenous drug use)?
- Has the patient had any previous blood transfusions?

Family history

- Any family history of liver disease (e.g. Wilson's disease, α_1-antitrypsin deficiency, hepatitis B infection)?

- Any family history of neurological symptoms (e.g. Parkinsonian or dystonic symptoms in Wilson's disease)?
- Any family history of diabetes mellitus (consider haemochromatosis)?

Drugs
- What medication is the patient taking? Any recent medication changes? Is the patient taking any herbal remedies?
- Is the patient taking any illegal, especially intravenous, drugs?

Alcohol
- What is the patient's daily/weekly consumption? Does the patient ever drink beer, wine, spirits, etc.?
- Use the **CAGE** questions:
  - Ever tried to **C**ut down?
  - Have people **A**nnoyed you by criticising your drinking?
  - Ever felt **G**uilty about alcohol consumption?
  - Ever drink early in morning (**E**ye-opener)?

Examination
- Is the patient well or unwell?
- Are there any signs of encephalopathy (e.g. confusion, coma, liver flap [asterixis])?
- Check hepatic foetor/smell of alcohol
- Any fever?
- Any melaena?
- Any signs of chronic liver disease:
  - spider naevii
  - palmar erythema
  - Dupuytren's contracture
  - clubbing
  - leuconychia
  - bruising
  - wasting
  - excoriations (suggesting obstructive jaundice)
  - gynaecomastia
  - jaundice
  - parotid enlargement
  - testicular atrophy
  - reduced body hair
  - abdominal distension.
- Is the liver palpable? Check size (percussion), border (regular/irregular) and if tender.
- Any peripheral oedema?
- Any signs of portal hypertension?
- Any superficial venous dilatation or caput medusa?
- Is there splenomegaly or ascites (shifting dullness to percussion)?

Specific clinical findings
Wilson's disease
- Kayser–Fleischer rings
- Neurological features: Parkinsonism, dystonia
- Sunflower cataracts

Haemochromatosis:
- 'Bronze' pigmentation
- Diabetes mellitus
- Arthritis
- Cardiac failure

Important clinical questions
- Are there signs of **chronic** liver disease?
- Are there pointers to the aetiology of the liver failure?
- How severe is the liver failure?

Inflammatory bowel disease

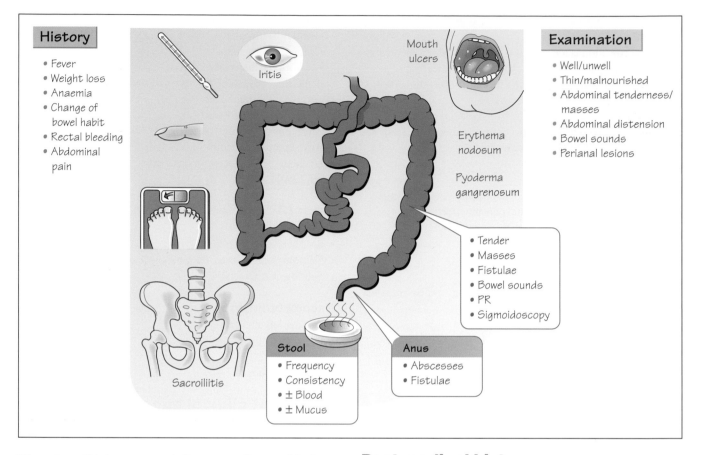

History
- Fever
- Weight loss
- Anaemia
- Change of bowel habit
- Rectal bleeding
- Abdominal pain

Iritis

Mouth ulcers

Erythema nodosum

Pyoderma gangrenosum

Examination
- Well/unwell
- Thin/malnourished
- Abdominal tenderness/ masses
- Abdominal distension
- Bowel sounds
- Perianal lesions

- Tender
- Masses
- Fistulae
- Bowel sounds
- PR
- Sigmoidoscopy

Sacroiliitis

Stool
- Frequency
- Consistency
- ± Blood
- ± Mucus

Anus
- Abscesses
- Fistulae

Ulcerative colitis is a recurrent inflammatory disease of the large bowel that includes involvement of the rectum. Crohn's disease is a similar chronic inflammatory disease of any part of the gut but with preferential involvement of the terminal ileum and ileocaecal region. Ulcerative colitis and Crohn's disease can present with local manifestations such as diarrhoea, abdominal pain, blood per rectum; with systemic symptoms such as weight loss or anaemia; or with associated symptoms such as iritis, pyoderma gangrenosum or sacroiliitis. Inflammatory bowel disease has a prevalence of 200/100 000; the incidence of new cases is 15/100 000 per year.

History
- When did the patient's bowel habit change? What is the frequency of stools? What is the consistency: any blood or mucus?
- Does the patient have abdominal pain? If so, where? What is its relationship to defaecation?
- Does the patient have mouth ulcers or perianal disease?
- Does the patient have a fever, weight loss, anorexia or symptoms of anaemia?
- Does the patient have iritis or sacroiliitis?
- Does the patient have any food allergies/intolerances?
- During severe attacks are symptoms suggestive of hypovolaemia/acute abdomen?
- Has there been any alteration in symptoms? Beware of an increased incidence in carcinoma after 5–10 years of active disease.

Past medical history
- What was the patient's previous response to treatments/operations/bowel resection, colostomies/ileostomies?
- Has the patient had any endoscopies/biopsies?
- Has the patient had any associated diseases (e.g. ulcerative colitis and sclerosing cholangiitis)?

Drugs
- Is the patient taking any corticosteroids, local or systemic?
- Is the patient taking immunosuppressants: azathioprine, cyclosporin, anti-TNF antibodies?
- Does the patient smoke or drink alcohol?

Family and social history
- Any family history of inflammatory bowel disease?
- Does the disease interfere with life (ability to work, etc.)?

Examination
- Is the patient well or unwell?
- Is the patient thin and/or poorly nourished?
- Are there any signs of pyoderma gangrenosum?
- Does the patient have: iritis, anaemia, clubbing, arthropathy, abdominal distension or abdominal tenderness or fistulae?
- Check bowel sounds.
- Perform a rectal examination.

88 Splenomegaly/hepatosplenomegaly

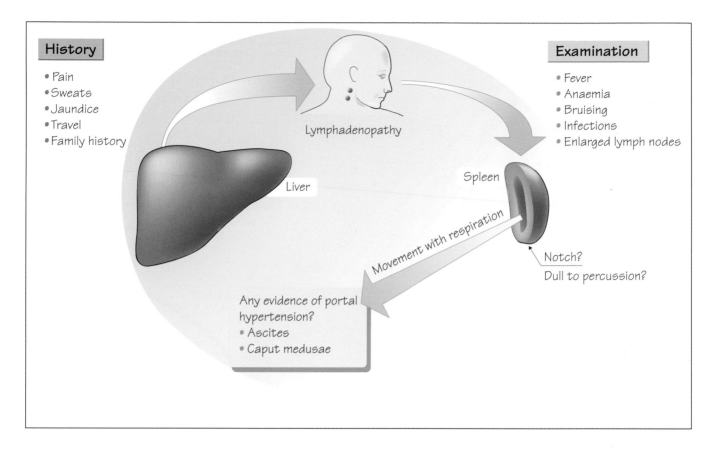

History
- Pain
- Sweats
- Jaundice
- Travel
- Family history

Lymphadenopathy

Examination
- Fever
- Anaemia
- Bruising
- Infections
- Enlarged lymph nodes

Liver

Spleen

Movement with respiration

Notch?
Dull to percussion?

Any evidence of portal hypertension?
- Ascites
- Caput medusae

Enlargement of the spleen and/or liver is usually detected by clinical examination. Symptoms of pain, discomfort or abdominal distension may occur but are unusual.

It is a very important finding in any patient with fever, anaemia or other unexplained illness.

History
- Any local abdominal pain, discomfort or distension?
- Are there any features suggesting haematological disease (e.g. easy bruising or bleeding symptoms of anaemia, infections, sweats or fevers)?
- Are there any features suggesting liver disease and, in particular, portal hypertension (e.g. jaundice, abdominal distension, etc.)?
- Are there any features of current infection (e.g. fever, rigors or jaundice suggesting infections such as malaria or glandular fever)?

Past medical history
- Any history of haematological disorders (e.g. lymphoma, leukaemia)?
- Any history of liver disease?
- Has the patient had any infective conditions (e.g. malaria)?
- Any personal history of inherited metabolic conditions (e.g. Gaucher's disease)?

Family history
Ask about any family history of inherited metabolic conditions (e.g. Gaucher's disease)?

Examination
- Is there anaemia, bruising, petechiae, polycythaemia, jaundice or lymphadenopathy?
- Does the patient have a fever?
- Are there signs of chronic liver disease and portal hypertension?
- Are there signs of infective endocarditis?
- Examine the patient for splenomegaly. Start from the right iliac fossa. Is there an edge? If so, does it move diagonally with respiration? Any overlying resonance to percussion? Is it tender? You need to distinguish from other masses that may be palpable in the left upper quadrant, such as an enlarged kidney (e.g. polycystic kidney), enlarged left lobe of liver or gastric and colonic malignancy.
- If either the spleen or liver is enlarged it is crucial to examine for enlargement of the other organ (i.e. is there hepatosplenomegaly)?

Acute abdomen

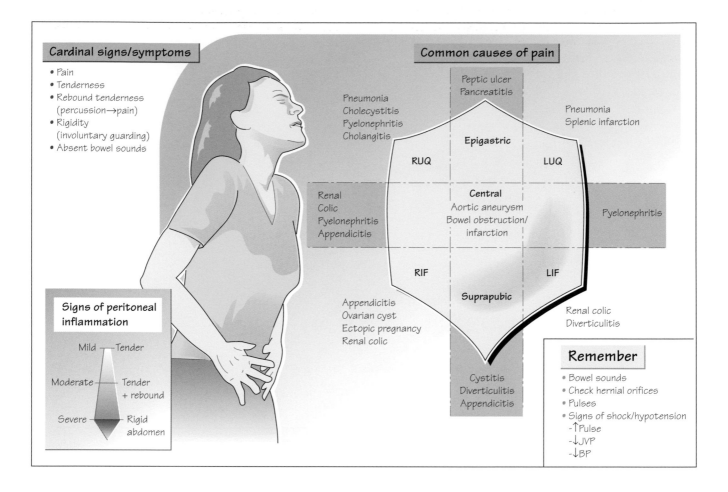

Cardinal signs/symptoms

- Pain
- Tenderness
- Rebound tenderness (percussion→pain)
- Rigidity (involuntary guarding)
- Absent bowel sounds

Signs of peritoneal inflammation

Mild — Tender

Moderate — Tender + rebound

Severe — Rigid abdomen

Common causes of pain

Pneumonia
Cholecystitis
Pyelonephritis
Cholangitis

Peptic ulcer
Pancreatitis

Pneumonia
Splenic infarction

Epigastric

RUQ   LUQ

Renal
Colic
Pyelonephritis
Appendicitis

Central
Aortic aneurysm
Bowel obstruction/infarction

Pyelonephritis

RIF   LIF

Suprapubic

Appendicitis
Ovarian cyst
Ectopic pregnancy
Renal colic

Renal colic
Diverticulitis

Cystitis
Diverticulitis
Appendicitis

Remember

- Bowel sounds
- Check hernial orifices
- Pulses
- Signs of shock/hypotension
  - ↑Pulse
  - ↓JVP
  - ↓BP

The term acute abdomen implies a presentation with the sudden onset of abdominal pain with features on examination of tenderness, guarding and rebound tenderness. It most commonly arises from intra-abdominal pathologies, such as perforated peptic ulcer, pancreatitis, perforated diverticulum, perforated appendix, ruptured aneurysm, ischaemic bowel or trauma. However, rarely, extra-abdominal disease, such as pneumonia, myocardial infarction or acidosis, can mimic the acute abdomen.

History

- When did pain start? Where did it start and has it moved? Does it radiate (e.g. to back, loin or chest)?
- Did the pain start suddenly or gradually?
- Have there been any accompanying symptoms: nausea, vomiting, constipation, back pain, haematemesis or melaena?
- What exacerbates the pain: movement, travel to hospital in the ambulance, breathing, coughing?
- When were the bowels last open? When was flatus last passed?

Past medical history

- Any history of indigestion, abdominal pain or abdominal operations?

- Any known aortic aneurysm, peptic ulcers, diverticular disease or pancreatitis?
- Consider the patient's fitness for general anaesthesia.

Drugs

- Is the patient using NSAIDs?
- Does the patient have any known allergies?

Family history

Any family history of rare metabolic causes of abdominal pain (e.g. porphyria, familial Mediterranean fever)?

Examination

- Is the patient well or unwell? If unwell, give oxygen and resuscitate with intravenous fluids.
- Is the patient shocked or confused?
- Does the patient look pale/anaemic?
- Is the patient in pain? Is the patient keeping very still?
- Check pulse, BP and postural hypotension.
- Check respiratory rate: any tachypnoea?
- Check JVP.
- Perform a chest examination and consider pneumonia (especially basal).

- Inspect the abdomen for distension or masses.
- Any skin discoloration, bruising (Grey–Turner's sign [flanks], Cullen's sign [periumbilical])?
- Gently palpate. Is there rigidity/tenderness? Is there an area of maximal tenderness? Any guarding? Any rebound tenderness?
- Is the aorta palpable? Are peripheral pulses present?
- Check the patient for herniae.
- Check the liver/spleen/kidneys are palpable.
- Auscultate: are bowel sounds absent or high pitched? Are there signs of bruits?
- Perform a rectal examination.
- Urine: check for haematuria. Use dipstick test for haematuria and leucocytes.

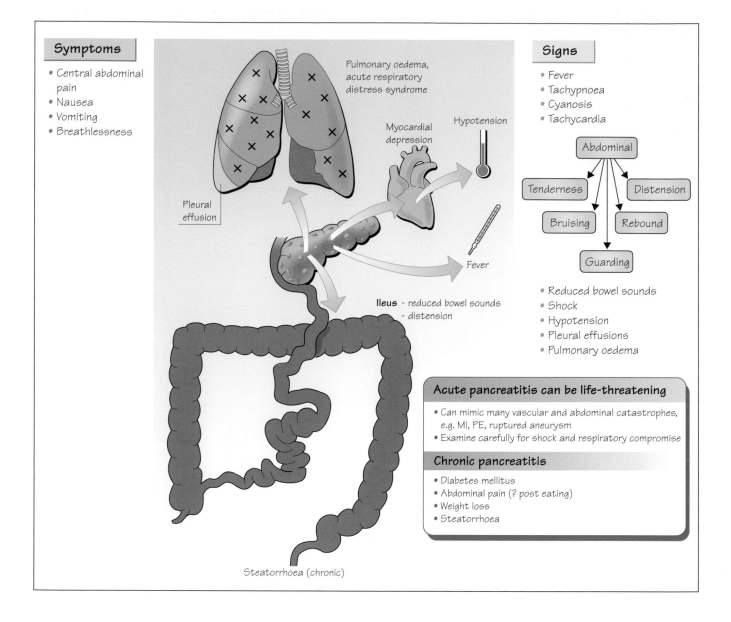

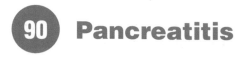

Symptoms

- Central abdominal pain
- Nausea
- Vomiting
- Breathlessness

Pulmonary oedema, acute respiratory distress syndrome

Hypotension

Myocardial depression

Pleural effusion

Fever

Ileus - reduced bowel sounds
- distension

Steatorrhoea (chronic)

Signs

- Fever
- Tachypnoea
- Cyanosis
- Tachycardia

Abdominal

Tenderness   Distension

Bruising   Rebound

Guarding

- Reduced bowel sounds
- Shock
- Hypotension
- Pleural effusions
- Pulmonary oedema

Acute pancreatitis can be life-threatening

- Can mimic many vascular and abdominal catastrophes, e.g. MI, PE, ruptured aneurysm
- Examine carefully for shock and respiratory compromise

Chronic pancreatitis

- Diabetes mellitus
- Abdominal pain (? post eating)
- Weight loss
- Steatorrhoea

Pancreatitis is an inflammatory condition of the pancreas that is provoked most commonly by gallstones or alcohol. If severe there can be massive inflammation, necrosis and sequestration of fluid with resultant shock and respiratory distress. Acute pancreatitis most commonly presents with severe abdominal pain. It can mimic many other important conditions, such as myocardial infarction, ruptured aortic aneurysm or any cause of an acute abdomen, such as perforated peptic ulcer. Chronic pancreatitis may produce malabsorption with weight loss and steatorrhoea.

History

• When did the pain start? Where did it start and is there any radiation? If so does it radiate to the back? Is it accompanied by vomiting? Are there any other symptoms? Is the pain precipitated by food?

• Are there any respiratory symptoms (especially shortness of breath)?

• Are there any other GI symptoms: nausea, vomiting, constipation?

Past medical history

• Are there any previous episodes of pancreatitis?
• Any history of known alcohol abuse?
• Is there a history of gallstones?
• Are there any signs of hyperlipidaemia?

Drugs

• Ask about drugs that can precipitate pancreatitis (e.g. azathioprine).
• Obtain a careful history of alcohol consumption.

Examination

- The examination should focus particularly on the presence of respiratory difficulties, shock and hypovolaemia.
- Is the patient well or unwell? Patients with severe pancreatitis can be very severely ill with shock, sepsis syndrome and respiratory failure.
- Are there any signs of diabetes mellitus?
- Does the patient have a fever?
- Is the patient pale, shocked? Check for tachycardia and hypotension. Is there a postural fall in BP?

- Check the respiratory rate. Are there any signs of respiratory distress? Check for pulmonary oedema: any crackles, pleural effusions?
- Is the patient jaundiced? Any other evidence of alcohol excess or chronic liver disease?
- Check the abdomen. Is it tender or rigid? Is the patient guarding? Is there rebound tenderness? Are there absent bowel sounds?
- Is there bluish discoloration of flanks (Grey–Turner's sign) or periumbilical area (Cullen's sign)?

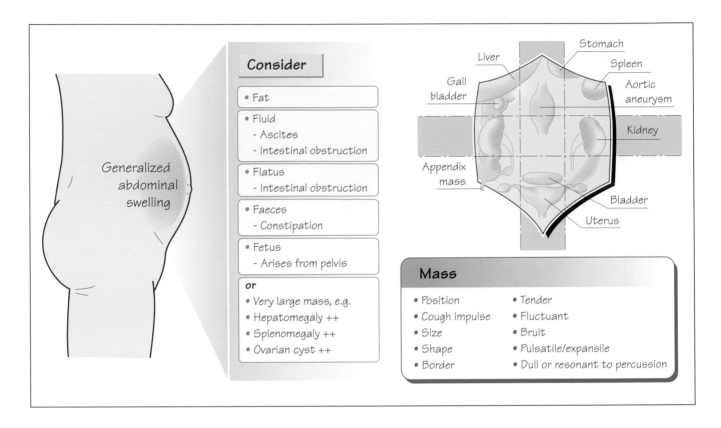

Abdominal masses may be noticed by the patient or be discovered incidentally during clinical examination or during investigation of symptoms, such as weight loss, change in bowel habit, anaemia or rectal bleeding.

History
• When was the mass first noticed and by whom?
• Any pain, discomfort?
• Any systemic features: weight loss, anorexia, fever?
• Any features of bowel obstruction (abdominal pain, distension, vomiting, constipation? Any changes in bowel habit?
• Any haematemesis, melaena or rectal bleeding?

Past medical history
• Ask about previous illnesses, especially abdominal disorders/operations.
• Is there any history of herniae or abdominal aortic aneurysm?

Family history
Any family history of bowel cancer or polycystic kidney disease?

Examination
• Is the patient well or unwell?
• Is the patient comfortable or in pain?
• Any evidence of weight loss, jaundice, anaemia, lymphadenopathy (especially Virchow's node)?
• Inspect the abdomen: is there an obvious mass? If so, is it increased on coughing?

• Palpation: check size, shape, position, border, tender, fluctuant, consistency and pulsatile/expansile.
• Auscultate: check bruit and succussion splash.
• Ascites present?
• Examine for liver, spleen, kidneys, aorta and herniae.
• Perform rectal, genitalia and vaginal examinations.

Herniae
A hernia is the protrusion of an organ or other structure through the wall that normally contains it. Abdominal herniae present as a lump which may be reduced with direct pressure and have an expansile cough impulse or as localized discomfort. They may be irreducible or may become obstructed and strangulated.
• Abdominal herniae may be:
  • inguinal (Either direct, pushing through the posterior wall of the inguinal canal and rarely strangulate or indirect, passing through the internal inguinal ring. They appear from above and medial to the pubic tubercle, can descend into the scrotum and are more common in men than women.)
  • femoral (Appear through the femoral canal below and lateral to the pubic tubercle, frequently strangulate and are more common in women than men.)
  • or more rarely umbilical, epigastric, spighelian, obturator or incisional.
• In examining a patient with a suspected hernia it is often helpful to get the patient to stand and to cough. Is the swelling reducible? Is it tender? Any features of bowel obstruction?

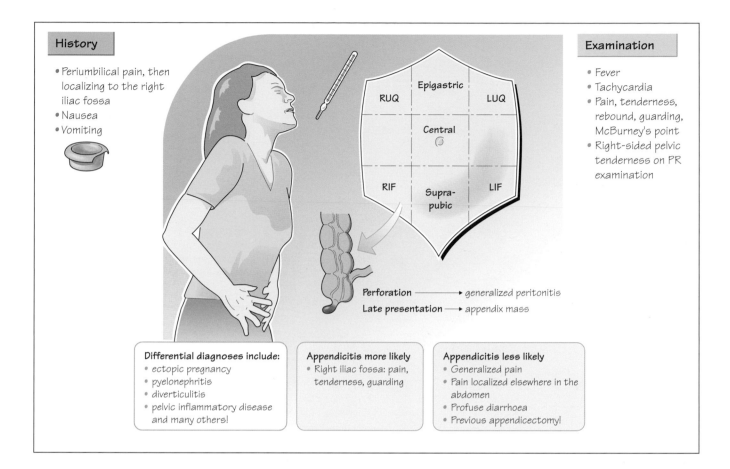

History
- Periumbilical pain, then localizing to the right iliac fossa
- Nausea
- Vomiting

Examination
- Fever
- Tachycardia
- Pain, tenderness, rebound, guarding, McBurney's point
- Right-sided pelvic tenderness on PR examination

Perforation ⟶ generalized peritonitis
Late presentation ⟶ appendix mass

Differential diagnoses include:
- ectopic pregnancy
- pyelonephritis
- diverticulitis
- pelvic inflammatory disease and many others!

Appendicitis more likely
- Right iliac fossa: pain, tenderness, guarding

Appendicitis less likely
- Generalized pain
- Pain localized elsewhere in the abdomen
- Profuse diarrhoea
- Previous appendicectomy!

Appendicitis is an acute inflammatory condition of the appendix in association with luminal obstruction and bacterial infection. It usually presents with abdominal pain. Classically the pain is initially diffuse and periumbilical, subsequently localizing to the right iliac fossa. However, other presentations with generalized pain, diarrhoea, vomiting or fever can occur. It can be very difficult to distinguish from other causes of abdominal pain. It is the commonest surgical emergency and can occur at any age. It has an incidence of 120/100 000 per year (although this may be falling).

History
- Where is the pain? What is the pain like? When did it start? Where?
- Has the pain moved? Where is the worst pain?
- Are there any other symptoms: vomiting, fever, anorexia, diarrhoea, dysuria or vaginal discharge?
- Could the patient be pregnant? Is the patient sexually active?

At what stage is her menstrual cycle and are there any problems with menstruation?
- Are there any urinary symptoms?
- Have there been previous episodes?
- Any previous appendicectomy (!)?

Examination
- Is the patient well or unwell? Is the patient in pain or comfortable? Is the patient lying still or moving uneasily?
- Is the patient febrile?
- Is the patient flushed?
- Check for tachycardia and hypotension.
- Check the abdomen: is there tenderness? If so, where is the area of maximal tenderness: McBurney's point? Is there rigidity, guarding, rebound mass, bowel sounds?
- Perform a rectal examination. Is there pain in right iliac fossa or locally?
- Perform a vaginal examination.

93 Asthma

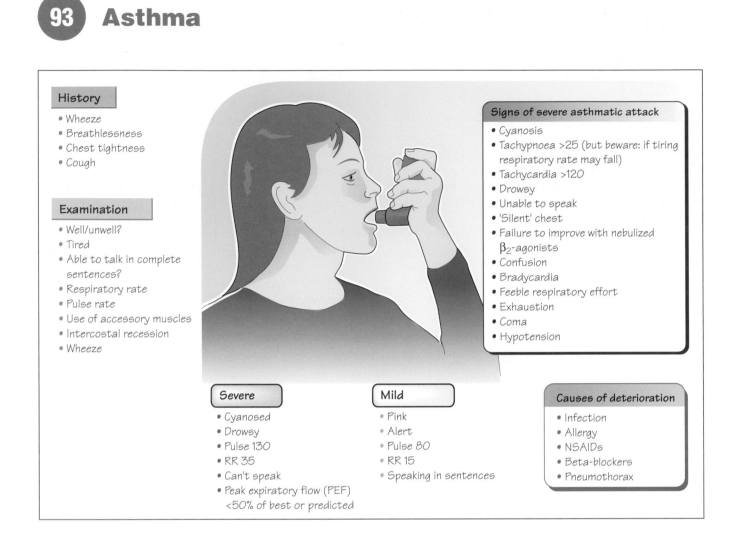

History
- Wheeze
- Breathlessness
- Chest tightness
- Cough

Examination
- Well/unwell?
- Tired
- Able to talk in complete sentences?
- Respiratory rate
- Pulse rate
- Use of accessory muscles
- Intercostal recession
- Wheeze

Signs of severe asthmatic attack
- Cyanosis
- Tachypnoea >25 (but beware: if tiring respiratory rate may fall)
- Tachycardia >120
- Drowsy
- Unable to speak
- 'Silent' chest
- Failure to improve with nebulized β_2-agonists
- Confusion
- Bradycardia
- Feeble respiratory effort
- Exhaustion
- Coma
- Hypotension

Severe
- Cyanosed
- Drowsy
- Pulse 130
- RR 35
- Can't speak
- Peak expiratory flow (PEF) <50% of best or predicted

Mild
- Pink
- Alert
- Pulse 80
- RR 15
- Speaking in sentences

Causes of deterioration
- Infection
- Allergy
- NSAIDs
- Beta-blockers
- Pneumothorax

Asthma is a very common condition characterized by episodic breathlessness and wheeze. Other symptoms such as cough also occur. The patient often describes their chest as feeling tight. It has a prevalence of at least 5%. The symptoms of asthma tend to be variable, intermittent, worse at night and provoked by triggers including exercise. Consider the diagnosis of asthma in any patient with episodic or variable wheeze, shortness of breath, chest tightness, or cough.

History
- What precipitated the attack: respiratory tract infection, exercise, allergen, aspirin/NSAIDs or cold air?
- What are the symptoms: wheeze (usually diffuse, polyphonic, bilateral and particularly expiratory), cough and breathlessness?
- Any unusual features present (severe chest pains, haemoptysis)?
- What has been the response to therapy (inhalers, nebulizers, corticosteroids)? Do they monitor their peak expiratory flow rate?
- When assessing the patient with severe asthma a calm and reassuring approach can be very therapeutic.

Past medical history
- Any previous admissions for asthma?

- Has the patient ever been artificially ventilated for asthmatic attack?
- Is the patient's sleep disturbed by asthma?
- What is the patient's usual exercise tolerance?
- Has the patient taken any days off work/school due to asthma?
- Does the patient have any other features of atopy (e.g. eczema/rhinitis)?
- Any diurnal variation in symptoms? (NB. Early morning deterioration is common.)
- Are there any associated diseases (e.g. bronchopulmonary aspergillosis, Churg–Strauss syndrome)?

Family and social history
- Assess the impact of the disease on the patient's life.
- Is there a family history of asthma/atopy?
- What is the patient's occupation? Any deterioration of asthma at work/relief at weekends? (There are specific occupational causes of asthma.)

Drugs
- What is usual treatment: inhalers, nebulizers, corticosteroids (inhaled or oral) or aminophylline?

- Do drugs show any precipitation of asthma (e.g. beta-blockers, aspirin)?
- Does the patient smoke?
- Does the patient have any allergies (e.g. to antibiotics, animals, pets or house dust mite)?

Examination

- If the patient is unwell administer oxygen by mask.
- Is the patient cyanosed?
- Is the patient distressed, frightened, able/unable to talk (complete sentences), tired or exhausted?
- Is there wheezing? (Distinguish from inspiratory stridor.) (NB. In severe asthma the chest may be 'silent' with little ventilation.)
- Any sputum? If so, what colour? Is it in plugs?
- What is the patient's respiratory rate?
- Check the patient's pulse rate.
- Check the patient's peak expiratory flow.
- In the well patient, examine his/her inhaler technique.
- Is there use of accessory muscles, intercostal recession?
- Consider pneumonia or pneumothorax as a cause of deterioration.
- Is there pulsus paradoxus? (NB. May be absent in severe attack.)
- Pulsus paradoxus (exaggerated decrease in BP on inspiration) can occur in severe asthma but may be absent in a severe attack and can also occur in pericardial tamponade, hypovolaemic shock, right ventricular failure and pulmonary embolism.

Other causes of breathlessness and wheeze

- Pulmonary oedema
- COPD
- Stridor
- Anaphylaxis

Patients at risk of developing fatal asthma

- Previous near fatal asthma, e.g. previous ventilation or respiratory acidosis.
- Previous admission for asthma especially in the last year.
- Requiring three or more classes of asthma medication.
- Heavy use of β_2-agonist.
- Repeated attendances at A&E for asthma care.
- Particularly if combined with adverse behavioural or psychosocial features.
- **NB. In an acute attack measure peak expiratory flow, pulse oximetry and perform arterial blood gases to determine Pao_2 and $Paco_2$. $Sao_2 < 92\%$, $Pao_2 < 8kPa$ and normal $Paco_2$ (4.6–6.0 kPa) or elevated $Paco_2$ are signs of a life-threatening attack.**

Evidence

The British Thoracic Society Guidelines. British guidelines on the management of asthma. *Thorax* 2003; **58** (Suppl. I): 1–94.

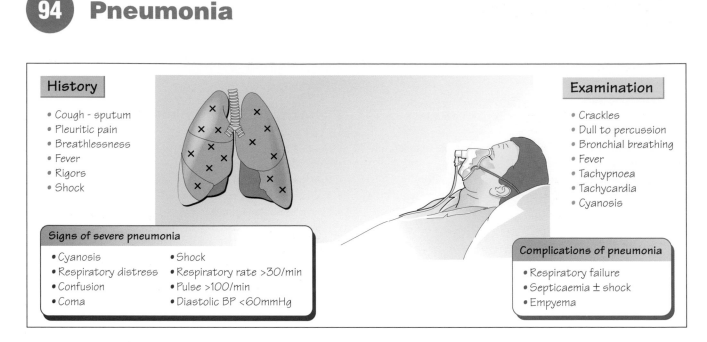

History

- Cough - sputum
- Pleuritic pain
- Breathlessness
- Fever
- Rigors
- Shock

Examination

- Crackles
- Dull to percussion
- Bronchial breathing
- Fever
- Tachypnoea
- Tachycardia
- Cyanosis

Signs of severe pneumonia

- Cyanosis
- Respiratory distress
- Confusion
- Coma
- Shock
- Respiratory rate >30/min
- Pulse >100/min
- Diastolic BP <60mmHg

Complications of pneumonia

- Respiratory failure
- Septicaemia ± shock
- Empyema

Pneumonia is a common illness of pulmonary infection acquired in the community or in hospital.

History

The symptoms of pneumonia may be local with a productive cough, breathlessness or pleuritic pain. The cough may be productive of sputum (often green) or contain blood (classically the rusty coloured sputum of pneumococcal pneumonia). There may be systemic symptoms, such as fatigue, anorexia, myalgias, fever and rigors. If severe, pneumonia may present with respiratory failure, shock or confusion.

The patient may have an underlying respiratory disease such as COPD or asthma, or be immunosuppressed due to drugs, HIV, neutropaenia or recent influenza. Other important aetiologies include aspiration, reduced coughing due to chest wall pain (e.g. rib fracture, postoperation) and bronchial obstruction due to tumour.

It is important to bear in mind that several serious illnesses may be difficult to distinguish from pneumonia including pulmonary embolus and pulmonary oedema.

Although the majority of pneumonias are caused by bacteria, such as *Streptococcus pneumoniae*, it is important to also consider more atypical pathogens, such as *Legionella*, *Mycoplasma* or *Mycobacterium tuberculosis*.

Examination

• As in any ill patient, it is vital to maintain the airway, ensure that breathing is adequate, provide supplemental oxygen and ensure circulatory adequacy.
• Is there respiratory distress (rapid shallow breathing, intercostal recession, fatigue)? Signs of cyanosis, respiratory distress, confusion, coma or shock imply a severe pneumonia requiring urgent treatment and resuscitation.
• A respiratory rate greater than 30 breaths/minute, a tachycardia > 100 b.p.m. and a temperature > 37.8°C increase the likelihood of pneumonia.

• In the chest focal consolidation may produce dullness to percussion, reduced breath sounds, bronchial breathing, and coarse crackles. It is important to recognize that severe pneumonia may be present and seen on a chest X-ray without such clinical findings. The sputum should be examined, and a chest X-ray and arterial blood gases are essential investigations.

Evidence

The **CURB-65** score can assess severity of pneumonia with a point each for:
• **C**onfusion
• **U**rea > 7 mmol/L
• **R**espiratory rate > 30/minute, low systolic (< 90 mmHg) or diastolic (≤ 60 mmHg)
• **B**lood pressure
• Age > **65** years at initial hospital assessment.
This enabled patients to be stratified according to increasing risk of mortality:

Score	Mortality (%)
0	0.7
1	3.2
2	3.0
3	17.0
4	41.5
5	57.0

Lim WS, van der Eerden MM, Laing R *et al*. Defining community acquired pneumonia severity on presentation to hospital: an international derivation and validation study. *Thorax* 2003; **58**: 377–82.

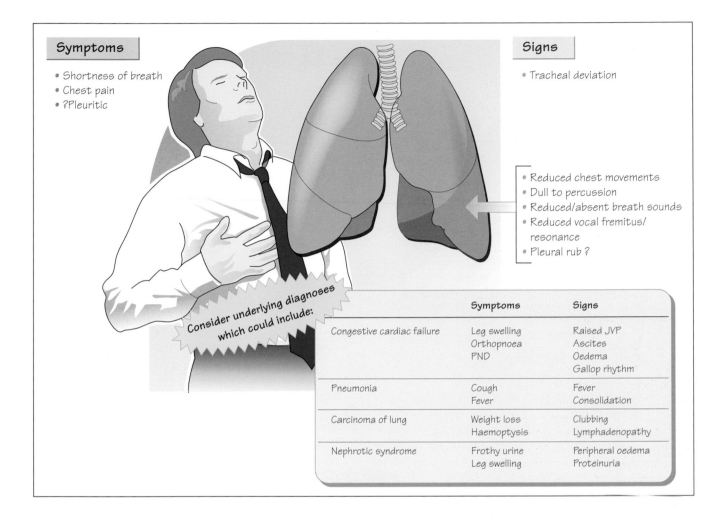

	Symptoms	Signs
Congestive cardiac failure	Leg swelling Orthopnoea PND	Raised JVP Ascites Oedema Gallop rhythm
Pneumonia	Cough Fever	Fever Consolidation
Carcinoma of lung	Weight loss Haemoptysis	Clubbing Lymphadenopathy
Nephrotic syndrome	Frothy urine Leg swelling	Peripheral oedema Proteinuria

Symptoms

- Shortness of breath
- Chest pain
- ?Pleuritic

Signs

- Tracheal deviation

- Reduced chest movements
- Dull to percussion
- Reduced/absent breath sounds
- Reduced vocal fremitus/resonance
- Pleural rub ?

Consider underlying diagnoses which could include:

Pleural effusion is the abnormal accumulation of fluid in the pleural space. Pleural effusion may present with shortness of breath, chest pains or due to symptoms of the underlying condition. The commoner causes include: congestive cardiac failure, pneumonia (?empyema), carcinoma of lung, lung metastases, mesothelioma, pulmonary embolus or nephrotic syndrome.

History

- When were the breathlessness, chest pains first noticed?
- What is the patient's exercise tolerance (breathless at rest, mild exertion, etc)?
- Are there any other symptoms suggesting one of the above aetiologies?
- Is there cough, haemoptysis, orthopnoea, paroxysmal nocturnal dyspnoea or peripheral oedema? Are there symptoms suggestive of malignancy elsewhere?
- Take a full smoking history (previous, current or passive) and gather a full occupational history (any asbestos exposure)?

Examination

- Does the patient look well or unwell?

- Is the patient in respiratory distress? Is the patient breathless at rest? (Treat with oxygen and consider drainage of the pleural effusion if unwell.)
- Is there clubbing? Is the patient thin, cyanosed, anaemic or jaundiced?
- Are chest movements symmetrical? Is the trachea central? Is percussion equal and resonant? Does the patient's breath sound present and symmetrical? Is there a pleural rub?
- Classically, a large unilateral pleural effusion produces reduced chest movements on the affected side, causes deviation of the trachea away from the affected side, with dullness (stony) to percussion and reduced (or absent) breath sounds on the affected side.
- Are there any signs of congestive cardiac failure (e.g. raised JVP, peripheral oedema or ascites)?
- Are there any signs of pneumonia (e.g. fever, productive cough or consolidation)?
- Are there any features suggestive of malignant disease (e.g. recent weight loss, haemoptysis or clubbing)?

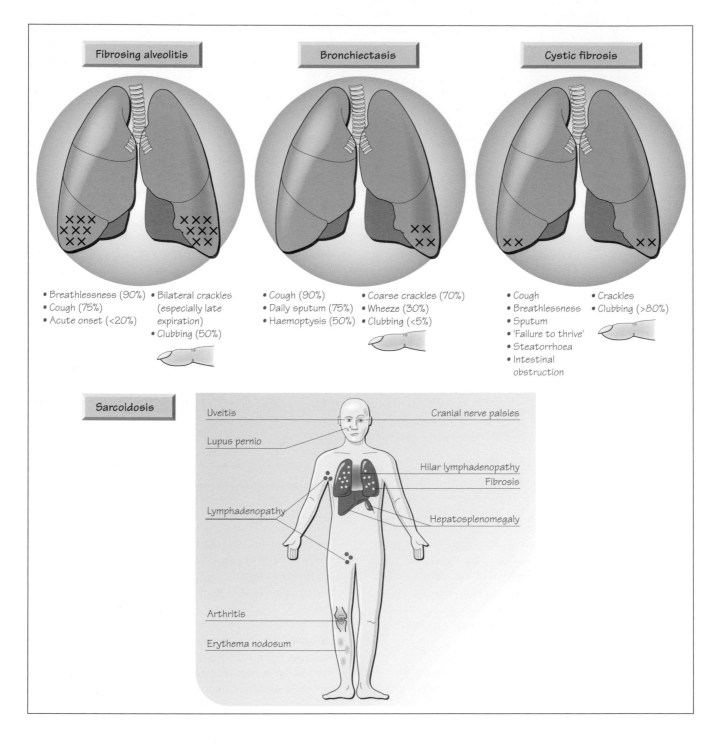

Fibrosing alveolitis

- Breathlessness (90%)
- Cough (75%)
- Acute onset (<20%)
- Bilateral crackles (especially late expiration)
- Clubbing (50%)

Bronchiectasis

- Cough (90%)
- Daily sputum (75%)
- Haemoptysis (50%)
- Coarse crackles (70%)
- Wheeze (30%)
- Clubbing (<5%)

Cystic fibrosis

- Cough
- Breathlessness
- Sputum
- 'Failure to thrive'
- Steatorrhoea
- Intestinal obstruction
- Crackles
- Clubbing (>80%)

Sarcoidosis

- Uveitis
- Lupus pernio
- Lymphadenopathy
- Arthritis
- Erythema nodosum
- Cranial nerve palsies
- Hilar lymphadenopathy
- Fibrosis
- Hepatosplenomegaly

Fibrosing alveolitis
History
Fibrosing alveolitis is characterized by inflammatory cells in the alveolar and interstitium together with pulmonary fibrosis. Patients with fibrosing alveolitis present with a gradually progressive shortness of breath, although more acute presentations can occur. There may be exertional dyspnoea and cough. There may be a history of exposure to allergens (e.g. extrinsic allergic alveolitis and bird fancier's lung) or of an associated disease, such as rheumatoid arthritis. Other classifications of interstitial lung disease have emerged recently based upon histological and radiographic findings. These include usual interstitial pneumonitis (UIP), non-specific interstitial pneumonitis (NSIP), bronchiolitis obliterans-organizing pneumonia (BOOP), respiratory bronchiolitis associated interstitial lung disease (RB-ILD), desquamative interstitial pneumonitis (DIP) and lymphocytic interstitial pneumonitis (LIP). However, the features on history and examination tend to be similar. Patients classically present with exercise-limiting breathlessness as their primary complaint. Many also have a troublesome non-productive cough. Bilateral basal crackles are prominent in all types of idiopathic interstitial pneumonia. Clubbing can be seen in all patients. A prolonged expiratory phase or wheezing is suggestive of RB-ILD or concomitant chronic obstructive pulmonary disease. Some respond well to treatment with steroids (e.g. NSIP, BOOP, RB-ILD and DIP) whilst others do not (e.g. UIP).

Past medical history
• Ask about other associated diseases (e.g. rheumatoid arthritis, scleroderma).
• A full drug history is vital and may reveal agents that can cause pulmonary fibrosis (e.g. amiodarone) and should detail treatments received, such as corticosteroids and other immunosuppressants.

Family and social history
The occupational history may reveal dust or allergen exposure (e.g. farmer's lung). The extent of disability should be sought, as should any hobbies or pets that might lead to allergen exposure.

Examination
• The classical features are clubbing and 'showers' of bilateral crackles.
• Is the patient breathless at rest or on exertion?
• Are there any signs of cyanosis?

Bronchiectasis
Bronchiectasis is a lung disease characterized by dilatation of bronchi that often become chronically infected. The classic symptom is of cough productive of purulent sputum. Many patients will have daily sputum production. There may also be haemoptysis and progressive deterioration in respiratory function. There may be winter exacerbations.

Past medical history
There may have been an underlying respiratory illness in childhood, such as pneumonia, whooping cough or TB. There are also rare inherited disorders with immotile cilia (Kartagener's = bronchiectasis and dextrocardia, defective cilia) or α_1-antitrypsin deficiency, and patients with immunodeficiency may present with bronchiectasis.

Examination
The commonest clinical finding is the presence of crackles on auscultation. In some patients wheeze may be audible. Clubbing may occur but is rare.

Cystic fibrosis
Cystic fibrosis is an inherited disorder usually presenting in childhood or adolescence with bronchiectasis. Other presentations include malabsorption due to pancreatic insufficiency with steatorrhoea, intestinal obstruction, rectal prolapse and failure to thrive.

Past medical history
• Any relevant previous hospital admissions?
• Any antibiotic treatments and any known colonization with antibiotic resistant organisms?
• Any treatments including postural drainage and chest physiotherapy and lung/heart–lung transplants?

Family history
Cystic fibrosis is autosomal recessive and so one in four siblings would be affected on average.

Examination
• Is the patient well or poorly nourished?
• Any indwelling line for antibiotic treatment?
• Any clubbing?
• Are there signs of respiratory distress?
• Does the patient have a productive cough?
• Rarely there may be signs of chronic liver disease.

Sarcoidosis
Sarcoidosis is a multisystem granulomatous condition that can affect many areas of the body but most commonly involves the lung. Presentations can be with breathlessness or incidentally noted hilar lymphadenopathy or fibrosis on chest X-ray. Other organs affected can include the skin (lupus pernio and erythema nodosum), joints (polyarthralgia), the eyes (uveitis) the CNS (neurosarcoid), or enhanced vitamin D hydroxylation can lead to hypercalcaemia.

Carcinoma of the lung

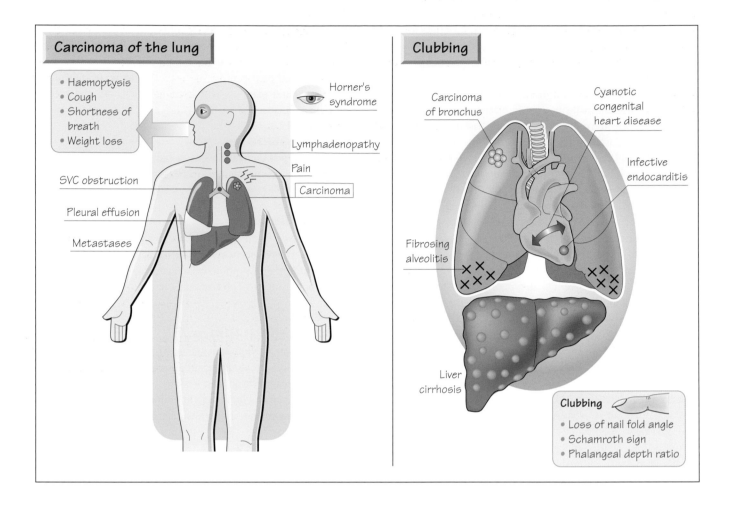

Carcinoma of the lung is the commonest fatal malignancy. It may present with symptoms due to local disease, due to metastases or due to the systemic effects of malignancy or be found incidentally during chest X-ray examination.

History

- *Symptoms of local disease:*
  - haemoptysis
  - cough
  - chest pain
  - wheeze
  - shortness of breath
  - Horner's syndrome (ptosis, miosis, reduced sweating)
  - pleural effusion
  - superior vena caval obstruction (headache, dilated veins, facial oedema?)
  - clubbing
  - lymphadenopathy
  - voice change (recurrent laryngeal nerve palsy)
  - chest X-ray abnormality.
- *Systemic symptoms of malignancy:*
  - weight loss
  - anorexia
  - fever
  - endocrine manifestations (e.g. Cushing's syndrome, SIADH)
  - hypercalcaemia.
- *Symptoms of metastases:*
  - jaundice
  - hepatic pain
  - skin lesions.
- Are there any symptoms suggesting secondary spread or other primary tumour?

Past medical history

- Enquire about the patient's smoking history.
- Ask about exposure to asbestos.
- Has the patient undergone any radiotherapy and/or chemotherapy?
- Ask about occupational history/exposure.
- Ask about respiratory function and other cardiorespiratory disease (if pneumonectomy/lobectomy contemplated).
- Enquire about any other primary malignancies.

Examination

• What is the general condition of the patient: thin/well nourished, anaemic, jaundiced? Consider their possible fitness for operative resection (e.g. test ability to climb stairs).
• Check the patient's voice (is it hoarse)? Check the patient's cough (is it 'bovine')?
• Is there clubbing? (One-third of patients with lung carcinoma are clubbed.)
• Does the patient's nails show nicotine stains?
• Does the patient have any radiotherapy tattoos?
• Check for respiratory signs (respiratory distress, cyanosis and tachypnoea).
• Perform a chest examination. Any pleural effusion, crackles, unequal air entry or lobectomy scar?
• Check for lymphadenopathy.

Rare complications

• Pericardial effusion.
• Horner's syndrome (ipsilateral ptosis, miosis, anhydrosis).
• Wasting of small muscles of the hand (invasion of brachial plexus).
• Pancoast tumour (apical tumour producing upper limb pain due to brachial plexus invasion and commonly Horner's syndrome).
• SVC obstruction (venous dilatation, facial swelling/oedema, fixed engorgement of neck veins, suffusion of eyes).

• Peripheral neuropathy, myopathy, dermatomyositis.
• Metastatic spread (e.g. hepatomegaly, skin nodules).

Clubbing

• Clubbing is the loss of the nail-fold angle due to thickening of the nail bed and is associated with a variety of important medical conditions. There may be increased sponginess of the nail bed and increased curvature of the nail. (It coincides rarely with hypertrophic pulmonary osteoarthropathy, which produces a painful swelling of the wrists.)
• Common causes:
  • carcinoma of bronchus
  • fibrosing alveolitis
  • cyanotic congenital heart disease
  • infective endocarditis
  • cirrhosis of the liver
  • congenital.
• Look especially for any respiratory signs or symptoms. The main concern is underlying carcinoma of the lung.

Evidence

Myers KA & Farquhar DR. Does this patient have clubbing? *JAMA* 2001; **286**: 341–7.

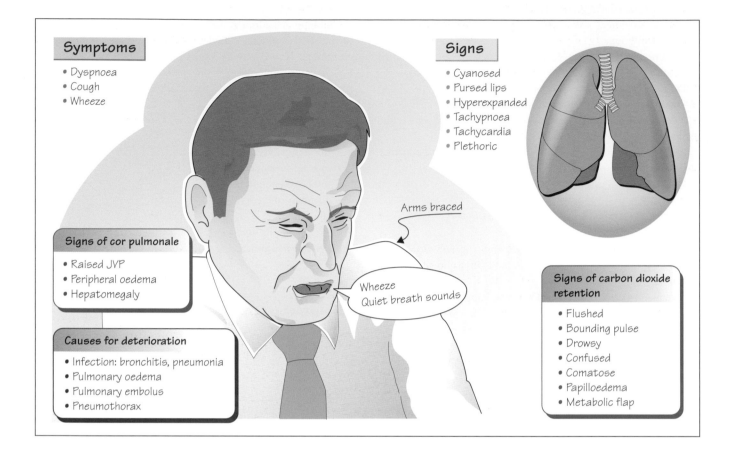

Symptoms

- Dyspnoea
- Cough
- Wheeze

Signs of cor pulmonale

- Raised JVP
- Peripheral oedema
- Hepatomegaly

Causes for deterioration

- Infection: bronchitis, pneumonia
- Pulmonary oedema
- Pulmonary embolus
- Pneumothorax

Signs

- Cyanosed
- Pursed lips
- Hyperexpanded
- Tachypnoea
- Tachycardia
- Plethoric

Arms braced

Wheeze
Quiet breath sounds

Signs of carbon dioxide retention

- Flushed
- Bounding pulse
- Drowsy
- Confused
- Comatose
- Papilloedema
- Metabolic flap

COPD is a disease characterized by a progressive airflow limitation caused by an abnormal inflammatory reaction. It encompasses diseases such as chronic bronchitis and emphysema and is most commonly due to smoking. The dominant symptom in COPD is feeling breathless, often noticed initially on exertion. There is often cough, which may be productive of sputum and wheeze. The symptoms commonly progress with increasing breathlessness and reduced exercise tolerance. There are exacerbations, commonly attributed to infection, during which there is increased breathlessness, cough, wheeze and sputum production. It usually occurs in those patients over 45 years of age. (Chronic bronchitis = sputum production on most days for 3 months of 2 successive years.) COPD has a prevalence of over 2%.

In some patients with COPD there may be loss of hypercapnic respiratory drive and thus reliance upon hypoxic stimulation of ventilation. Uncontrolled administration of oxygen can lead to the loss of stimulation of ventilation by hypoxia and to increased and dangerous hypercapnia (carbon dioxide retention).

There is usually a history of smoking (if not the diagnosis should be questioned and/or other aetiologies sought).

History

- How long has the patient felt breathless? When does the patient feel breathless: at rest or on exertion?

- What can the patient do before feeling short of breath? How far can the patient walk?
- Does the patient cough? If so, is there any sputum, how much and what colour?
- Is the patient wheezy? If so, when?
- How long has the patient been as bad as this?
- What seemed to trigger it?
- Does the patient get chest pain or breathless when lying down?
- Has the patient ever been ventilated? Has the patient ever been hospitalized? (If so, what were the baseline spirometry and blood gases?)

Past medical history

- Ask about any previous respiratory conditions (e.g. asthma, TB, carcinoma of the bronchus, bronchiectasis or emphysema).
- Enquire about any other cardiac or respiratory conditions.
- Has there been any episodes of pneumonia?
- Ask about any symptoms of sleep apnoea (daytime sleepiness, snoring). Is there winter deterioration?

Drugs

- Ask about the patient's response to treatments: corticosteroids, nebulizers, home oxygen? Does the patient use home oxygen? If so, for how many hours a day does he/she use it?

- Establish the patient's smoking history (previous [packs a day/years], current and passive).

Family and social history

- What is the patient's occupational history (pneumoconiosis)?
- Any family history of chronic breathing problems (consider α_1-antitrypsin deficiency)?
- What is the extent of the patient's disability? What is the patient's exercise tolerance? How far can the patient walk? Is the patient able to get out of the house? Can the patient climb the stairs? Where is the patient's bed/bathroom, etc.? Who does the patient's shopping, washing, cooking, etc.?

Examination

- Is the patient well or unwell? Is the patient distressed, anxious, able to speak (able to complete sentences)?
- Patients often sit upright and may brace themselves with their arms.
- Is the patient breathless at rest or on minimal exertion (e.g. getting onto couch)?
- Is the patient cyanosed (plethoric [polycythaemia])?
- Is the patient using oxygen, nebulizers or inhalers?
- Check the patient's respiratory rate and pulse rate.
- Any sputum? If so, what colour? Any blood (haemoptysis)?
- Any audible wheeze or stridor?
- Any purse-lipped breathing? Prolonged expiratory phase?
- Any use of accessory muscles (intercostal recession or tracheal tug)?
- What is the maximum laryngeal height? (Distance between the top of the thyroid cartilage and the suprasternal notch at end expiration < 4 cm is a sign of COPD.)
- Any hyperexpansion?
- Are the respiratory movements symmetrical?
- Are there any scars?
- Is the trachea central?
- Is the JVP elevated?
- Check heart sounds. Are there any signs of cor pulmonale?
- If the JVP is elevated check right ventricular heave. Any signs of hepatomegaly or peripheral oedema?
- Check breath sounds (commonly quiet, distant). Any added crackles, wheeze or rub?
- Check percussion: Any dullness?
- Are there any signs of carbon dioxide retention (bounding pulse, flushed, drowsy, confused, coma)?

Table 98.1 Differential diagnosis of chronic obstructive pulmonary disease (COPD).

COPD
Mid-life onset
Slowly progressing symptoms
Long history of smoking

Asthma
Early onset
Varying symptoms
Symptoms during the night/early morning
Presence of allergy, rhinitis and/or eczema
A family history
Airflow limitation that is largely reversible

Congestive heart failure
Fine basal crackles on auscultation
Dilated heart on chest radiography
Pulmonary oedema
Volume restriction not airflow limitation on pulmonary function tests

Bronchiectasis
Large volume of purulent sputum
Coarse crackles/clubbing

Tuberculosis
Onset at all ages
Lung infiltrate on chest radiography
Microbiological confirmation
High local prevalence of TB

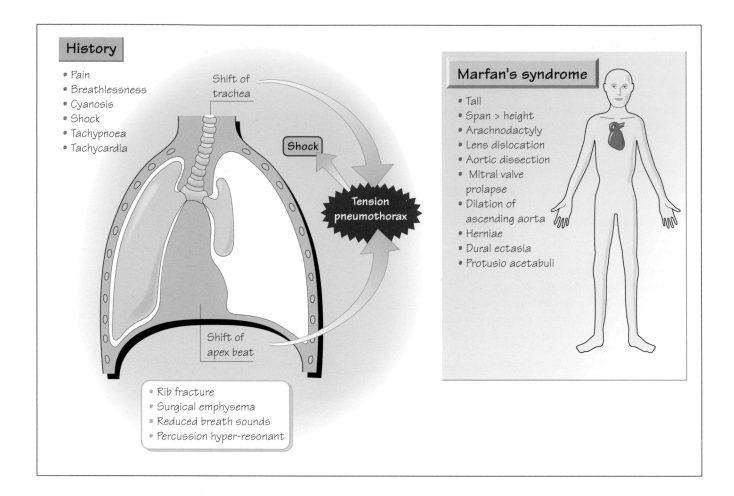

History
- Pain
- Breathlessness
- Cyanosis
- Shock
- Tachypnoea
- Tachycardia

Shift of trachea

Shock

Tension pneumothorax

Shift of apex beat

- Rib fracture
- Surgical emphysema
- Reduced breath sounds
- Percussion hyper-resonant

Marfan's syndrome
- Tall
- Span > height
- Arachnodactyly
- Lens dislocation
- Aortic dissection
- Mitral valve prolapse
- Dilation of ascending aorta
- Herniae
- Dural ectasia
- Protusio acetabuli

Pneumothorax is air in the pleural space. It can occur in the context of chronic respiratory disease, such as asthma or COPD, with pleural disease (such as mesothelioma), when a patient is being ventilated, following trauma, with connective tissue disease (such as Marfan's syndrome) or be idiopathic (classically occurring in tall, young men). It can complicate any invasive procedure of the chest, such as central venous cannulation. It should be considered in any patient with a sudden onset of breathlessness.

History

Pneumothorax commonly presents with a sudden onset of sharp chest pain. It may be accompanied by breathlessness.

A tension pneumothorax may arise in which there is increasing accumulation of air in the pleural space that cannot escape, producing mediastinal shift and in which shock and cyanosis may develop rapidly. It is a reversible cause of cardiac arrest.

Past medical history

- Any previous pneumothorax?

- Any known respiratory disease?
- Does the patient have diagnosed Marfan's syndrome?
- Smoking considerably increases the incidence of idiopathic pneumothoraces.

Examination

- Is the patient unwell, in need of supplemental oxygen and urgent/immediate aspiration of the pneumothorax?
- Are there any signs of shock, especially hypotension?
- Is the patient in pain?
- Is the patient distressed?
- Is the patient tachypnoeic?
- Are there signs of cyanosis?
- Classically, the affected side is hyperresonant to percussion with reduced breath sounds. (However, such clinical signs may be absent even with significant pneumothorax.)
- Could there be a tension pneumothorax? Consider this possibility in any unwell patient with chest pain and breathlessness.
- In the unwell, breathless patient, chest X-rays may be necessary to exclude a pneumothorax.

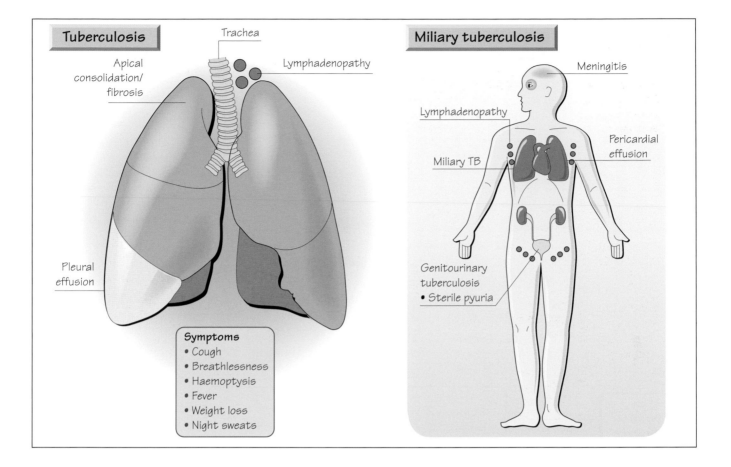

Infection with *Mycobacterium tuberculosis* can present with local effects anywhere in the body or with systemic effects of chronic infection.

History
• A high index of suspicion is required especially in the immunosuppressed or those from endemic areas.
• *Local symptoms:* cough, breathlessness, haemoptysis, lymphadenopathy, rash (e.g. lupus vulgaris), chest X-ray abnormality or GI disturbance.
• *Systemic effects:* fever, night sweats, anorexia or weight loss.
• Tuberculosus meningitis tends to have a greater duration of illness, headache, fever and greater incidence of cranial nerve palsies than bacterial meningitis.

Past medical history
• Any exposure to patients with TB?
• Is the patient immunosuppressed (corticosteroids/HIV)?
• Has the patient had previous chest X-rays showing abnormalities?
• Any history of BCG vaccination or Mantoux tests?
• Any history of diagnosed TB?

Drugs
Has the patient had any treatment for TB? If so, what agents were used, what was the duration of the treatment, what was the patient's compliance with the treatment and was there any observed therapy?

Family and social history
• Any family or social history of TB?
• Ask about alcohol consumption, intravenous drug use and foreign travel.

Examination
• TB may produce local chest signs, systemic signs, or if miliary TB has developed many parts of the body may be affected producing, e.g., meningitis, skin lesions, retinal lesions, spinal osteomyelitis (Pott's disease) or genitourinary TB.
• Is there pyrexia, anaemia or jaundice?
• Any lymphadenopathy?
• Does the patient appear thin or malnourished?
• Any tracheal deviation?
• Look for any apical lung signs (any fibrosis)?
• Any pleural effusion?
• Any pyuria (sterile)?
Suspect TB in any patient with chronic fever, weight loss, unexplained respiratory symptoms or lymphadenopathy.

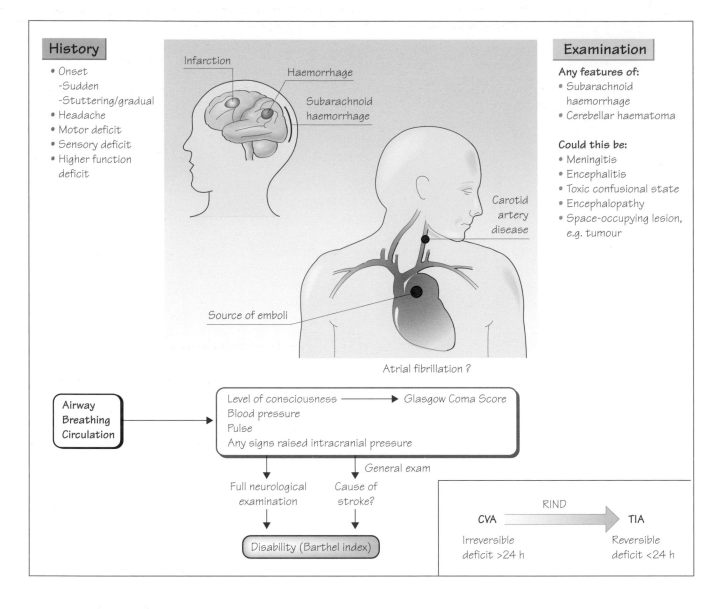

History

- Onset
  - Sudden
  - Stuttering/gradual
- Headache
- Motor deficit
- Sensory deficit
- Higher function deficit

Infarction

Haemorrhage

Subarachnoid haemorrhage

Carotid artery disease

Source of emboli

Atrial fibrillation ?

Examination

Any features of:
- Subarachnoid haemorrhage
- Cerebellar haematoma

Could this be:
- Meningitis
- Encephalitis
- Toxic confusional state
- Encephalopathy
- Space-occupying lesion, e.g. tumour

Airway
Breathing
Circulation

Level of consciousness → Glasgow Coma Score
Blood pressure
Pulse
Any signs raised intracranial pressure

General exam

Full neurological examination

Cause of stroke?

Disability (Barthel index)

RIND

CVA → TIA

Irreversible deficit >24 h

Reversible deficit <24 h

Stroke represents a sudden neurological deficit due to a disturbance of the CNS blood supply. The underlying pathologies are usually haemorrhage or thromboembolism. The incidence is 0.2% of the population per year rising to 1% in people over 75 years of age.

The onset of the deficit is usually sudden and often corresponds to the area of brain supplied by a specific blood vessel. If the deficit resolves completely within 24 hours it is termed a TIA. The deficits can range from trivial to deep unresponsive coma depending upon the area of the CNS involved.

History

- The cardinal feature is sudden onset (usually over seconds) of neurological deficit (e.g. weakness, numbness, dysphasia, etc.).
- When was the deficit first noticed? Did it develop suddenly or gradually?
- What symptoms were noticed: weakness, numbness, diplopia, dysphasia or falls?
- Any sensory neglect?
- Any accompanying symptoms: headache, nausea, vomiting or fitting?
- Any other recent neurological defects (e.g. TIAs or amaurosis fugax)?
- Any witnesses to the event?
- Any subsequent problems (e.g. aspiration, damage from fall)?
- Has the patient had any recent falls or head trauma (consider subdural/extradural haematoma)?
- What is the extent of disability and are there any functional consequences?
- Assess the activities of daily living with, e.g., Barthel's Index of Daily Living (Table 101.1).

Table 101.1 Barthel's Index of Daily Living.

Activity	Score
Feeding	0 = unable 1 = needs help cutting, spreading butter, etc., or requires modified diet 2 = independent
Bathing	0 = dependent 1 = independent (or in shower)
Grooming	0 = needs help with personal care 1 = independent face/hair/teeth/shaving (implements provided)
Dressing	0 = dependent 1 = needs help but can do about half unaided 2 = independent (including buttons, zips, laces, etc.)
Bowels	0 = incontinent (or needs to be given enemas) 1 = occasional accident 2 = continent
Bladder	0 = incontinent, or catheterized and unable to manage alone 1 = occasional accident (< once every day) 2 = continent
Toilet use	0 = dependent 1 = needs some help, but can do something alone 2 = independent (on and off, dressing, wiping)
Transfers (bed to chair and back)	0 = unable, no sitting balance 1 = major help (one or two people, physical), can sit 2 = minor help (verbal or physical) 3 = independent
Mobility (on level surfaces)	0 = immobile or < 50 yards 1 = wheelchair independent, including corners, > 50 yards 2 = walks with help of one person (verbal or physical) > 50 yards 3 = independent (but may use any aid; e.g. stick) > 50 yards
Stairs	0 = unable 1 = needs help (verbal, physical, carrying aid) 2 = independent
Total	= /20

The total score can be useful as an estimate of dependence. As a rough guide, a score of 14 is often compatible with the level of support found in a residential home; a total score of 10 may just be compatible with discharge home with maximum support and a carer in attendance.

Past medical history

• Any previous stroke, TIA, amaurosis fugax, collapses, fits or subarachnoid haemorrhage?
• Any known vascular disease (e.g. carotid stenoses, coronary atherosclerosis, peripheral vascular disease)?
• Any known bleeding or clotting tendency?
• Any possible embolic source (e.g. atrial fibrillation, prosthetic valve, carotid stenosis, carotid or vertebral dissection)?
• Any history of hypertension, hypercholesterolaemia or smoking?

Drugs

• Is the patient taking anticoagulants (e.g. warfarin) or antiplatelet agents (e.g. aspirin)?
• Has the patient taken any recent thrombolytics?

Family and social history

• Any family history of stroke?
• Establish the patient's smoking and alcohol history.

Examination

• Is the patient well or unwell?
• Ensure the airway is preserved and protected. This may require positioning in the recovery position or even intubation. Give oxygen and ensure that breathing and circulation are maintained.
• Check the conscious level: use the Glasgow Coma Score (see Chapter 33).
• Assess speech: check the patient's comprehension of commands and listen to the patient speaking. If there seem to be difficulties, ask the patient to name specific objects. Ask the patient to repeat a phrase after you.
• Is there dysarthria or dysphasia (receptive or expressive)?
• Assess the patient's posture.
• Is the patient normal/hemiplegic/decerebrate/decorticate?
• Undertake a full neurological examination. In particular are there any focal neurological deficits (e.g. weakness of one side).
• Check tone. This may be normal or reduced early on following a stroke producing an upper motor neurone lesion, but usually tone subsequently increases abnormally.
• Is power reduced? If so, is this in 'pyramidal distribution' (i.e. flexors stronger in arms, extensors in legs)?
• Is co-ordination impaired? Are there any features of cerebellar lesion?
• Are reflexes reduced or increased? As for tone, this may be normal or reduced early on following an upper motor neurone lesion, but usually reflexes subsequently increase abnormally.
• Are there any cranial nerve deficits?
• Do the neurological signs point towards a lesion in a particular part of the CNS or the interruption of a particular arterial supply?
• Assess the degree of disability with Barthel's Index of Daily Living (Table 101.1).

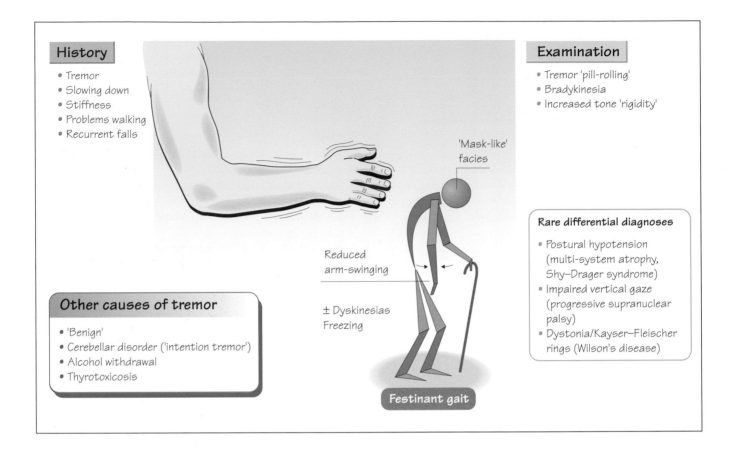

History
- Tremor
- Slowing down
- Stiffness
- Problems walking
- Recurrent falls

Examination
- Tremor 'pill-rolling'
- Bradykinesia
- Increased tone 'rigidity'

'Mask-like' facies

Reduced arm-swinging

± Dyskinesias
Freezing

Rare differential diagnoses
- Postural hypotension (multi-system atrophy, Shy–Drager syndrome)
- Impaired vertical gaze (progressive supranuclear palsy)
- Dystonia/Kayser–Fleischer rings (Wilson's disease)

Other causes of tremor
- 'Benign'
- Cerebellar disorder ('intention tremor')
- Alcohol withdrawal
- Thyrotoxicosis

Festinant gait

Parkinsonism is a clinical syndrome characterized by tremor, slow movements and increased tone. This may be seen in idiopathic Parkinson's disease or with other aetiologies, such as anti-dopaminergic drugs and Wilson's disease. It may present with difficulties with walking, tremor, recurrent falls or general deterioration. The classical features are a 'pill-rolling' tremor (4–8 Hz), increased tone ('lead-pipe') (which together with tremor may produce 'cog-wheel' rigidity) and bradykinesia (slowness of movements).

The tremor is usually most obvious at rest, improving with movement and sleep. The patient may appear slow to initiate movement and speech, find difficulty in performing rapidly alternating movements and the increased tone may become more prominent with movements of the opposite limb. There may be a 'mask-like' expression with reduction in facial expression and blinking. It has a prevalence of 0.5% of the population in people over 65 years of age.

History
- When were difficulties with walking/tremor, etc., first noticed? Were they noticed by the patient or by other people?
- Have there been falls? Has the patient had difficulty turning in bed? Do they have difficulties getting out of a chair, writing (e.g. micrographia), opening jars?
- What is the patient unable to do that they would like to?

- What are the functional consequences of the patient's impairment?

Past medical history
Check the history of any associated conditions (e.g. Wilson's disease or other neurological diseases, carbon monoxide poisoning).

Drugs
- Has there been administration of anti-dopaminergic drugs, such as neuroleptics?
- Has the patient received treatment with, e.g. levodopa? What was the response? Does improvement vary with time after the dose? Are there manifestations of drug side-effects (e.g. dyskinesias, or confusion)?

Examination
- Examine the patient's face, posture and gait.
- How far can the patient walk? Can he/she walk heel–toe? Can he/she turn? Can he/she get up from a chair? Can he/she climb stairs?
- Any tremor? If so, where? Is it increased or decreased with motion?
- Any rigidity (of limbs, of trunk)?
- Is there bradykinesia? Can the patient perform rapidly alternating movements?

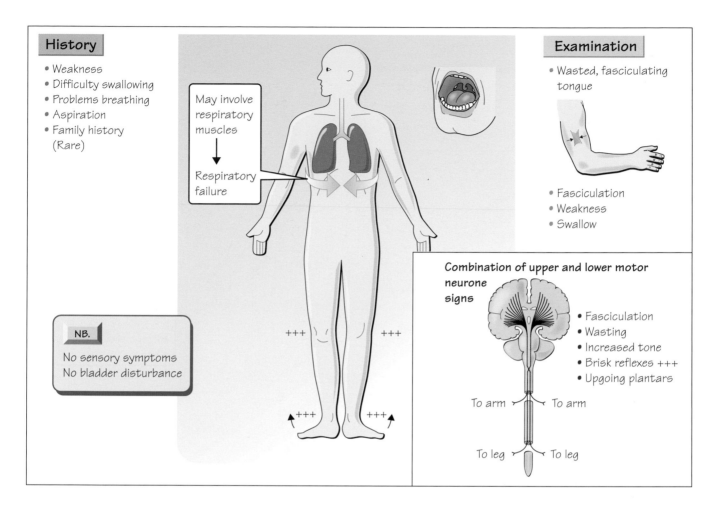

History
- Weakness
- Difficulty swallowing
- Problems breathing
- Aspiration
- Family history (Rare)

May involve respiratory muscles → Respiratory failure

NB.
No sensory symptoms
No bladder disturbance

Examination
- Wasted, fasciculating tongue
- Fasciculation
- Weakness
- Swallow

Combination of upper and lower motor neurone signs
- Fasciculation
- Wasting
- Increased tone
- Brisk reflexes +++
- Upgoing plantars

To arm   To arm
To leg   To leg

Motor neurone disease is an illness characterized by progressive degeneration of upper and lower motor neurones; it usually presents with gradual development of weakness affecting the tongue, bulbar muscles and limbs. This can produce difficulty in swallowing, slurring of speech, walking difficulties and, eventually, respiratory weakness and aspiration pneumonia. In contrast to other neurological disorders, e.g. multiple sclerosis, there are no sensory symptoms or signs. Incidence (and death rate) is 2/100 000 per year.

History
- When were the symptoms first noticed? What were they? Have they fluctuated or worsened?
- What treatments have been tried? Any need for ventilatory support? Has the patient had a tracheostomy? Are there any symptoms of aspiration pneumonia?
- What are the functional consequences? What is the patient's mobility? Does the patient utilize mobility aids (e.g. wheelchair)? Can the patient feed or wash him/herself?
- If there is significant dysarthria, written communication may

be required. However, when obtaining a history, above all, patience is required.

Family history
Very rarely there is a family history of motor neurone disorder.

Social history
- What is the patient's occupation? Can the patient still work? How is he/she supported practically?
- How have the patient and relatives adjusted to the diagnosis?

Examination
- The cardinal features are combined upper and lower motor neurone signs without any sensory findings.
- Any dysarthria?
- Examine the tongue: is it wasted, fasciculating or spastic?
- Are there difficulties with swallowing/aspiration?
- Is there increased tone or limb weakness?
- Are the reflexes brisk and plantars upgoing?
- Ensure there are no significant sensory abnormalities.

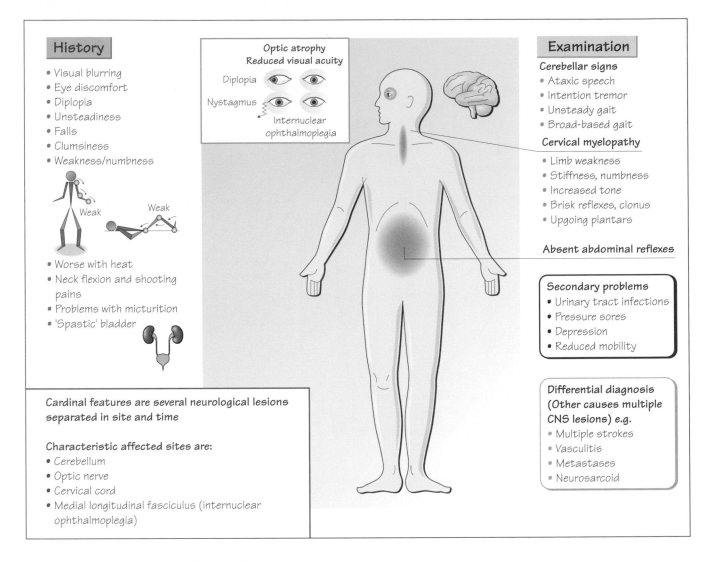

History

- Visual blurring
- Eye discomfort
- Diplopia
- Unsteadiness
- Falls
- Clumsiness
- Weakness/numbness

Weak   Weak

- Worse with heat
- Neck flexion and shooting pains
- Problems with micturition
- 'Spastic' bladder

Cardinal features are several neurological lesions separated in site and time

Characteristic affected sites are:
- Cerebellum
- Optic nerve
- Cervical cord
- Medial longitudinal fasciculus (internuclear ophthalmoplegia)

Optic atrophy
Reduced visual acuity
Diplopia
Nystagmus
Internuclear ophthalmoplegia

Examination

Cerebellar signs
- Ataxic speech
- Intention tremor
- Unsteady gait
- Broad-based gait

Cervical myelopathy
- Limb weakness
- Stiffness, numbness
- Increased tone
- Brisk reflexes, clonus
- Upgoing plantars

Absent abdominal reflexes

Secondary problems
- Urinary tract infections
- Pressure sores
- Depression
- Reduced mobility

Differential diagnosis
(Other causes multiple CNS lesions) e.g.
- Multiple strokes
- Vasculitis
- Metastases
- Neurosarcoid

Multiple sclerosis is a chronic neurological condition characterized by CNS demyelination that causes a wide range of deficits at different times and in different sites throughout the CNS. Whilst any location in the CNS can be affected, there are particular sites that are more commonly affected, such as the optic nerve, the cerebellum and the cervical cord. The disease may be slowly progressive or marked by relapses and remissions. It has a prevalence of 100/100 000 but there is marked geographical variation.

History

- When did the patient first notice any symptoms? What were they? How did they progress? Did they improve, gradually worsen or recur?
- Has there been visual blurring, eye discomfort (e.g. optic neuritis)?
- Any unsteadiness, falling or intention tremor (e.g. cerebellar)?
- Is there weakness, numbness, stiffness, jerky movements or problems walking (e.g. cervical myelopathy)?

- Are there problems with micturition or defaecation?
- Do hot baths exacerbate symptoms?
- Does neck flexion produce shooting pains (Lhermitte's symptom, which can also be found in cervical spondylosis or B_{12} deficiency)?
- Are there any abnormalities of mood: euphoria or depression?
- What can the patient not do? What is the patient's mobility? Does the patient use a stick or wheelchair, etc.?

Past medical history

- Any previous episodes, visual disturbance, weakness, numbness or unsteadiness, etc.?
- Any associated problems (e.g. UTIs, bed sores, depression)?

Drugs

- Any treatments received and any effects (e.g. corticosteroids, interferon)?
- Any specific treatments for spasticity (e.g. baclofen)?

Family and social history

- Any family history of neurological illness?
- What is the patient's occupation? How has the illness affected his/her work, family, relationships, etc.?
- What support does the patient receive?
- What modifications have been made to the patient's home?

Examination

- Is there evidence of neurological lesions at several sites within the CNS?
- Perform a full neurological examination with particular focus on:
  - *Optic nerve.* What is the visual acuity? Is there normal colour vision, pupillary reaction, appearance of an optic disc (e.g. papillitis, optic atrophy)?
  - *Cerebellar function.* Examine gait, posture and co-ordination (e.g. finger–nose). Any intention tremor or dysdiadochokinesis? Is speech classically abnormal? Is there 'scanning speech' or nystagmus? Is there internuclear ophthalmoplegia (failure to adduct eye on lateral gaze with nystagmus of the abducting eye)?
  - *Limbs.* Are there signs of upper motor neurone dysfunction (e.g. increased tone, reduced power in 'pyramidal' distribution, brisk tendon reflexes, absent abdominal reflexes, upgoing plantar responses)? Are there sensory deficits?
- What are the functional consequences of the patient's impairments?
- Consider other consequences, such as secondary infections (e.g. pneumonia, UTI or bed sores). Is there fever, tachycardia, tachypnoea, etc.?
- Consider the differential diagnosis of multiple CNS lesions:
  - multiple CVAs in young adults from illnesses such as phospholipid antibody syndrome
  - metastases
  - cerebral vasculitis
  - SLE
  - neurosarcoid
  - CADASIL (cerebral autosomal dominant arteriopathy with subcortical infarcts and leukoencephalopathy)
  - meningovascular syphilis
  - HTLV1 infection
  - Lyme disease
  - paraneoplastic cerebellar ataxia
  - genetic disorders of myelin, such as the leukodystrophies.

105 Peripheral neuropathy

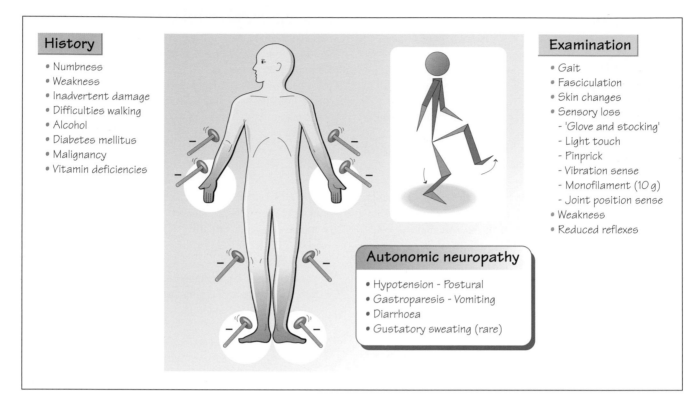

History
- Numbness
- Weakness
- Inadvertent damage
- Difficulties walking
- Alcohol
- Diabetes mellitus
- Malignancy
- Vitamin deficiencies

Examination
- Gait
- Fasciculation
- Skin changes
- Sensory loss
  - 'Glove and stocking'
  - Light touch
  - Pinprick
  - Vibration sense
  - Monofilament (10 g)
  - Joint position sense
- Weakness
- Reduced reflexes

Autonomic neuropathy
- Hypotension - Postural
- Gastroparesis - Vomiting
- Diarrhoea
- Gustatory sweating (rare)

Peripheral neuropathy may present with motor or sensory symptoms usually affecting the hands and feet initially. There are a large number of potential causes of which diabetes mellitus, alcohol excess, malignancy, medication, vitamin deficiencies and inherited causes are the commonest.

History
- What are the symptoms: numbness, 'pins and needles', weakness, foot dragging/slapping, tripping, inadvertent damage (e.g. burns because of sensory deficit) or muscle wasting?
- When did they start? Are they progressive?
- What are the functional consequences (e.g. difficulty in walking, holding knife, writing, etc.)?
- Are there any symptoms of associated conditions (e.g. diabetes mellitus, malignancy)?

Past medical history
Ask about any significant medical conditions, especially diabetes mellitus, malignancy, vasculitis or other neurological conditions.

Drugs
Is the patient taking any medications (e.g. vincristine)?

Family and history
Any family history of neuropathy (e.g. Charcot–Marie–Tooth disease)?

Social history
- Has there been any unusual occupational exposure to potential neurotoxins (e.g. lead)?
- Are there any home adaptations or use of walking aids, etc.?

Examination
- Perform a full general and neurological examination for signs of diabetes, malignancy, etc.
- Examine gait, is it high stepping and stamping?
- Examine symptomatic areas.
- Inspect: is there wasting, abnormal posture, trophic skin changes, fasciculation or scarring?
- Check tone: is it normal or reduced?
- Is power reduced? If so, to which muscle groups? Does it conform to a particular peripheral nerve distribution or is there generalized peripheral weakness of hands ± feet?
- Is co-ordination impaired?
- Examine reflexes: are they normal or reduced?
- *Examine sensation:*
  - light touch (Any impairment? If so, what is the distribution: 'glove and stocking', dermatomal, peripheral nerve or nerve root distribution?)
  - pin prick
  - vibration sense
  - joint position sense
  - deep pain
  - hot/cold
  - monofilament (10 g).

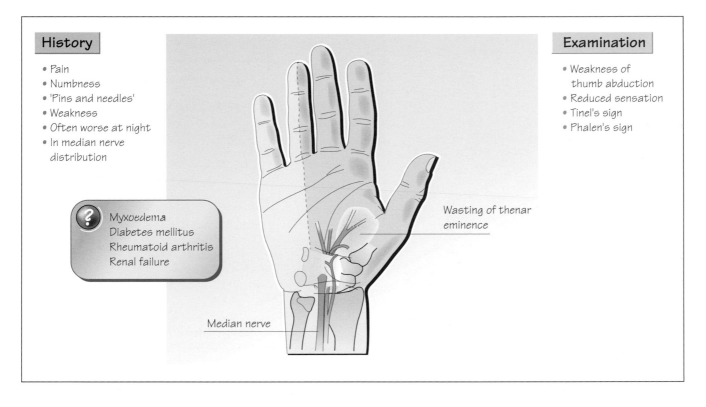

History
- Pain
- Numbness
- 'Pins and needles'
- Weakness
- Often worse at night
- In median nerve distribution

?
Myxoedema
Diabetes mellitus
Rheumatoid arthritis
Renal failure

Examination
- Weakness of thumb abduction
- Reduced sensation
- Tinel's sign
- Phalen's sign

Wasting of thenar eminence

Median nerve

This syndrome, the result of compression of the median nerve in the carpal tunnel, is the commonest example of entrapment neuropathy. It usually presents with symptoms of pain, numbness and/or weakness of the affected hand due to compression of the median nerve at the wrist.

History
- The patient may describe numbness, 'pins and needles' and weakness of the affected hand. The condition may be bilateral and produces symptoms in the palmar surface of the thumb, first, middle and median side of the ring fingers. It is often worse at night and pain may extend along the arm.
- There may be associated conditions, such as diabetes mellitus, rheumatoid arthritis, renal failure and myxoedema.
- Are there symptoms of entrapment neuropathy elsewhere or of an underlying peripheral neuropathy?

Examination
- Any weakness and wasting of the thenar eminence?
- Any weakness of thumb abduction and/or opposition?
- Is there reduced sensation in the palmar surface of the hand?

- Tinel's sign (eliciting symptoms with percussion over the carpal tunnel) or Phalen's sign (eliciting symptoms with flexion at the wrist) may be present.
- Examine the patient for other sites of neuropathy (e.g. mononeuritis multiplex).
- Symptoms may be due to carpal tunnel syndrome without objective neurological signs, and confirmation with electrophysiological testing may be required.

Evidence

Symptoms of pain in the median nerve distribution and weakness of thumb abduction are the most predictive signs and symptoms for electromyographic diagnosis of carpal tunnel syndrome. Phalen's and Tinel's signs, thenar atrophy and sensory testing abnormalities are of less diagnostic value.

D'Arcy CA & McGee S. Does this patient have carpal tunnel syndrome? *JAMA* 2000; **283**: 3110–7.

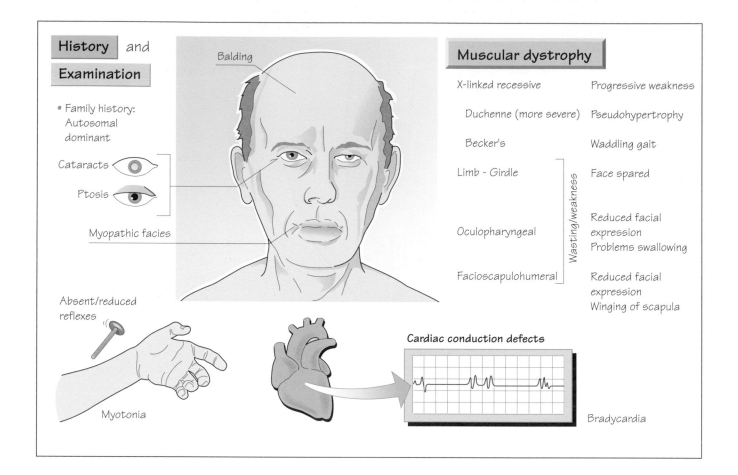

History and Examination

• Family history: Autosomal dominant

Cataracts

Ptosis

Myopathic facies

Balding

Absent/reduced reflexes

Myotonia

Cardiac conduction defects

Bradycardia

Muscular dystrophy

X-linked recessive	Progressive weakness
Duchenne (more severe)	Pseudohypertrophy
Becker's	Waddling gait
Limb - Girdle	Face spared
Oculopharyngeal	Reduced facial expression / Problems swallowing
Facioscapulohumeral	Reduced facial expression / Winging of scapula

Wasting/weakness

Myotonic dystrophy (dystrophia myotonica)

Myotonic dystrophy is an inherited autosomal dominant condition. There is muscular weakness and wasting which can produce a rather 'drooping expression'. Myotonia may be present, which may be apparent due to the delay in the patient releasing his/her grip upon shaking hands. It can be demonstrated by a delay in opening and closing fists repetitively or by difficulty in opening eyes after tight closure. The other features include frontal balding, ptosis, cataracts and cardiac conduction defects.

Muscular dystrophy

The muscular dystrophies are inherited muscle disorders characterized by progressive muscle wasting and weakness of variable distribution and severity. There may be wasting of muscles, pronounced weakness and significant disability, sometimes progressing to respiratory failure. The muscular dystrophies can be subdivided into several groups according to the distribution of predominant muscle weakness (Table 107.1). In several types the heart can be seriously affected, occasionally in the absence of clinically significant weakness.

Table 107.1 The inheritance and clinical features of muscular dystrophies.

Type of muscular dystrophy	Inheritance	Typical features
Duchenne's	X-linked recessive	Wasting Weakness Pseudohypertrophy Requires wheelchair by 12 years Death from respiratory failure < 30 years
Becker's	X-linked recessive	Less severe than Duchenne's Wasting Weakness Onset by 12 years Problems walking in their twenties Death during their forties or fifties
Emery–Dreifuss	X-linked, autosomal recessive and autosomal dominant forms	Contractures Muscle wasting especially proximal upper limbs, distal in lower limbs Cardiomyopathy
Distal	Autosomal dominant Autosomal recessive	Late onset (in their forties) Early onset (before their thirties) Distal wasting and weakness
Facioscapulohumeral	Autosomal dominant	Weakness of facial and shoulder girdle muscles
Oculopharyngeal	Autosomal dominant	Ptosis, weakness of extraocular muscles Dysphagia, onset in their twenties
Limb girdle	Autosomal dominant and recessive forms	Progressive limb girdle weakness, some forms with cardiac involvement

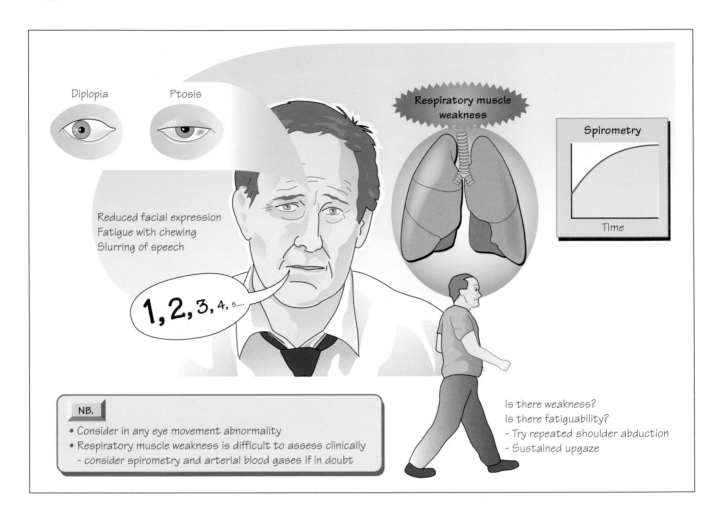

This is an autoimmune condition in which antibodies to the acetylcholine receptor result in weakness. It may present insidiously with increasing weakness, producing symptoms such as double vision (diplopia), difficulty swallowing or the drooping of eyelids (ptosis). Sometimes more dramatic presentations can occur with respiratory failure. It has a prevalence of 15/100 000 with a new case incidence of 1/100 000 per year.

History
• What has the patient or other people noticed?
• When is the weakness most marked: after activity; towards the end of day? Is there fatigue?
• Has there been double vision or drooping of eyelids? Are there problems with speech, swallowing or breathing?

Past medical history
• Any other autoimmune conditions?
• Any thymoma or thymectomy?

Drugs
Has the patient received any treatment; immunosuppression, anti-cholinergics or plasmapheresis?

Examination
• Any muscular weakness? Examine after repetitive movements.
• Examine eye movements. Look for ptosis, abnormal eye movements. Examine prolonged up-gaze. Orbicularis oculi fatigue may be observed on gentle eye closure; after complete initial closure of the eyelids, they separate within seconds and the white of the sclera starts to show (positive 'peek sign').
• Is the patient's speech normal or weakening with prolonged speech? Ask the patient to count to 100.
• Reflexes and sensation are normal. (In the related myaesthenic syndrome associated with small cell lung cancer [Eaton–Lambert syndrome] there is proximal weakness and hyporeflexia, and repeated muscle contraction may lead to increased strength.)
• If there is any suggestion of respiratory symptoms or weakness, assess respiratory function with spirometry and arterial blood gases.

109 Cerebellar disorders

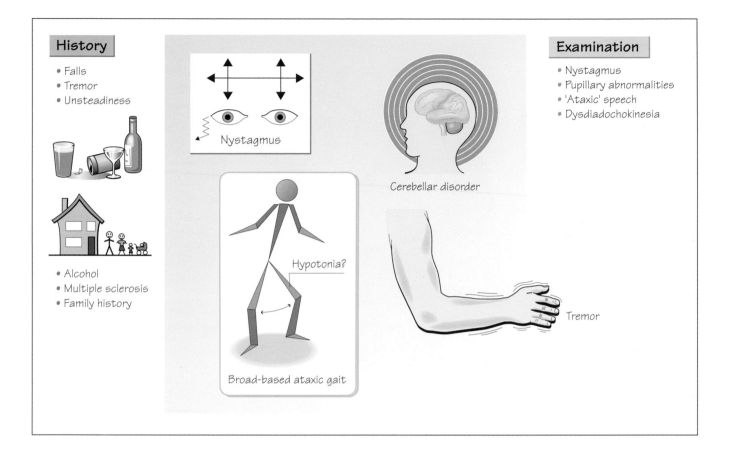

History
- Falls
- Tremor
- Unsteadiness

- Alcohol
- Multiple sclerosis
- Family history

Nystagmus

Hypotonia?

Broad-based ataxic gait

Cerebellar disorder

Tremor

Examination
- Nystagmus
- Pupillary abnormalities
- 'Ataxic' speech
- Dysdiadochokinesia

Cerebellar disorders may present with falls, unsteadiness, tremor or nystagmus. There are many possible causes of disease affecting the cerebellum, including ischaemic or haemorrhagic stroke, tumours, demyelination, alcohol excess and Wernicke's encephalopathy.

History
- When were symptoms first noticed? What were they? Did they have sudden or gradual onset? Are there any other associated neurological symptoms?
- Can the patient walk? If so, how far can the patient walk? Have there been falls? Any unsteadiness?
- Any tremor? If so, is it worse on intention?
- Are there any symptoms of raised intracranial pressure (e.g. headaches)?

Past medical history
- Any previous history of multiple sclerosis, stroke or primary tumours?
- Any previous history of alcohol abuse?

Family and social history
Any family history of cerebellar disorders (e.g. Friedreich's ataxia)?

Drugs
Ask about the patient's alcohol intake.

Examination
- Examine the patient's gait: is it classically unsteady and broad based?
- Any papilloedema or optic atrophy?
- Any evidence of disease in other parts of the CNS (e.g. consider multiple sclerosis)?
- Any evidence of alcohol excess (consider alcohol-induced cerebellar atrophy, acute intoxication or Wernicke's encephalopathy)?
- Are there any abnormalities of eye movements or pupils? Any signs of nystagmus?
- Is the tone in limbs classically reduced? (NB. This may be difficult to distinguish from normal.)
- Is tremor worse on intention (e.g. on finger–nose testing or 'past-pointing')?
- Any inability to perform rapidly alternating movements (dysdiadochokinesis)?
- Examine for signs of alcohol abuse and other neurological signs.

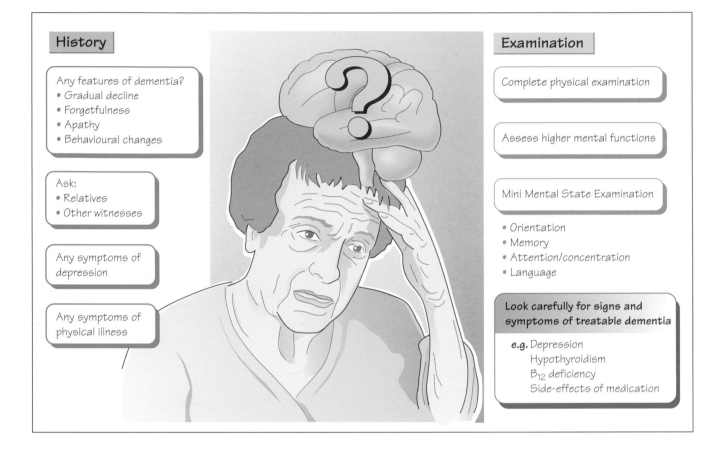

Within the figure:

History

Any features of dementia?
• Gradual decline
• Forgetfulness
• Apathy
• Behavioural changes

Ask:
• Relatives
• Other witnesses

Any symptoms of depression

Any symptoms of physical illness

Examination

Complete physical examination

Assess higher mental functions

Mini Mental State Examination

• Orientation
• Memory
• Attention/concentration
• Language

Look carefully for signs and symptoms of treatable dementia

e.g. Depression
Hypothyroidism
B_{12} deficiency
Side-effects of medication

Dementia is characterized by acquired losses of cognitive and emotional abilities severe enough to interfere with daily functioning and quality of life. It is common with a prevalence of 1% at 60 years of age; roughly doubling in incidence every 5 years thereafter. It usually presents with a gradual decline in cognitive ability. It may be noticed during assessment of another illness, or because of memory difficulties or behavioural changes described by the patient or relatives. There are important treatable causes of dementia: it should be distinguished from acute confusional states and attempts should be made to define the precise cause.

History

• What problems have been reported? Who reported them: the patient, relatives, friends or other professionals? Obtain objective evidence.
• Have there been difficulties with memory, disorientation, concentration and apathy? Are there functional or social consequences (isolation, malnutrition, etc.)? Any change in personality?
• Was there any obvious precipitant, such as head injury?
• Was there any sudden deterioration? Were there any precipitants to this (e.g. changes in medication, other illnesses or changes in environment)?
• Has there been a gradual or a stepwise decline?

• Are there any features of depression? (Beware of pseudodementia.)
• Are there any features of hypothyroidism?
• Are there any features suggesting physical illness?
• Are there any unusual neurological features (e.g. ataxia, weakness, myoclonus, headaches or symptoms of neuropathy)?

Past medical history

• Any other illnesses, particularly atheromatous disease and its risk factors?
• Any other neurological conditions?

Drugs

• Is the patient taking any medications, especially tranquillizers, sedatives, etc.?
• Is the patient taking any treatments for dementia (e.g. cholinesterase inhibitors)?
• Any signs of alcohol abuse?

Family and social history

• Any family history of dementia (consider rare inherited causes such as Huntington's disease)?
• Establish a complete description of social circumstances, carers, support and family.

Examination

- Carry out a complete physical examination.
- Give particular consideration to hypothyroidism, other illnesses and potential causes of acute confusional states.
- Perform a full neurological examination.
- Look for primitive reflexes: grasp, pout and palmo-mental reflex.
- Check higher mental functions.
- *Check orientation:*
  - Ask the patient their age, name, the time, the date, the location.

Table 110.1 Mini Mental Status Examination.

	Score
Orientation	
1 Ask the patient 'What is the year, season, date, day, month?'	/5
2 Ask the patient 'Where are you?' (Country, county, town, place, floor [or ward]?)	/5
Memory registration	
3 Tell the patient that you want him/her to remember something for you, then name three unrelated objects (speak clearly and slowly). Ask the patient to repeat the three objects (score 3 points if correct the first time, 2 points if correct the second time and 1 point if correct the third time). Ask patient to keep the three things in mind	/3
Attention and concentration	
4 Ask the patient to take seven from 100, then seven from the result, and so on for five subtractions. Score 1 point for each correct answer *or* Ask the patient to spell 'world' backwards, and score 1 point for each correct letter	/5
Memory recall	
5 Ask the patient to recall the three objects from test 3	/3
Language	
6 Show the patient two familiar objects (e.g. a pen, a watch) and ask him/her to name them	/2
7 Ask the patient to repeat a sentence after you 'No if's, and's or but's'	/1
8 Ask the patient to follow a three-stage command (e.g. 'Please take this paper in your left hand, fold it in half and put the paper on the floor.')	/3
9 Ask the patient to read and follow a written instruction (e.g. 'Close your eyes'.)	/1
10 Ask the patient to write a simple sentence. The sentence should contain a subject and a verb and should make sense	/1
11 Ask the patient to copy a picture of intersecting pentagons	/1
Total score	**/30**

A score below 24 indicates probable cognitive impairment. A score below 17 indicates definite cognitive impairment.

- *Check language:*
  - Is the patient left- or right-handed?
  - Get the patient to talk: ask the patient an open question (e.g. ask them to describe the room in detail).
- *Check memory:*
  - Immediate recall. Ask the patient to repeat the names of three objects (e.g. cat, book, rose and then again 5 minutes later).
  - Recent memory. Ask the patient about recent events and ask him/her to recall the three memorized objects.
  - Remote memory. Ask the patient about school, work history, childhood, etc.
- *Check comprehension:*
  - Ask the patient to repeat simple phrases.
  - Ask the patient to name simple objects.
  - Assess test reading and writing ability.
  - Ask the patient to perform a task (e.g. show how you would comb your hair).
- *Mood:*
  - Assess the patient's mood and look for any features of psychiatric illness, particularly depression.
- Document the assessment with a Mini Mental Status Examination (Table 110.1). There are problems with the sensitivity of this test (e.g. false-negatives in highly educated persons) and its specificity (e.g. false-positives in persons with sensory or motor impairment, independent of their true cognitive abilities).

Causes of dementia
Common causes of dementia

Common causes include:
- Alzheimer's disease (common, dominant memory impairment with gradual decline)
- vascular dementia (stepwise course?)
- Pick's disease (prominent frontal lobe signs, disinhibition, primitive reflexes)
- dementia with Parkinsonism (e.g. Lewy body dementia which may also feature visual hallucinations and fluctuating cognitive loss)
- normal pressure hydrocephalus (gait disorder, urinary incontinence and cognitive decline)
- Creutzfeldt–Jakob disease (rare, rapid decline, myoclonus [though this can be seen in other dementias]).

Treatable causes of dementia

Treatable causes include:
- hypothyroidism
- vitamin B_{12}, thiamine deficiency
- cerebral vasculitis
- neurosyphilis
- hydrocephalus
- depression
- frontal lobe meningioma
- medication related
- AIDS.

NB. Acute confusional states may mimic dementia.

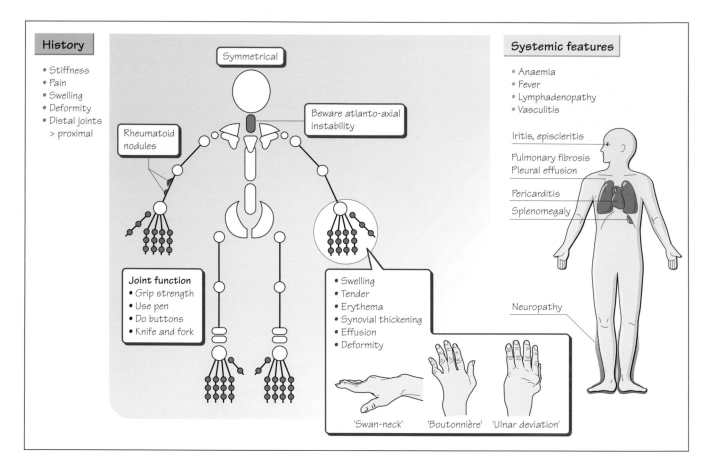

Rheumatoid arthritis is a symmetrical, deforming peripheral arthropathy. This is a common disorder that affects women more frequently than men. Initially symptoms are of joint stiffness and swelling but, as the condition progresses, there may be substantial joint deformity and systemic features. It is the commonest inflammatory arthropathy with a prevalence of 1.5%.

History
• Which joints are affected? Commonly, wrists, fingers, elbows, shoulders, knees and the atlanto-axial joint are affected.
• Any pain? If so, when and where?
• Is there stiffness, swelling or deformity? Commonly there is morning stiffness lasting for more than 1 hour.
• What are the functional consequences? What can the patient no longer do (e.g. walking distance, able to dress, transfer)?
• Are there any systemic features: malaise, weight loss or symptoms of anaemia?
• Are any other systems involved? Is there iritis, symptoms of anaemia, ankle swelling (nephrotic syndrome), breathlessness (pulmonary fibrosis?)?

Past medical history
• What has been the pattern of the disease? What joints are affected? What is the activity of the inflammation? Any other organ involvement?

• What treatments has the patient received? Has the patient had any joint replacement surgery, medication, physiotherapy or other aids?
• Any history of other autoimmune disorders?

Drugs
• What medication has the patient received and with what side-effects (e.g. corticosteroids [Cushingoid], methotrexate [pulmonary fibrosis], penicillamine, gold [nephrotic syndrome]), anti-TNF treatments?
• What is the patient's current medication?
• Does the patient have any allergies, intolerances or side-effects from the medication?

Family and social history
• Any family history of autoimmune diseases?
• How has the disease affected work, family, spouse and children?
• Have there been adaptations to improve mobility, etc.?

Examination
• Is the patient well or unwell? Is the patient anaemic or breathless?
• Inspect all the joints. Is there swelling, tenderness to palpation, erythema, synovial thickening, joint effusion, reduced range of

movement, ankylosis, subluxation, deformity? In active disease joints are warm, have synovitis and pain on movement.

- The classical patterns of deformity in the hands are:
  - ulnar deviation of the fingers
  - 'Swan-neck' (extension at PIP, flexion at DIP)
  - Boutonnière deformities (flexion at PIP, extension at DIP)
  - 'Z-thumb' (subluxation of first MCP joint with compensatory hyperextension of IP joints).
- Consider the possibility of atlanto-axial joint instability and take measures to protect the neck if possible.
- Are there rheumatoid nodules?
- Is there evidence of vasculitis (e.g. nail-fold infarcts)?
- Look for systemic complications of rheumatoid arthritis (e.g. anaemia, lymphadenopathy).

- Check for CVS signs: conduction disturbances, cardiac failure, perciarditis, increased incidence coronary disease?
- Check for respiratory system signs: pulmonary fibrosis, pleural effusion?
- Check for splenomegaly?
- Examine for neurological signs: carpal tunnel syndrome, cervical cord compression, peripheral neuropathy?
- Check for renal signs: any proteinuria secondary to, for example, amyloid?
- Check for eye signs: iritis, episcleritis?
- Look for complications of therapy (e.g. Cushingoid [corticosteroids]).
- Examine the patient for functional abilities (e.g. doing up buttons, brushing hair, writing, etc.).

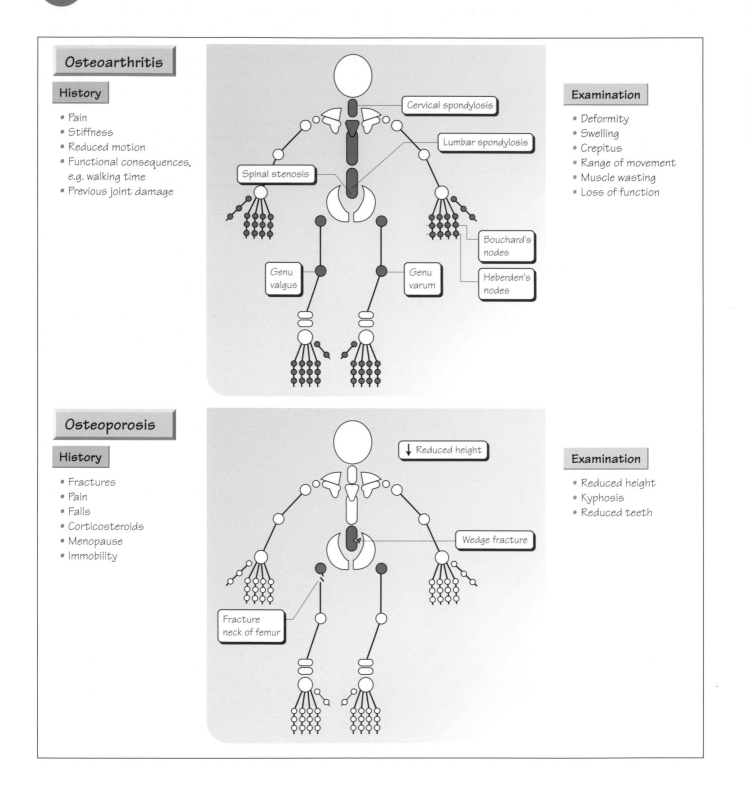

112 Osteoarthritis and osteoporosis

Osteoarthritis

History

- Pain
- Stiffness
- Reduced motion
- Functional consequences, e.g. walking time
- Previous joint damage

Examination

- Deformity
- Swelling
- Crepitus
- Range of movement
- Muscle wasting
- Loss of function

Cervical spondylosis

Lumbar spondylosis

Spinal stenosis

Bouchard's nodes

Heberden's nodes

Genu valgus

Genu varum

Osteoporosis

History

- Fractures
- Pain
- Falls
- Corticosteroids
- Menopause
- Immobility

Examination

- Reduced height
- Kyphosis
- Reduced teeth

↓ Reduced height

Wedge fracture

Fracture neck of femur

Osteoarthritis

Osteoarthritis is characterized by joint pain, tenderness, limitation of movement, crepitus and local inflammation without systemic inflammation. Osteoarthritis is very common, particularly with increasing age. The joints most commonly affected are the hips, knees and fingers.

History

• What joints are affected? What are the symptoms: pain, ache, stiffness, reduced mobility?
• Pain is often aching and deep and may improve with rest. Pain can radiate widely away from the affected joint. Symptoms classically worsen in cold, damp weather.
• What alleviates/exacerbates the symptoms?
• Ask about any previous joint injury, congenital joint abnormality, metabolic/endocrine disorders (e.g. acromegaly, haemachromatosis) and previous inflammatory or septic arthritis.
• Are there any features of inflammatory arthritides (e.g. early morning stiffness, fever, etc.)?
• Are there any other skeletal disorders (e.g. osteoporosis, previous fractures), gout or neurological disease (e.g. diabetic neuropathy producing Charcot's joints)?

Past medical history

• Any other serious illnesses?
• Any joint replacement surgery?

Drugs

Is the patient taking any medication such as NSAIDs?

Family and social history

• What is the patient's occupational history?
• Ask about the extent of disability and functional problems.

Examination

• Are there any signs of systemic illness (e.g. fever, weight loss)?
• Examine affected joints for deformity, tenderness, crepitus, reduced range of movement and functional impairment. Joint involvement is usually symmetrical.
• Particularly examine the hands, knees, hips and spine.
• Examine for Heberden's nodes (osteophytes in sides of distal interphalangeal joints) and, less commonly, Bouchard's nodes (hypertrophy in PIP joints) and squaring of the thumb.

Osteoporosis

Osteoporosis is a condition characterized by reduced bone density. It occurs more commonly in patients with advancing age, female sex, low weight, smoking, early menopause, corticosteroids, hypercalciuria, prolonged immobility and malabsorption. There is an increased incidence in patients with conditions such as thyrotoxicosis, rheumatoid arthritis and hyperparathyroidism, and in those with a family history of osteoporosis. It may present with bone fractures, often following minimal trauma. Common fracture sites include the femoral neck, pubic rami, crush fractures of the vertebra and the wrist. It may manifest with reducing height. Fractures in the elderly, particularly of the hip, are very common and associated with very high rates of mortality (up to 30% in the 6 months following a hip fracture).

Past medical history

• Has the patient sustained fractures. Where? When? Following what trauma?
• Has bone mineral density been assessed?
• Consider timing of menopause, use of oestrogens, corticosteroids.
• Consider other medical and surgical conditions including renal disease, endocrine disorders (such as thyrotoxicosis, hyperparathyroidism), rheumatioid arthritis, eating disorders, prolonged immobilization, gastrectomy, small bowel resection, intestinal bypass and organ transplants.

Family history

• Any family history of osteoporosis, multiple fractures, renal calculi?

Drugs

Consider the use of drugs that might enhance the risk of osteoporosis, e.g. corticosteroids and those used to treat osteoporosis such as bisphosphonates, oestrogens, androgens, vitamin D, calcitonin. Ask about dietary calcium intake and vitamin supplements.

Examination

• Examine patient's weight and height.
• Are there signs of weight loss, malnutrition, poor dentition?
• Are there signs of Cushing's disease?
• Are there signs suggesting vertebral collapse)? e.g. Is there reduced lower-rib pelvis distance? Is there kyphosis?
• Consider the presence of features placing the patient at greater risk of falls, e.g. poor eyesight, Parkinsonism.

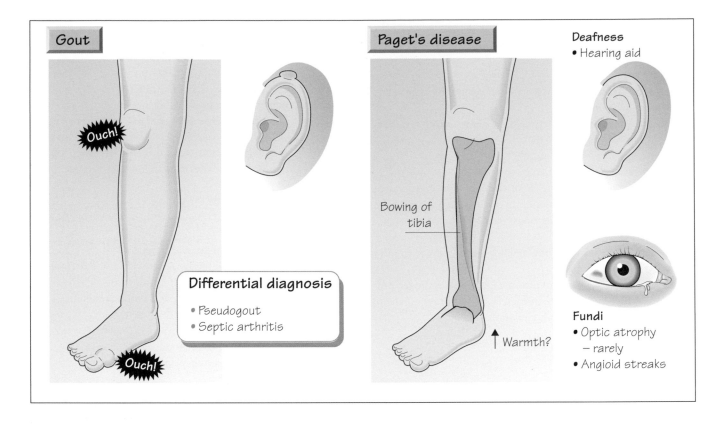

Gout

Differential diagnosis
- Pseudogout
- Septic arthritis

Ouch!

Ouch!

Paget's disease

Bowing of tibia

↑ Warmth?

Deafness
- Hearing aid

Fundi
- Optic atrophy – rarely
- Angioid streaks

Gout

Gout presents with an intensely painful, inflamed joint due to urate crystal deposition. The most commonly affected joint is the first metatarsophalangeal joint but others such as the knee and ankle can also be affected. The prevalence is 0.1%.

History

- The patient would present with an acute painful, red joint—often the great toe.
- It may be difficult to walk because of pain or even to bear a bed sheet on foot.
- Episodes often last from a few days to a few weeks.
- Are there any systemic symptoms (e.g. fever or rigors) which should prompt consideration of septic arthritis?
- Gout affects men more than women (10 : 1) and most commonly in middle age.
- Early onset suggests renal disease and/or enzymatic disorder.

Past medical history

- Any previous attacks or myeloprolferative/lymphoproliferative disease?
- Any renal impairment or renal calculi?

Family history

Is there a strong family history that might suggest the rare genetic abnormalities of purine metabolism?

Drugs

- Is the patient using any allopurinol, NSAIDs or colchicine for treatment?
- Some drugs are associated with an increased incidence of gout (e.g. cyclosporin, diuretics).

Examination

- Does the patient have a painful, inflamed reddened joint?
- Rarely there are gouty tophi, particularly on the patient's ear.
- The differential diagnosis includes pseudogout (pyrophoshate crystal deposition) and septic arthritis. It may be necessary to undertake investigations such as joint aspiration to establish diagnosis.

Paget's disease

This disorganized remodelling of particular areas of bone can present with abnormal shape and enlargement of bones such as the tibia or the skull. This can produce pain, deformity or be recognized as a cause of a raised alkaline phosphatase. Rarely, it produces cranial nerve palsies and, e.g., deafness. Very rarely (if ever) Paget's disease is a cause of high output cardiac failure or it can undergo sarcomatous change. It may have a prevalence of > 3% in people over 55 years of age, but the vast majority of people with the disease are asymptomatic.

114 Ankylosing spondylitis

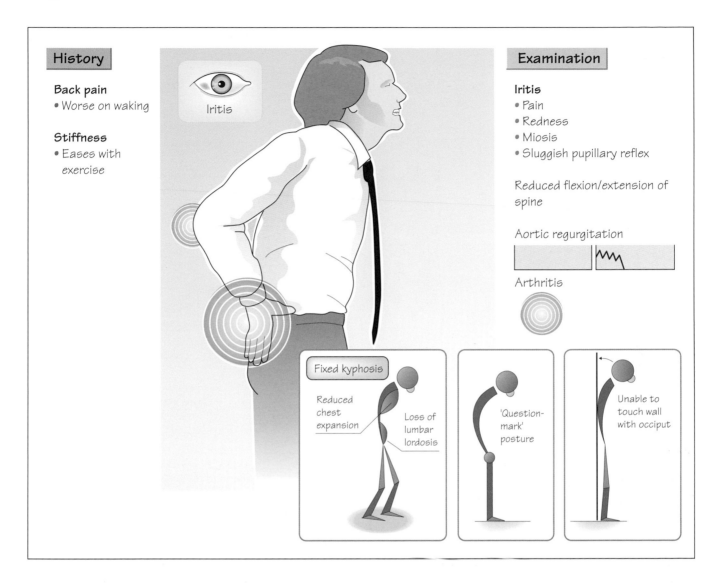

History

Back pain
• Worse on waking

Stiffness
• Eases with exercise

Iritis

Examination

Iritis
• Pain
• Redness
• Miosis
• Sluggish pupillary reflex

Reduced flexion/extension of spine

Aortic regurgitation

Arthritis

Fixed kyphosis

Reduced chest expansion

Loss of lumbar lordosis

'Question-mark' posture

Unable to touch wall with occiput

This is an inflammatory arthritis that particularly affects the axial skeleton (spine and sacro-iliac joints). It may present with back stiffness, pain and arthralgia of knees or hips. It is much more common in men than women and usually presents in the second to fourth decade. It has a prevalence of 100/100 000, increasing to 1–2% of the 6% of the population who have HLA-B27.

History
• What joints are affected? Is there pain, stiffness or a fixed deformity? What are the functional consequences?
• Are there any symptoms of iritis or cardiac failure?

Past medical history
Any history of reponse to treatment: physiotherapy, NSAIDs?

Family history
There is 10–20% prevalence of ankylosing spondylitis in adult first-degree relatives who have inherited HLA-B27.

Examination
• If the symptoms are long standing and severe, check for flexed posture with marked limitation of movements of the spine.
• Does the patient have a reduced ability to touch his/her toes? Measure the distance.
• The range of motion of the lumbar spine can be assessed using the Schober test. Identify level of posterosuperior iliac spine. mark midline at 5 cm below iliac spine and at 10 cm above iliac spine. Following maximal flexion of the spine remeasure the distance between the marks. Normal flexion increases the distance by at least 5 cm.
• Are there any deformities in other joints (especially the knees and hips)?
• Is respiratory expansion impaired? (Rarely, there is apical fibrosis.)
• Rarely there is iritis or aortic regurgitation.

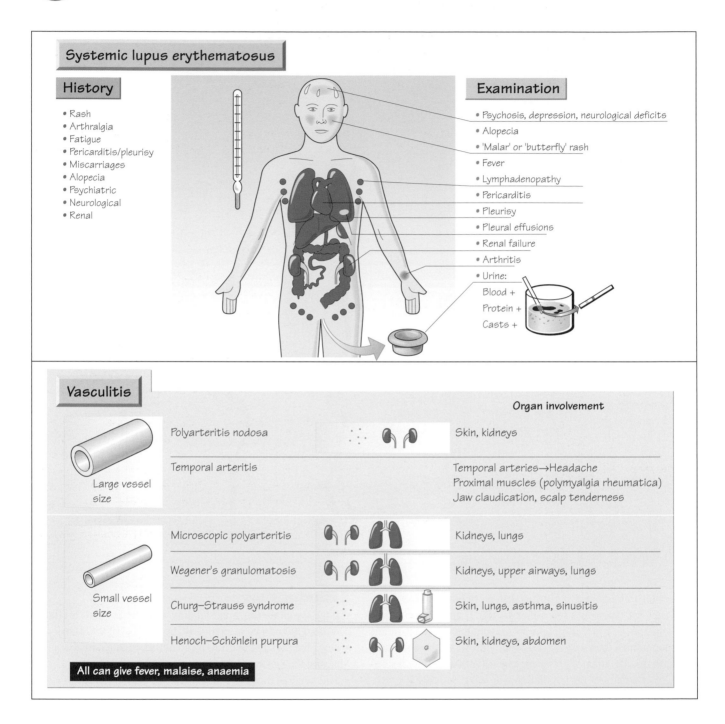

Systemic lupus erythematosus

History

- Rash
- Arthralgia
- Fatigue
- Pericarditis/pleurisy
- Miscarriages
- Alopecia
- Psychiatric
- Neurological
- Renal

Examination

- Psychosis, depression, neurological deficits
- Alopecia
- 'Malar' or 'butterfly' rash
- Fever
- Lymphadenopathy
- Pericarditis
- Pleurisy
- Pleural effusions
- Renal failure
- Arthritis
- Urine:
  Blood +
  Protein +
  Casts +

Vasculitis

			Organ involvement
Large vessel size	Polyarteritis nodosa		Skin, kidneys
	Temporal arteritis		Temporal arteries→Headache Proximal muscles (polymyalgia rheumatica) Jaw claudication, scalp tenderness
Small vessel size	Microscopic polyarteritis		Kidneys, lungs
	Wegener's granulomatosis		Kidneys, upper airways, lungs
	Churg–Strauss syndrome		Skin, lungs, asthma, sinusitis
	Henoch–Schönlein purpura		Skin, kidneys, abdomen

All can give fever, malaise, anaemia

Systemic lupus erythematosus

SLE is a systemic autoimmune disorder. It is characterized by the presence of anti-nuclear antibodies. It is capable of producing manifestations in many organs and hence can present with very many symptoms and signs. Clinical presentations can include malar rash, arthralgia, alopecia, pericarditis, renal failure, neurological deficits or even psychiatric disturbances. It has a prevalence of 100/100 000.

History

• What symptoms has the patient experienced (e.g. malar rash [photosensitive], discoid rash [erythematous raised patches], athralgia/arthritis, fever, fatigue, pleuritic chest pains, pericarditis, ankle swelling, fits, oral ulcers)?
• What other organs have been affected?
• Has there been any thromboembolic events or recurrent miscarriages (consider associated anti-phospholipid syndrome)?
• Ask about renal and neurological diseases as these are of particular importance.

Past medical history

• Any renal disease or any other serious manifestations of SLE?
• Consider any history of thromboembolic events.
• Any other autoimmune conditions (e.g. hypothyroidism)?

Drugs

• Is the patient receiving treatment with immunosuppressants (e.g. corticosteroids, azathioprine)?
• Is the patient taking anti-coagulants: warfarin, aspirin?
• Beware of drug-induced lupus.

Family history

Any family history of lupus or another autoimmune disease?

Examination

The examination needs to be complete but with particular consideration to:
• rash
• fever
• anaemia
• alopecia
• lymphadenopathy
• oral ulcers
• joint swelling: effusion and tenderness
• tachypnoea: consider pulmonary hypertension, pulmonary emboli, renal failure with fluid overload, pleural effusions and pulmonary fibrosis
• BP: check for hypertension
• pericardial/pleural rubs
• ankle oedema
• neuropathy
• neurological deficit, including focal deficit and cognitive impairment
• psychiatric disturbance, especially psychosis
• urine: dipstick proteinuria, haematuria and casts.

Vasculitis

This is a term which describes the inflammation of blood vessels that occurs in several important conditions, such as polyarteritis nodosa, microscopic polyarteritis, Wegener's granulomatosis, Churg–Strauss syndrome, Henoch–Schönlein purpura and temporal arteritis.

In affecting blood vessels, these disorders can produce manifestations in many organs. Of particular importance are the development of characteristic skin changes, renal failure, neurological abnormalities and pulmonary involvement. A high index of suspicion is required for these rare diseases because of the variety of symptoms and signs that they may produce. Precise diagnosis may require tissue biopsy and autoantibody determination. The figure opposite illustrates the more common presentations for each.

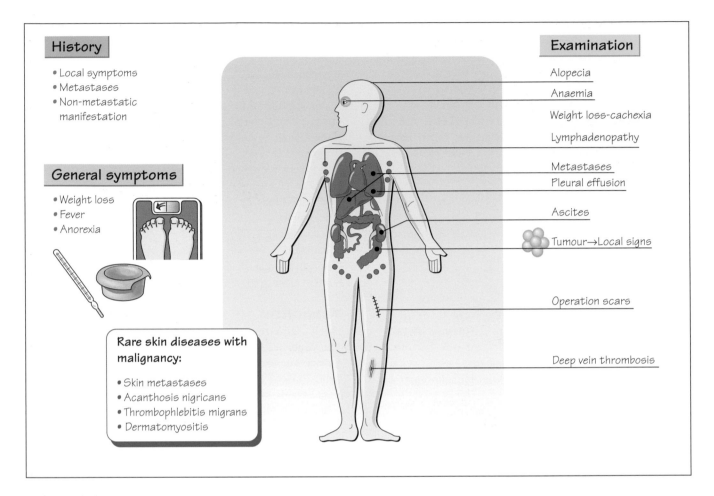

History

- Local symptoms
- Metastases
- Non-metastatic manifestation

General symptoms

- Weight loss
- Fever
- Anorexia

Rare skin diseases with malignancy:

- Skin metastases
- Acanthosis nigricans
- Thrombophlebitis migrans
- Dermatomyositis

Examination

Alopecia

Anaemia

Weight loss-cachexia

Lymphadenopathy

Metastases
Pleural effusion

Ascites

Tumour→Local signs

Operation scars

Deep vein thrombosis

Patients with malignant disease can present in a variety of ways due to local effects of the tumour, the effects of metastases, systemic effects (such as weight loss and malignancy) and non-metastatic effects due to hormone production or antibody generation.

History

- Are there local symptoms due to malignancy (change in bowel habit, haematemesis, haemoptysis or abdominal mass)?
- Are there any symptoms due to metastases (e.g. jaundice, enlarged lymph nodes)?
- Ask about systemic symptoms (fever, weight loss, anorexia, itch).
- Are there non-metastatic manifestations of malignancy (e.g. Cushingoid appearance, thromboembolism)?
- What is the patient's functional level?

Past medical history

- Any known malignancy, local spread or metastases?
- Any treatment or surgery?
- Any exposure to carcinogens (e.g. smoking, asbestos)?

Drugs

- Has the patient received chemotherapy, radiotherapy or hormonal therapy? If so, what were the side-effects?
- Is the patient taking any symptomatic treatments (e.g. analgesia)?

Family history

Any strong family history of particular cancers? Consider inherited cancer syndromes (e.g. von Hippel Lindau, *BRCA1*, etc.).

Social history

How has the patient and their family been affected by the illness? Are they coping? Are they receiving support, palliative care?

Examination

- Does the patient look well? Any recent weight loss?
- Does the patient have anaemia, jaundice or lymphadenopathy? Consider DVT and PE.
- Examine any known tumour. Look for lymphatic and metastatic spread, and non-metastatic manifestations (neuropathy, etc.).

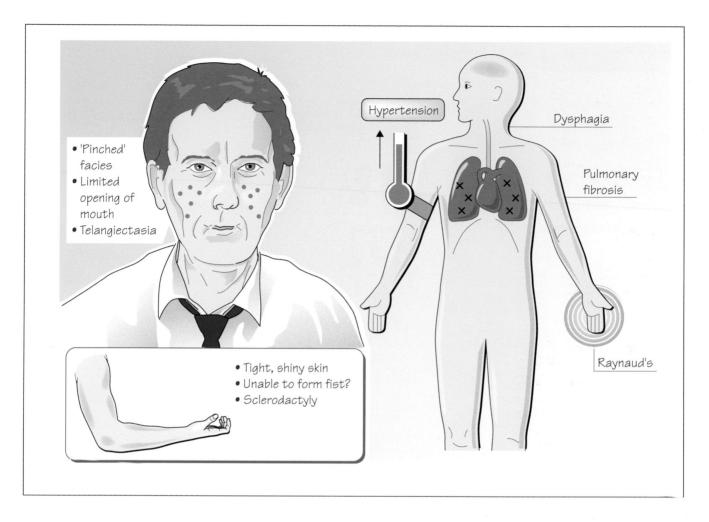

- 'Pinched' facies
- Limited opening of mouth
- Telangiectasia

- Tight, shiny skin
- Unable to form fist?
- Sclerodactyly

Hypertension

Dysphagia

Pulmonary fibrosis

Raynaud's

This is a condition also known as systemic sclerosis in which there is abnormally tight skin of the fingers and other areas, such as the mouth. It can produce difficulty in opening the mouth fully with a small aperture (microstomia) and the function of the hands can be impaired. There may also be difficulties swallowing and renal involvement. There is a prevalence of 20/100 000. There may be small localized areas of scleroderma without systemic involvement known as morphea. The systemic sclerosis may be limited (CREST) or diffuse in which skin changes are accompanied by systemic involvement.

History
- When were problems first noticed? What were the problems?
- Any difficulty with swallowing, breathing or use of the hands?
- Have there been symptoms of Raynaud's phenomenon?

Examination
- There is usually tight, shiny skin of the fingers, which may limit movement. There may be telangiectasia, calcinosis, limited opening of the mouth and tight facial skin.
- Check for hypertension.
- Is there pulmonary fibrosis?

CREST
Check for CREST:
- **C**alcinosis
- **R**aynaud's
- o**E**sophageal involvement
- **S**clerodactyly
- **T**elangiectasia.

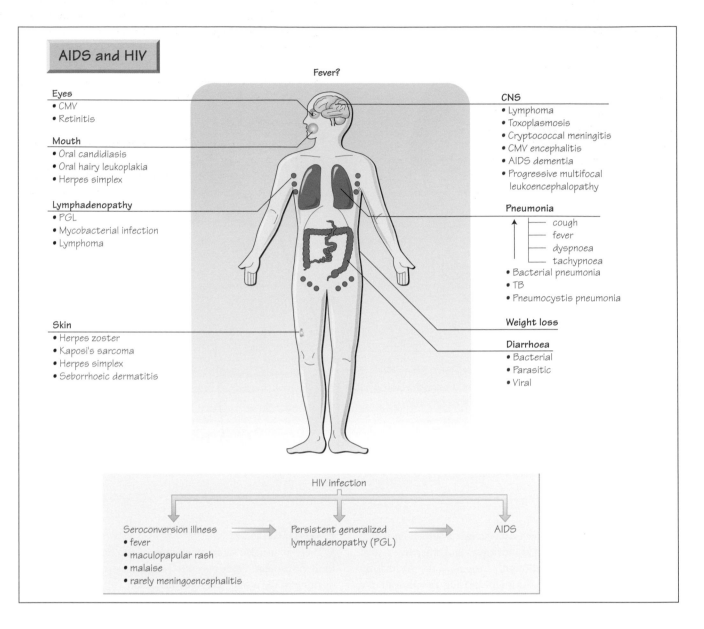

Acute HIV infection is usually asymptomatic but **seroconversion** 2–8 weeks later may be accompanied by a transient illness with fever, malaise, myalgia, maculopapular rash and, rarely, meningoencephalitis.

A period of aymptomatic infection then follows usually of 10 years or so during which up to one third of patients have **persistent generalized lymphadenopathy** (**PGL**) (lymph nodes > 1 cm at two or more extrainguinal sites). Later some patients develop constitutional symptoms (such as weight loss, diarrhoea, and fever) and night sweats may develop together with minor opportunistic infections (such as herpes zoster [shingles], tinea infections, seborrhoeic dermatitis and recurrent herpes simplex). This collection of symptoms and signs is sometimes known as **AIDS-related complex** (**ARC**).

AIDS itself is said to have developed when there is a depressed CD4$^+$ T-cell count and certain characteristic infections or neoplasms have occurred, which are listed below:

- candidiasis of bronchi, trachea, oesophagus or lungs
- cervical cancer, invasive
- coccidioidomycosis
- cryptococcosis, extrapulmonary
- cryptosporidiosis, chronic intestinal
- cytomegalovirus disease including retinitis
- encephalopathy, HIV-related
- herpes simplex: chronic ulcer(s) (> 1 month's duration); or bronchitis, pneumonitis, or oesophagitis
- histoplasmosis, disseminated or extrapulmonary
- isosporiasis, chronic intestinal
- Kaposi's sarcoma
- lymphoma, Burkitt's, immunoblastic or brain

- mycobacterial infection
- *Pneumocystis carinii* pneumonia
- pneumonia, recurrent
- progressive multifocal leukoencephalopathy
- *Salmonella* septicemia, recurrent
- toxoplasmosis of brain
- wasting syndrome due to HIV.

History

- Given this multitude of different infections and neoplasms there are many different ways in which the patient with HIV/AIDS can present.
- Consider the possible route by which the HIV infection may have been acquired: e.g. sexual, intravenous drug use, haemophilia, blood transfusion, needle stick injury.

- Consider the possibility that the patient may also have acquired other infections such as hepatitis B, TB or syphilis.
- Has the patient received antiretroviral agents? Have they had any side-effects? What has been the response of CD4 count and/or viral load? Opportunistic infections are unlikely to be responsible for any presentation if the CD4 count is well maintained.
- Are they receiving prophylactic agents, e.g. co-trimorazole for *Pneumocystis carinii* pneumonia?

Examination

- **A full general examination is essential in the care of patients infected with HIV.**
- There should be a particular focus on the presence of fever, lymphadenopathy, rash, mucous membranes, fundi and lungs.

Appendix: A self-assessment framework of communication skills in history and examination

This framework is designed to be used after you have seen a patient. It is adapted from the Calgary–Cambridge guide to the medical interview (Kurtz SM, Silverman JD & Draper J. *Teaching and Learning Communication Skills in Medicine*. Oxford: Radcliffe Medical Press, 2005). It can be used by yourself, by a colleague who was present at the interview or to assess a video of the interview.

Initiating the session
Did you:
- greet the patient (e.g. shake hands, smile, make eye contact) and obtain the patient's name?
- introduce yourself, your role and the nature of the interview? Did you confirm that the patient consented to this? Were you wearing a name badge?
- demonstrate respect and interest? Did you ensure the patient's physical comfort and privacy? Did you identify the reason(s) for the consultation? Did you establish that they were happy with the presence of others, e.g. relative, nurse, other students? If appropriate, did you establish the need for an interpreter?
- identify the patient's problems or the issues that the patient wished to address?
- begin with an appropriate opening question (e.g. 'What problems brought you to the hospital?' or 'What seems to be the trouble?')
- listen attentively to the patient's opening statement, without interruption or directing the patient's response?
- focus mainly on the patient's presenting problem(s) during the interview?
- confirm the list of problems and screen for further problems (e.g. 'You've mentioned headaches and tiredness, is there anything else troubling you . . . ?')

Gathering information
Did you:
- encourage the patient to tell the story of his/her problem(s) from when it first started to the present in his/her own words and clarify the reason for presenting now?
- use open and closed questioning technique, beginning with open questions and later moving appropriately to closed?
- listen attentively, allowing the patient to complete statements without interruption and leaving space for the patient to think before answering or to continue after pausing?
- facilitate the patient's responses verbally and non-verbally by using encouragement, silence, repetition, paraphrasing and interpretation?
- pick up on verbal and non-verbal cues (body language, speech, facial expression, affect)?
- clarify the patient's statements that were unclear or needed amplification (e.g. 'Tell me what you mean by light headed?')?
- periodically summarize to verify your own understanding of what the patient has said and invite the patient to correct interpretation or to provide further information?

- use concise, easily understood questions and comments, and avoid or adequately explain jargon?
- establish dates and the sequence of events?
- actively determine and appropriately explore:
  - patient's ideas (i.e. beliefs regarding cause)?
  - patient's concerns (i.e. worries) regarding each problem?
  - patient's expectations (i.e. goals, what help the patient had expected for each problem)?
  - effects: how each problem affects the patient's life?
- encourage the patient to express his/her feelings?

Providing structure
Did you:
- summarize at the end of each line of inquiry to confirm understanding before moving on to the next section?
- structure the interview in a logical sequence?
- attend to timing and keep the interview focused?

Building relationship
Using appropriate non-verbal behaviour
Did you:
- demonstrate appropriate non-verbal behaviour:
  - eye contact, facial expression?
  - posture, position and movement?
  - vocal cues, e.g. rate, volume, tone?
- if reading or writing notes or using a computer, did you do so in a way that did not interfere with dialogue or rapport?
- demonstrate appropriate confidence?

Developing rapport
Did you:
- accept the legitimacy of the patient's views and feelings?
- use empathy to communicate understanding and appreciation of the patient's feelings or predicament, or overtly acknowledge the patient's views and feelings?
- provide support, express concern, understanding, willingness to help?
- deal sensitively with embarrassing and disturbing topics and physical pain, including when associated with physical examination?

Involving the patient
Did you:
- explain the rationale for questions or parts of the physical examination that could appear to be unclear?
- during the physical examination, explain what you were doing and ask permission?

Ending the interview
Did you:
- explain that the interview was now coming to an end?
- enquire if the patient had any questions or unresolved issues?

• explain to the patient what will happen next, or when you will see him/her again (e.g. 'I'm now going to tell the Registrar about you and then I'll return with her in 15 minutes and we'll explain what we think the problem is and what we need to do about it.')?

• Did you wash your hands before and after examining the patient?

Index

stethoscope
    auscultation *20*, 21
    disinfection 11
stings, allergies 15
straight leg raise 37, 51, *76*, *77*
Streptococcus pneumoniae 166
stridor *26*, 27
stroke 37, 176–177
    hypertension *78*
    mitral stenosis 118
    multiple sclerosis differential diagnosis *180*, 181
subacute combined degeneration of the cord
        (SACDOC) 84
subarachnoid haemorrhage 18, *60*, 61
    meningitis differential diagnosis 83
    polycystic kidney disease 148
subphrenic abscess 82
substance abuse, psychiatric assessment 49
suicide attempts 48, 100–101
swallowing
    myaesthenia gravis 186
    see also dysphagia
Swan–Ganz catheter 115
symphysis–fundal height disease 35
syncope 23, *110*, 111
    aortic stenosis 120
    pulmonary embolism 134
syphilis, tertiary 122
systemic disease
    joints 93
    skin conditions 42, 43
systemic lupus erythematosus *196*, 197

tachycardia *110*, 111
    appendicitis 163
    pancreatitis *160*, 161
temperature 18, 19
    intensive care unit patient 75
    MEWS 19
temporal arteritis 61, *196*, 197
temporal lobe *36*, 39
temporomandibular joint *40*, 41
tension pneumothorax 174
testes
    examination 30, 31, *152*, 153
    lumps *152*, 153
    torsion *152*
    tumours *152*
tetralogy of Fallot 125
thalassaemia 84
thenar atrophy 183
thinking, disorganized *88*, 89
thoracic spine *40*, 41, *76*, *77*
thrills 20, *24*, 25
throat, examination 46, 86
thromboembolism
    prosthetic cardiac valves 136
    stroke 176
thyroid, examination 46, *52*, 53
thyroid hormones 140, 141
    deficiency 143

thyrotoxicosis 68, *69*, 141
    osteoporosis 193
    palpitations 92
    signs/symptoms *141*
tilting disc prosthetic valve 136
Tinel's sign 183
tongue
    examination 46, *52*, 53
    motor neurone disease 179
transient ischaemic attack (TIA) 176, 177
trauma 106–107
    alcohol intoxication 108
    headache 61
    joint 93
    pneumothorax 174
travel history 16
    anaemia 84
    diarrhoea 63
    jaundice 81
tremor
    cerebellar disorders 187
    multiple sclerosis 180, 181
    Parkinson's disease 178
tricuspid regurgitation *24*, 25, 124
tricuspid stenosis *24*
trigeminal nerve *38*, 39
trochlear nerve *38*, 39
Troissier's sign 29
tuberculosis 175
    back pain *76*, *77*
    chronic obstructive pulmonary disease
        differential diagnosis *173*
    lymphadenopathy 86
Turner's syndrome 125

ulcerative colitis 156
unconscious patient *72*, 73
urinary calculi 98, 99
urinary incontinence *150*, 151
urinary symptoms 150–151
    female 32
urinary tract infection 82
    confusion 88
    dysuria 98
    urinary retention 150
urine
    abnormalities 47
    chest pain 57
    dipstick testing 31, 47, 98, 99, 149
    examination *28*, 29, 31, 47
    microscopy 98, 99, 149
    retention 150

vaginal examination 29
vaginal prolapse *32*, 33
    urinary incontinence *150*, 151
vagus nerve *38*, 39
varicocoele *152*
vasculitis *196*, 197
    multiple sclerosis differential diagnosis *180*,
        181

peripheral neuropathy 182
    rheumatoid arthritis *190*, 191
vasovagal attack *110*, 111
ventilation, hypoxic stimulation 172
ventricular failure
    left 116, 117, 119
    right 116, 117
ventriculoseptal defect 126–127
vestibulocochlear nerve *38*, 39
Virchow's node 29
visual acuity *44*, 45, 53
    multiple sclerosis *180*, 181
    red eye 94
visual field
    defects in acromegaly *144*
    testing *44*, 45, 53
visual system 44–45, *52*, 53
vital observations 18
    angina *112*, 113
    myocardial infarction *112*, 113
    postoperative fever *82*
    trauma *106*, 107
vitamin B_{12} deficiency 84, 85, *188*, 189
vitamin deficiencies, peripheral neuropathy
        182
vomiting 62–63
    appendicitis 163
    blood 65
    differential diagnosis *64*
    dizziness 95
    examination 63
    intestinal obstruction *62*, 64
    meningitis 83

walking
    cerebellar disorders 187
    see also gait
Weber's test *38*, 39, *46*
Wegener's granulomatosis *196*, 197
weight loss 68, *69*
    cough 87
    differential diagnosis *69*
    dysphagia *66*, 67
    HIV/AIDS *200*
    malignant disease 198
Wernicke's encephalopathy *108*, 109, 187
wheeze *26*, 27
    asthma 164
    breathlessness 96
    causes 164, 165
    chronic obstructive pulmonary disease 172
    fibrosing alveolitis 169
white coats, cleaning 11
William's syndrome 125
Wilson's disease 154, 155, 178
wounds
    infections in postoperative fever 82
    intensive care patient *74*, 75
wrist
    examination *40*, 41
    tenderness 27